The power of yoga

Yamini Muthanna

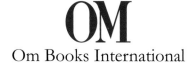
Om Books International

First published in 2015

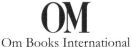

Om Books International

Corporate & Editorial Office
A-12, Sector 64, Noida 201 301
Uttar Pradesh, India
Phone: +91 120 477 4100
Email: editorial@ombooks.com
Website: www.ombooksinternational.com

Sales Office
107, Darya Ganj, New Delhi 110 002, India
Phone: +91 11 4000 9000
           2326 3363, 2326 5303
Fax: +91 11 2327 8091
Email: sales@ombooks.com
Website. www.ombooks.com

Editors: Dipa Chaudhuri, Ipshita Mitra
Design: Alpana Khare Graphic Design

ISBN: 978-93-83202-01-0

10 9 8 7 6 5 4 3 2 1

Printed in India

||AUM SHRI GURUBHYO NAMAHA||

Different schools of yoga interpret the teachings from Patanjali's *Yoga Sutra*s differently. This book does not intend to contradict any of these philosophies or techniques. As practitioners of yoga, we tend to explore, guided by the intricate maps bequeathed to us by great masters in their scholarly texts. The deeper we explore, the more we discover a plethora of practices, complex philosophies and contradictory teachings. In the circumstances, *The Power of Yoga* is a guide that helps you understand the basic principles and practice of Hatha Yoga.

Yoga asanas are the main focus of this book. The sequencing patterns of the asanas are determined by the principles of balance and counterbalance. A variety of sequences based on energy patterns are its highlight. Focusing on the arrangement of the chakras, the patterns are detailed to deal with a particular lifestyle-based issue. These patterns are categorised and illustrated for better understanding. The illustrations are based on the author's personal study and practice of yoga.

Yamini Muthanna
Yoga Acharya
YOGASTHALA
Bengaluru, Karnataka
India

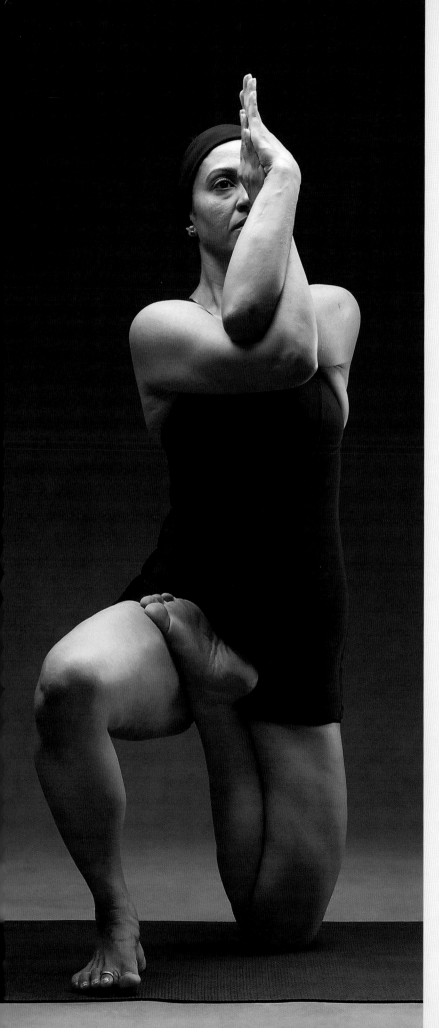

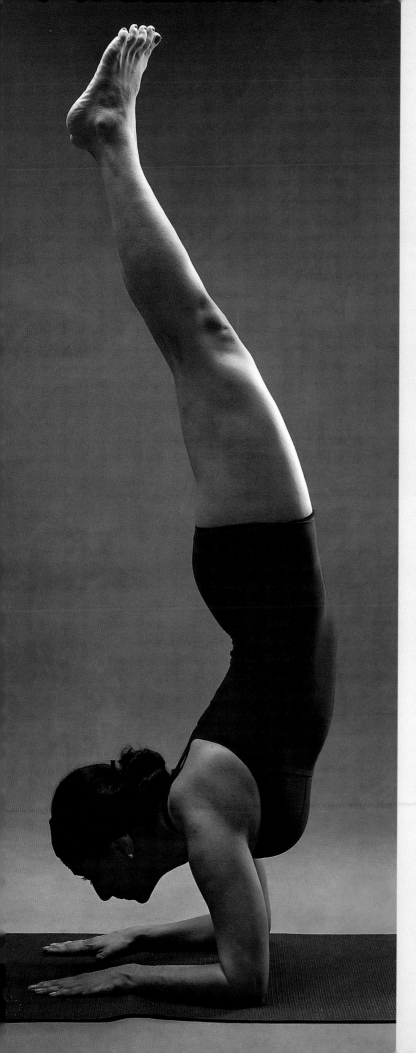

SECTION C: THE SEQUENCE MANUAL

Chapter 7

Chapter 8

Chapter 9

SECTION D: PRECAUTIONS

Chapter 10

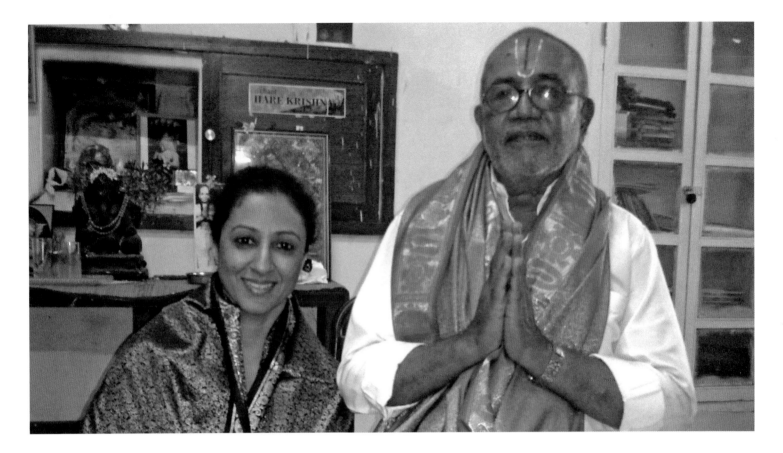

FOREWORD

I remember Yamini when she came to my Yoga Shala at Parakala Mutt, Mysore in 1988. A young, enthusiastic teenager, she was very eager to learn. Respectful and humble, she was a dedicated student who learnt the techniques of practising asanas to perfection, and within 6 months of starting her training, even won the All India Yoga Sports Championship, conducted by the Yoga International Sports Federation in 1989. Yamini is a talented, hard-working and determined individual. It is rewarding for me to see that she has grown to be a fine practitioner and teacher of yoga, training a number of students from all over the world in the skills and techniques of yoga asanas.

In *The Power of Yoga*, she has mentioned some aspects of the philosophy of yoga, which are important to understand. These provide a basic knowledge for those interested in taking up the practice of yoga seriously. This book certainly provides an impetus to the readers to further explore the finer aspects of this ancient practice.

Asanas are therapeutic in nature and should be performed with proper understanding, technique and care. They accelerate the power of healing. Regular practice of the asanas improves the overall health of the practitioner. Asanas are not a trivial exercise routine for weight loss, but a technique to liberate oneself from a disturbed mind and body to arrive at a balanced and composed state.

Yamini is an experienced practitioner of yoga. I am proud she has written this book. I wish this book all success and hope the readers will benefit from its content.

My blessings to Yamini and all the students of yoga who shall read this book and carry forward the rich legacy of our forbears .

B N·S·Jyengar

Yoga Visharadha B.N.S. IYENGAR (B.A.)
MYSORE

ACKNOWLEDGEMENTS

I bow to God and my elders for all the blessings and courage bestowed upon me.
I bow to the great Sage Patanjali for the *Yoga Sutras*.

‖ *Jeevamani Brajathpani*
Sasravishwambhara
Mandalaya Anantaya
Nagarajaya Namonamaha
Abaahu Purushakaram
Sanka Chakrasi Dharinim
Sahasrashirasamswetha
Pranamami Patanjalim ‖

‖ *Shri Gurubhyo Namaha*
Parama Rishibhyo Namaha ‖

(Adorned with the bright bead and effulgent jewels
Who spreads blessings with his thousand-hooded heads
To the bearer of the mandala
He who is finite
Salutations to the King of the Nagas
Whose upper body has a human form
Who holds a conch and a discus
Who is crowned by a thousand-headed cobra
I salute the scholarly sage Patanjali

(I bow in respect to my guru
I bow in respect to the great sage Patanjali)

I thank my guru, Yoga Visharadha (title given by the Maharaja of Mysore), Yoga Rathnakara Shri B.N.S. Iyengar and his most revered teacher, Shri T. Krishnamacharya for all that I have learnt in yoga till date. Guruji's patience and insistence on perfection deeply influenced my study, learning, practice and teaching. I feel his guiding hand during my yoga classes. I became his disciple in 1988 and shall always remain so.

My loving husband, Vinoo Muthanna and my children Rithwik Iyappa and Manya Thangamma have been a source of great energy and encouragement in all that I undertake. My parents, Capt. Chendrimada Machaiah and Sundari Machaiah, my parents-in-law, Kotera Chengappa and Radha Chengappa, have always made my endeavours propitious with their love and blessings. My gratitude, respect and love for all of them.

I would like to thank all my teachers, especially my Bharatanatyam Guru, 'Amma' Dr. Vasundhara Doraswamy (student of Shri Pattabhi Jois), an ardent practitioner of yoga herself, whose grace, hard-work, discipline and strength helped me overcome several obstacles in life and inspired me to venture into the path of yoga. Initially, she trained me in the skill, which led me to explore it further with Guruji.

I would like to thank Sudeep Gurtu, the fabulous photographer who, though not a practitioner of yoga, had to do many a 'Vinyasa', trying to photograph me. The shoot demanded extra time, patience and skill. We worked from morning to evening without a break, and little food, to get the beautiful results you see in this book. Aarti Rao Shetty, thank you for introducing me to Sudeep who made me feel comfortable during the shoot as I am camera shy.

I thank all my students whose keen interest, regular practice and constant feedback on various sequencing patterns have made this book possible. Special thanks to those who took time off their busy schedules and accompanied me on my shoots to ensure perfect alignment of the asanas and encouraged longer holds of the asanas until the photograph looked just right. Thank you very much Kiran Karunakaran, Cristina Hug, Rani Jairaj, Preetika Narang and Alan Hartman.

Ms. Parvati Menon and Ms. Rajitha Ghatkar provided the initial feedback on this book. Thank you both for your suggestions and support. They helped me to structure the book better.

Swarna and Ramakrishnan (Ramki) helped me connect with one of India's finest publishing houses, Om Books International. Placing the sequences and asana tips in the right order for easy reference was a challenging task, performed very ably by Swarna, especially with her 9-month-old son, Shiva, trying his best to co-operate with us while we worked. Swarna and Ramki also introduced me to Alpana Khare and Bikram Grewal without whose help, the book would have stayed in my notepad forever. I thank all of them profusely. Alpana's design of the book is for all of us to appreciate.

Finally, I would like to thank Ajay Mago, Dipa Chaudhuri and Ipshita Mitra of Om Books International for all that they did for *The Power of Yoga*.

ENCOUNTER WITH YOGA: MY STORY

My tryst with yoga started at the age of 18, when I saw a photograph of the winner of the International Yoga Championship, in the Yoga Nidrasana. With typical teenage enthusiasm, I said to myself, 'I can do this!' Thus I embarked on a journey with no idea of the treasure trove that was lying in wait for me! I walked into the Patanjali Yoga Shala at the Parakala Mutt one morning at 5:30 a.m. As I was climbing up the old wooden stairs of the temple building, I could hear wave upon wave of breathing sounds. At least 50 men must have been practising yoga in the hall. Guruji, Shri B.N.S. Iyengar, was adjusting a student doing Urdhva Dhanurasana. He gestured to me to proceed to the women's section which had barely 4 disciples! Upon joining us there, he asked me to recite along with him: 'Parama Rishibhyo Namaha, Shri Gurubhyo Namaha' (I bow in respect to the great sage Patanjali, I bow in respect to my guru). Then, after evoking with a sloka, the blessings of the great sage Patanjali – He who gave the universe the *Yoga Sutra*s – I started my first yoga class.

I was born in Virajpet, a picturesque town in Kodagu, and grew up in Hunsur, a small town 40 km from Mysore. My childhood had its share of ups and downs, as is common in most middle-class Indian homes. Responsibilities fell on my shoulders at an early age. At 17, with a professional secretarial course under my belt, I had to help support my loving family, a decision I will never regret. With a full time job, I completed my higher education through correspondence courses, getting my Master's in English Literature from Mysore Open University. But my days were filled with other activities: I was learning Bharatnatyam, classical music, and, of course, yoga. My day would start at 5:00 a.m. with a yoga session at the Yoga Shala in the morning, and finish late in the evening with studies, dance rehearsals, and regular Bharatanatyam performances. I do not know whether an average teenager today would find this 'cool' or 'fun', but for me, my life was full and power-packed!

My family and friends thought that I was overworked. No one, not even my mother, could keep track of my activities and schedule. Today when I look back, I sometimes wonder why there was never any stress involved in juggling so many activities and roles. In fact, I only recall the sense of sheer pleasure at being able to do everything. I suppose I felt that way because I never consciously searched for peace outside of myself or the circumstances around me. I found it in all the things that life offered me in my role as daughter, student, sister, friend, wife, mother, teacher of dance and yoga, stage artist... My journey goes on.

I started learning Ashtanga Yoga in 1988 under the able guidance of my revered Guruji, Shri B.N.S. Iyengar, at the Patanjali Yoga Shala, Parakala Mutt, Mysore. And I have been running a yoga-learning centre called Yogasthala for several years now. As an instructor, I enjoy weaving yoga practice into an interesting and challenging Vinyasa flow (sequence). I encourage my students to personalise their practice by helping them understand the benefits of each asana at every person's individual level. I pay attention to precision and mindfulness, alignment and breathing, to create a challenging and dynamic energy flow, emphasising strength, flexibility and balance. I firmly believe this helps in healing and detoxifying the body and mind at the deepest levels. I also pay attention to the theory of yoga and help interested students understand its deeper philosophical import.

As a teacher of yoga, my conviction stems from my personal practice that has enriched every aspect of my own life. My belief in this ancient knowledge system that has remarkable modern relevance and applicability underlines my passion and commitment to it. I hope to guide as many students as I possibly can to attain their highest potential of mental, physical and spiritual harmony through yoga.

The Power of Yoga is the culmination of a deep desire to share my study, experience and practice with those who wish to harness yoga to enhance the quality of their lives.

CHAPTER 1
WHY YOGA

It can be daunting to choose from a myriad, ever-evolving fitness systems at our disposal. While these diverse regimens cater to generic requirements, they do not necessarily take into account individual constitutions and the special needs that arise from specific lifestyles or work styles.

Each of us is unique in our own way, conditioned by genetic predisposition, social environment, profession and so on. These catalysts in turn, shape our distinctive personalities. Personality types not only determine the way we approach life, but also influence our choice of healthcare.

However, whether we are introverted, extroverted, laid back or high-strung, we must understand the pressing need to focus on mental development alongside physical development in our troubled and stressful lives.

The need to deal with the discomfort caused by stress, makes the practice of yoga an ideal and viable option. Yoga is not just a physical exercise routine, but a combination of our physical, mental and spiritual faculties. It is universally acknowledged that this ancient practice seeks to strengthen mental dimensions through physical stances called asanas or postures and breathing techniques or Pranayama.

This book suggests a practice to prepare ourselves to be alert and aware of the ever-changing circumstances of life. Contrary to popular belief, yoga is not an archaic or arcane path that only rishis and yogis choose to tread. Instead, it remains incredibly relevant to our modern lives. In fact, yoga can help negotiate the many ups and downs of everyday living, big and small. What sets yoga apart from other fitness systems is its focus on the mind, body and spirit. Yoga stimulates glands, facilitates cell replacement, improves blood circulation, increases flexibility, detoxifies the system, stalls ageing, keeps you energetic, calms the mind, strengthens the body and helps you connect with the deeper self – all without making you sweat!

But you might wonder how this centuries-old practice can be applied to the frenzied paced of our times. Amazingly sufficient, yoga offers each person an exclusive sequence of asanas to specifically suit his or her day's schedule, nature of work, mood and stress levels. For instance, if you are scheduled to make an important work presentation, a couple of asanas could be sequenced to help you to calm the nerves and concentrate better at the task on hand.

A sequence of asanas and Pranayama, practised towards directing the mind for a purpose, activates certain nerve points governed by energy centres within the body called chakras. These chakras are aligned along the length of the spine and networked to various auxiliary chakras which control the body's reflexes and alert the mind.

The good news is that you don't have to travel far and wide to set out on this powerful journey towards self-empowerment. You can start your quest right here with this book, which aims to provide committed practitioners with a customised build-up, leading to a positive mind, a fit body and overall good health. Ultimately, a well-planned yoga practice is not about an exercise routine, but about living healthily, happily and mindfully in your real world.

HOW TO USE THIS BOOK (Q&A)

WHAT IS THE PURPOSE OF THIS BOOK?
The purpose of this book is to help understand and sequence variations from the thousands of recorded yoga asanas, to form a practice flow within a limited time span to suit a particular lifestyle and, more importantly, a particular state of physical, mental and emotional issues that a practitioner would like to address.

HOW TO USE THIS BOOK?
The key section of the book 'The Sequence Guide' aims to aid people practise asanas to cope better with the day-to-day schedules characterised by various situations. It comprises 21 practice patterns, where each asana is presented in a photograph. It also has an easy-to-use matrix for quick referencing while doing the practice, thus ensuring an uninterrupted Vinyasa.

The rest of the book deals with deeper aspects of yoga including its philosophy, chakras, bandhas, mudras, Pranayama, and more. It also cautions the reader about various injuries that could occur due to faulty practice and lack of technical knowledge. It helps understand the benefits and contra-indications of each asana and also the author's tips on getting the alignment right in each asana.

It is recommended to do a thorough reading of Sections A, B and D, before approaching Section C: The Sequence Guide. Each section has been explained in detail later.

ON WHAT BASIS ARE THESE SEQUENCING PATTERNS FORMED?

The sequencing of asanas is based on the author's experience of therapeutic yoga teaching over several years. Encouraged by the positive results from various students, this book is an attempt to structure an interesting daily practice of yoga, suitable for our current lifestyle.

CAN I APPLY THESE SEQUENCES TO OVERCOME SPECIFIC CONCERNS?

To address specific issues is the main aim of this book. It is important to understand the concern that you would want to address in your practice. You may find the answers in this book.

WHO CAN USE THIS BOOK?

This book can be used by beginners, enthusiasts and serious practitioners. However, it is recommended that the asanas are performed under the watchful eyes of a good teacher / guru.

IS THIS BOOK PRIMARILY ABOUT SEQUENCING OF ASANAS?

The main subject of the book is sequencing of asanas. The book will also introduce you to an understanding of the deeper meaning of yoga, a meaning that all those who practise yoga know exists but do not quite know how to internalise.

IS THE BOOK THEORETICAL OR INSTRUCTIONAL?

The explanation in this book is simple. The aim is to make the vast ocean of knowledge as accessible and relevant as possible to all. The book has a section on the author's own journey into yoga, the process of understanding its philosophy, discipline and benefits. The sequencing of asanas is primarily instructional in nature, making this a practical book as well.

Section A: Introduction

This section is about the Philosophy of Yoga, the Mind and the Ashtanga Principles. This would serve as a good foundation to ensure long-term mindful practice.

Section B: Instructional Guide

This section deals with topics such as planning personal practice; understanding each asana's benefits and its contra-indications; the deeper elements of asanas – chakras, nadis, mudras, bandhas and Pranayama.

Section C : The Sequence Manual

This is the core of the book, which aims to help programme the reader's yoga practice for the day, keeping in mind the various issues or maladies in focus. I have included a few of my personal tips for each asana to help the reader get in and out of it systematically following the right technique.

Section D: Precautions

Here the author briefly introduces the muscle groups of our body, states the probable causes for injury of each group and also the precautions one needs to take in case of such injuries, including avoiding of certain asanas. This is a very important aspect of yoga practice as it helps understand and monitor the healing process of any injury and makes the body alert and strong to avoid injury in future.

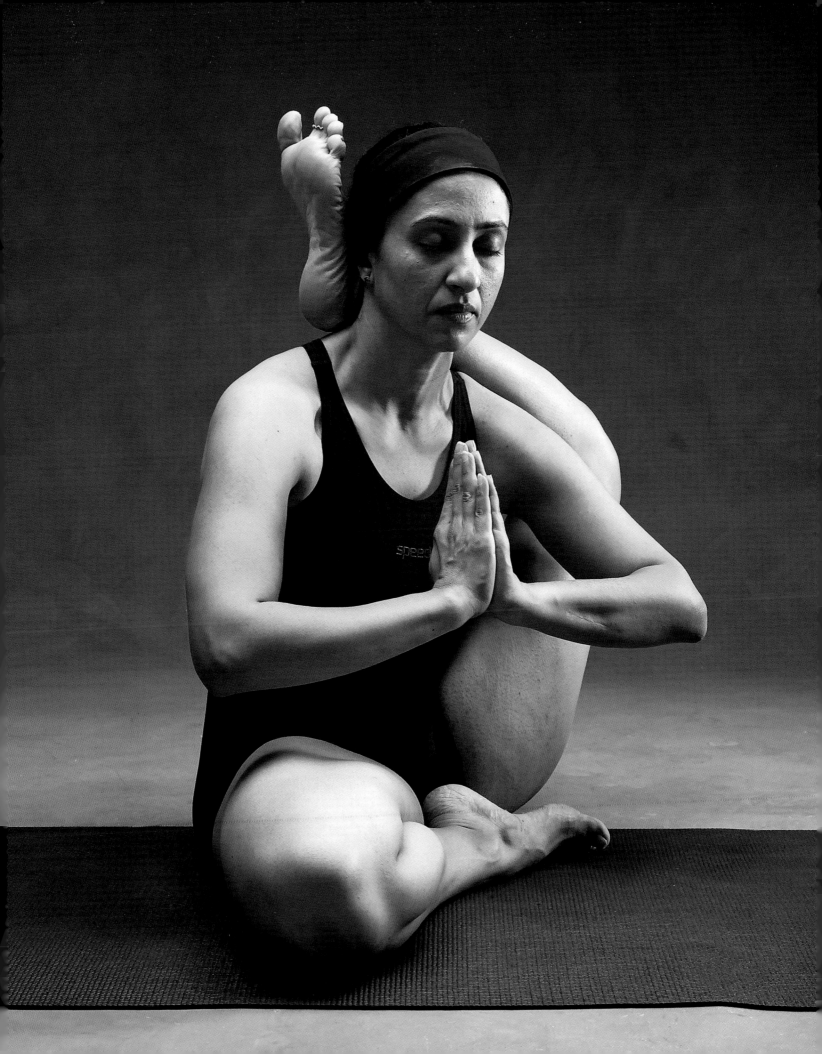

CHAPTER 2

UNDERSTANDING THE PHILOSOPHY OF YOGA

Yoga was first mentioned in the Indian Scriptures, The Vedas – 'The source of knowledge in ancient India'. These classical texts are composed of extremely terse and self-contained aphorisms or sutras. 'Sutra' literally means threads of knowledge. The idea of it being in this form is that each individual's blossoming thoughts are bound to form a garland of complex philosophy. These aphorisms by their very nature invite a host of commentaries and annotations for their appropriate comprehension for the learner. This has been the tradition of ancient Indian scholasticism.

Patanjali's *Yoga Sutra*s outline the sovereign path of yoga. Composed of 195 aphorisms, the sutras form a tapestry of knowledge derived from many yogic traditions, and are structured around 4 chapters:

CHAPTER 1: SAMADHI PADA (STATE OF UNION)

With 51 sutras, this chapter talks about the State of Union with the Ultimate Soul, and delineates the different hurdles, kinds of thought patterns the seeker is likely to encounter in the quest to understand the true consciousness of the soul, and how to overcome them.

CHAPTER 2: SADHANA PADA (PRACTICE)

The 55 sutras in this chapter describe the approach towards a disciplined and regular yoga practice. They establish the aim of yoga as a purpose to control thought patterns (chitta vritti). Also, the practice of Ashtanga Yoga is prescribed as an effective tool for devicing an action plan to attain the goal of controlling and disciplining the mind, body and the senses.

CHAPTER 3: VIBHUTI PADA (POWERS)

The 56 sutras of this chapter speak of the Powers of Sadhana or disciplined practice. They portray the accomplishments that are a result of regular yoga practice. The practices which have been stressed upon are the final 3 limbs of Ashtanga Yoga – dharana (concentration), dhyana (meditation), and samadhi (contemplation), which are touched upon in the forthcoming chapters.

CHAPTER 4: KAIVALYA PADA (BLISS)

The 34 sutras in this chapter deal with the impressions left by our endless cycles of birth. They speak of the ultimate goal towards detachment of maya or worldly desires, portraying the yogi as an entity who has gained independence from all bondages and achieved the absolute ananda or bliss.

The philosophy of yoga is important as the basis of the study and practice of yoga depends on the level of the practitioner's understanding of it.

UNDERSTANDING THE MIND

From my own study and experience, I sense that the central doctrine of the philosophy of yoga is that 'nothing exists beyond the mind and its consciousness'. Therefore, it is important to understand the nature and elusiveness of the mind. External factors influencing day-to-day life have considerable impact on the health of our mind, body and spirit. To gain freedom from this perplexity is the objective of this philosophy. It indicates a process that culminates in withdrawal or detachment from all false sources of knowledge, while inculcating an inner sense of balance and tranquility.

According to the philosophy of yoga, the mind can fall under any of the following 5 categories:

A. Kshipta, or distressed. In this state, the mind is disturbed, lacks judgement, is hyperactive, and is unable to ignore external stimuli.
B. Mugdha, or confused and perplexed. This state is characterised by inertia, lethargy, sluggishness and ignorance.
C. Vikshipta, or distracted. In this state, the mind is inconsistent, unable to reflect and turbulent, and dwells either in the past or future.

The causes for the above three states of mind include sickness, incompetence, doubt, delusion, fatigue, overindulgence, confusion, lack of perseverance, and regression.

D. Ekagra, or deep concentration
E. Nirudha, or the balanced state of mind

Ekagra and Nirudha are achieved when the mind is calm, undisturbed and still. Such a mind is ready to meditate, and there is clarity in understanding the nature of self.

According to the text, the aim of the philosophy of Ashtanga Yoga is to train the mind to be focused (ekagra) and balanced (nirudha) from being disturbed (kshipta), stupefied (mugdha) or inconsistent (vikshipta).

UNDERSTANDING ASHTANGA YOGA

Ashtanga Yoga or the 'Eight-limbed Yoga' is based on eight principles: yama, niyama, asana, Pranayama, Pratyahara, dharana, dhyana and samadhi. These constitute the eight stages for achieving Nirudha or a balanced state of mind.

These stages liberate a person from physical and mental distress, and put him / her on the path to peace. These sutras provide guidelines; they are not rigid rules. They offer the framework, but how we adapt that to our life is for us to discover. Ashtanga Yoga is not a set of asanas but principles or limbs which forms the basis of a yoga sadhana / practice.

YAMA: MORAL RESTRAINTS

Yama, the first principle of Ashtanga, deals with our interaction with the external world. This must ideally be conducted through non-violence (ahimsa), truthfulness (satya), honesty (asteya), celibacy (brahmacharya) and non-covetousness (aparigraha).

NIYAMA: FIXED PRACTICES

Niyama, the second principle of Ashtanga, governs our interaction with ourselves in our internal world, through a process of self-regulation. Patanjali lists 5 pathways to achieve this: through purity of thought (soucha), contentment (santosha), austerity (tapas), self-reflection (swadhyaya), and meditation (ishwar pranidhana).

ASANAS: POSTURES

Asanas, the third principle in the yoga system are practised to achieve physical discipline. They are performed to ensure that every muscle, nerve and gland of the body is healthy, strong and in perfect condition in order to keep the body free from disease and fatigue. The regular practice of asanas helps develop agility, balance, endurance and vitality.

PRANAYAMA: REGULATION OF LIFE FORCE / BREATH

The fourth principle, is Pranayama, deals with the science of breathing. It is said that a yogi's life is not measured by the number of days, but by the number of breaths. A variety of rhythmic breathing patterns are practised to maintain the health of the respiratory system. Proper and focused breathing fosters a calm mind and a conscious spirit. As desires and distractions in the mind are stilled, the mind is set free and becomes ready for concentration.

PRATYAHARA: WITHDRAWAL OF SENSES OR STILLING THE MIND FOR THE PURPOSE OF SELF-ANALYSIS

The fifth principle is the stage of self-examination. This stage is a process of the study of the self and of the objects that the senses tend to pursue, and the process of weeding out unwanted thoughts and actions, to progress towards a stage that leads to 'peace of mind', a pre-requisite to meditation.

DHARANA: DETERMINED MIND CONTROL

The sixth principle is that of Dharana, the practice of concentrating on a single-point goal. This stage is about stilling the mind and controlling the thoughts to achieve complete absorption.

DHYANA: STATE OF BALANCED MIND

The seventh principle is that of Dhyana or meditation and is pivotal for all those who practise yoga. Once you reach this stage in the practice, it becomes effortless for the mind to ward off all distractions and move towards the mystical state of union with the universal consciousness.

SAMADHI: ABSORPTION INTO A STATE OF PEACE

The eighth principle is the state of Samadhi. At this stage, the mind reaches the peak of meditation, where the body and the senses are completely at rest. However, the state of intelligence is at its most alert and beyond expression. It is believed that this is a state of indescribable joy and profound silence. Samadhi is believed to be the end of a seeker's or yogi's quest.

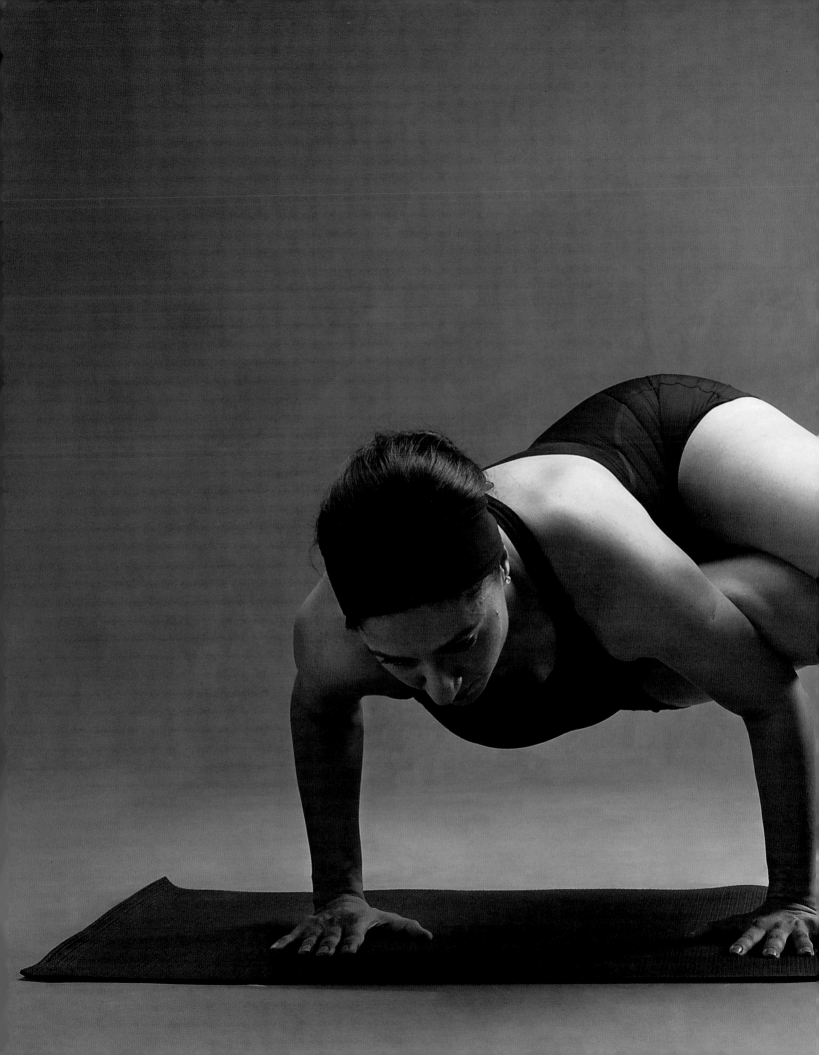

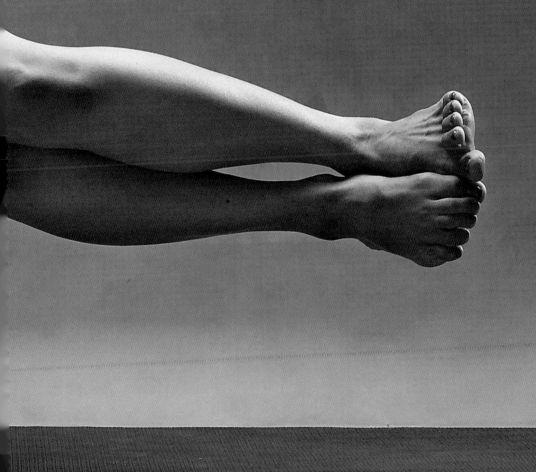

SECTION B
INSTRUCTIONAL GUIDE

CHAPTER 3
YOGA FOR PERSONAL PRACTICE

Before planning a yoga programme, it is essential to understand and determine the goals and purpose of your decision to practise yoga. The objectives may be different for each practitioner:

GENERAL
- To satisfy one's curiosity about yoga
- To train the body to be generally flexible
- To make yoga part of an exercise routine

SPECIFIC
- To balance mind and body
- To address specific ailments
- To maintaining organ functions

SPIRITUAL
- To practise breathing
- To arrive at self-understanding
- To conduct self-analysis
- To transform present lifestyle

While the objectives will differ from person to person, the goal of the entire yoga programme should be to achieve a 'balanced state of mind'.

PLANNING YOUR DAILY PRACTICE
An extensive asana practice session would be very time-consuming. It would be ideal to create short practices. However, care should be taken to ensure that all parts of the body are engaged and counterbalanced in each session.

The points to be considered for planning a session of yoga practice are:
- Selecting the asanas
- Practising asanas
- Breathing
- Combining the asanas

SELECTING ASANAS
The best way to select asanas for practice is to identify the categories that address the various groups of muscles. The muscles work usually in groups and not individually. Thus, an asana that stretches and exercises one muscle group is always countered with an asana that works in a reverse manner, releasing the strain.

PRACTISING ASANAS
There are two ways of practising an asana:
A. Repeating
B. Holding

Repetition involves moving the body into and out of the asanas from their starting point (Samasthiti). This action of repetition is considered to be the most effective way of releasing muscular and skeletal tightness. With this approach, heaviness of the body and mind, also known as the tamasic guna (turbulent or disturbed state) is released. It also helps in improving blood circulation and the flow of oxygen to all parts of the body.

Once the asanas are formed, the entire frame of the asana is held still. Powerful inhalation and exhalation are then practised while holding the asana. This manner of practising the asanas helps remove toxins from the body, creating a feeling of inner purification. This is also useful for overcoming the agitation of the mind and body (rajasic guna).

While the goal of the student is to achieve the final asana, each person will have individual resistant points that must be overcome gradually before the final asana is achieved.

GUNAS
Ancient Hindu texts classify human behaviour as being linked to three gunas or human tendencies. These tendencies also serve as a guide when assessing physical conditions and diets:

A. Sattvic, the tendency that relates to balance, serenity and purity in being
B. Rajasic, the tendency that relates to power and dynamism
C. Tamasic, the tendency that relates to turbulence and agitation (opposite of Sattvic), associated also with ignorance.

NOTE
Only specific asanas can be held for long periods of time for therapeutic reasons.

A student can select a sequence of asanas that could address a specific purpose for each day's practice session. When planning a sequence, it is important to incorporate asanas along with their opposing or reverse asanas.

BREATHING WHILE IN ASANA

Before trying to incorporate the proper method of breathing into the practice of asanas, it is important to know and understand your normal breathing pattern, and only then correct your breathing while practising asanas. Breathing in an asana could be challenging and difficult for a person whose breathing habits are normally faulty (Section B, Chapter 4).

Proper breathing is key to neutralising the effects of daily stress. It improves oxygen and blood circulation in the body and also strengthens the neuro-electrical system. Breath-control is a fast and effective way of breaking down anxiety, anger and depression. It is the most important aspect while in an asana as it enables us to draw focus and attention into the body and mind. Correct breathing also makes it easier to stretch and execute the asanas accurately. The proper chest and diaphragm expansion and contraction helps the spine become strong, supple and lubricated, which helps free the body into a fluid stretch.

The practice of yoga is meant to influence every aspect of our being and existence by awakening the koshas or subtle layers. The asanas strengthen and tone the physical body; Pranayama helps mastery over breath to regulate pranic energy – the life force, helps in meditation for a calm and steady mind, and finally aids in the process of self-study and introspection for developing inner knowledge. Yoga is a system that develops and integrates all parts of the being. It thus refines, condenses and elevates the experience of life.

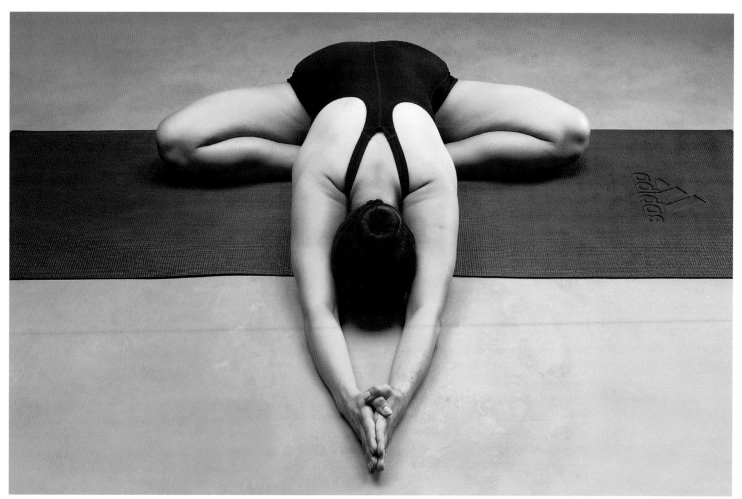

BADDHA KONASANA

DEEPER ASPECTS OF ASANA PRACTICE

Another classic text of yoga, the *Taittiriya Upanishad,* indicates that a human body has 5 koshas or subtle layers which lie one beneath the other, like the skin of an onion. These koshas make up our personality. The practice of yoga makes you aware of all the 5 koshas or sheaths by activating and rejuvenating the energy fields that hold the material body together.

1. ANNAMAYA KOSHA

This is the physical sheath which can be seen and touched – the vehicle in which our existence travels. Asana practice helps strengthen and maintain this kosha.

2. PRANAMAYA KOSHA

Within the annamaya kosha lies the pranamaya kosha or sheath of life energy. This governs the biological processes, from respiration to digestion and the circulation of blood.

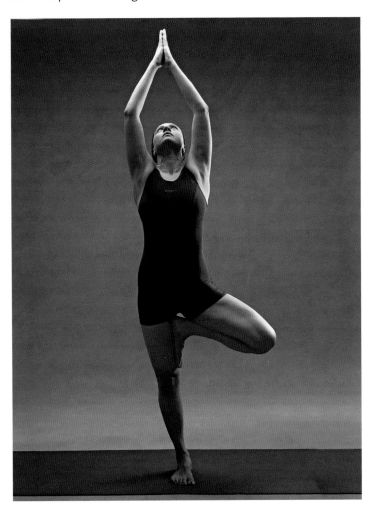

VRIKSHASANA

When the Pranamaya Kosha ceases to function, the entire functioning of the body starts to disintegrate. Pranayama practice replenishes the vitality of the Pranamaya Kosha.

3. MANOMAYA KOSHA

Beneath the Pranayama Kosha is the Manomaya Kosha or sheath made up of thought energy. This third kosha, made up of thought processes, is responsible for sensory and motor activities. The health of the Manomaya Kosha is enhanced by practising concentration, meditation and mantra meditation.

4. VIJNANAMAYA KOSHA

Deeper still lies another sheath, the Vijnanamaya Kosha, that comprises intellect, the power of judgement. It encompasses all the functions of the conscience. The path of development for this kosha comes from a conscious study of spiritual truths, their deep contemplation and incorporation into the core of the personality.

5. ANANDAMAYA KOSHA

Hidden at the core is the subtlest of sheaths, the Anandamaya Kosha, composed of pure joy. This is the most challenging kosha to reach and is said to be underdeveloped in most human beings.

DOSHAS

Our understanding of doshas (3 humors that govern our bodily functions) is derived from the science of Ayurveda. Doshas govern our psycho-biological functioning. There are three doshas in the body: Vata, Pitta and Kapha. Their constitution is present in every cell, tissue and organ of the body. When they are in balance, the body is in perfect health.

The three doshas are responsible for individual characteristics. They regulate bodily functions, both physical and emotional. Stress, improper diet, environmental conditions are some of the factors that cause an imbalance of the doshas.

In Ayurveda, Vata signifies the predominance of air, Pitta signifies the predominance of fire, and Kapha signifies the predominance of water. People have their dominating doshas, which give them their typical character. The other two also exist but are less prominent. Each person has a particular energy pattern which gives them their physical features, and mental and emotional characteristics.

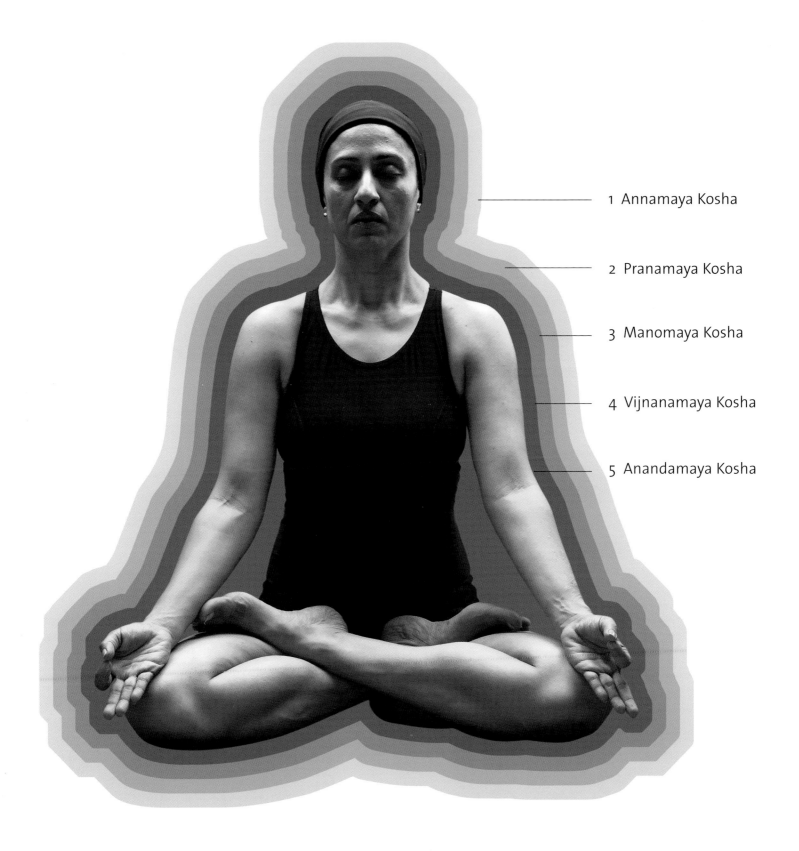

1 Annamaya Kosha

2 Pranamaya Kosha

3 Manomaya Kosha

4 Vijnanamaya Kosha

5 Anandamaya Kosha

CHAPTER 4
UNDERSTANDING SEQUENCE PRACTICE

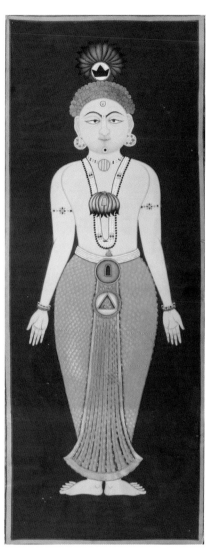

During the initial stages of yoga practice, the most common understanding is that yoga is a physical workout which involves getting into specific asanas. Some might even consider it as an approach to mental discipline, or a prelude to a meditation practice, a curious spiritual practice, etc. These are true as a practitioner experiences some of these effects, depending on the attitude of the person approaching the practice. As you progress, you will observe that yoga fosters the opportunity to grow an awareness of the inner self. In the beginning stages, you might only observe obvious physical features like body, muscle structure, bone structure but eventually you will start perceiving reactions, desires, emotion, behaviour patterns, etc. These results which are felt in the body are due to the awakening of certain energy points known as chakras.

To deal with particular lifestyle needs or issues, subtle patterns of energy flow require to be accurately channelised in the body. Specific chakras roused in a certain precise manner can form these patterns. Asanas help awaken these chakras and conscious sequencing of asanas will aid in developing these patterns of energy flow, which brings about the required positive change in health and attitude.

Understanding the basic features of each chakra, will help you practise with awareness.

CHAKRAS

SAHASRARA: CROWN CHAKRA

This chakra combines and integrates the powers of all the energy centres of the body. Physically, it is the crown which governs spirituality. Spiritually, it is the realisation of cosmic intelligence referred to as the Absolute Truth.

Element: No element is associated with this chakra.

Location: On the crown

Function: Spiritual and self-awareness

(The verb associated with this chakra is that of knowledge – 'I AM AWARE'.)

Gland: Its role may be envisioned as somewhat similar to that of the pituitary gland, which secretes hormones to communicate to the rest of the endocrine system and also connects to the central nervous system.

Parts of the body it governs:
* Cerebral cortex
* Central nervous system

Malfunction results: Depression, alienation, confusion, boredom, apathy and inability to learn or comprehend

Food: Fasting feeds this chakra

Colour: Violet

Symbol: Lotus with 1000 petals

Bija mantra / Seed mantra: 'Aum'

Yogic path: Meditation

Asanas: Inverted-head asanas like Shirsasana, Matsyasana

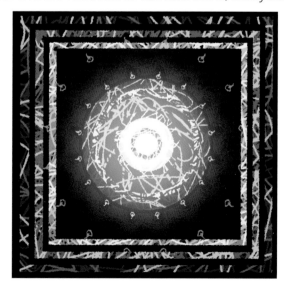

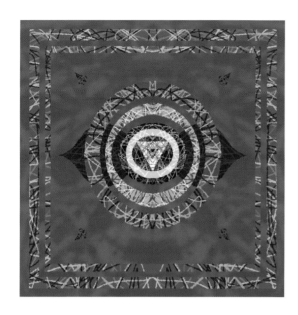

VISHUDDHA: THROAT CHAKRA

This chakra governs such issues as self-expression and communication. Physically, Vishuddha governs communication, emotionally it governs independence, mentally it governs fluent thought, and spiritually, it governs a sense of security.

Element: Akasha tatva (Ether, sound)

Location: Throat

Function: Communication and self-expression

(The verb associated with this could be 'I Speak'.)

Glands: Thyroid and parathyroid. Thyroid, a gland located in the throat area, which produces thyroid hormone, is responsible for growth and maturation.

Parts of the body it governs:

* Throat

Malfunction results: Physical problems including sore throat, stiff neck, colds, thyroids problem, hormonal issues and hearing difficulty

Food: Fruits

Symbol: Lotus with 16 petals

Colour: Pale blue or turquoise

Bija mantra / Seed mantra: 'Ham'

Yogic path: Mahamantra or chants

Asanas: Sarvangasana, Supta Vajrasana, Veerasana, Matsyasana

AJNA: BROW CHAKRA

This chakra governs knowledge and intuition. Physically, it is located in the centre of the forehead, and is usually referred to as the third eye. Spiritually this chakra gives the power of clairvoyance.

Element: Maha tatva (Mind, intelligence)

Location: Brow centre

Function: Seeing and intuiting

(The verb associated with this chakra could be 'I SEE / I UNDERSTAND'.)

Gland: Pineal gland. The pineal gland is a light-sensitive gland that produces the hormone melatonin which regulates sleep and awakening.

Parts of the body it governs:

* Forehead
* Sinus area

Malfunction results: Blindness, nightmares, sleeplessness, headache, blurred vision

Food: Vegetables (rich in vitamins), foods that are not spicy

Symbol: Lotus with 2 petals

Colour: White, indigo and deep blue

Bija mantra / Seed mantra: 'Aum'

Yogic path: Meditation and silence

Asanas: Seated yoga mudras, kriyas

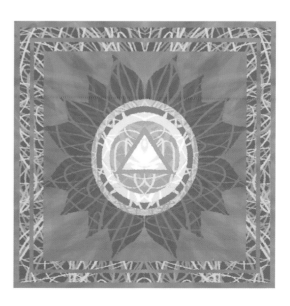

ANAHATA: HEART CHAKRA

This chakra governs the feelings that involve complex emotions, compassion, tenderness, unconditional love, equilibrium, rejection and well-being. Physically, it governs circulation and spiritually, it governs devotion.

Element: Vayu tatva (Air)

Location: Chest / Heart centre

Function: Love

(The verb associated with this chakra could be 'I FEEL LOVE / AFFECTION / COMPASSION'.)

Gland: Thymus. The thymus is an element of the immune system as well as part of the endocrine system. It produces the T Cells responsible for fending off disease.

Body parts it governs:

*   Lungs
*   Heart
*   Arms and Hands

Malfunction results: Asthama, High BP, heart and lung diseases

Food: Vegetables rich in Vitamin C

Symbol: Lotus with 12 petals

Colour: Green

Bija mantra / Seed mantra: 'Yam'

Yogic path: Pranayama

Asanas: Back-bending asanas, Ushtrasana, Dhanurasana

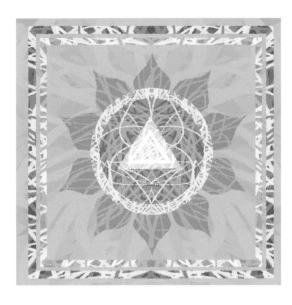

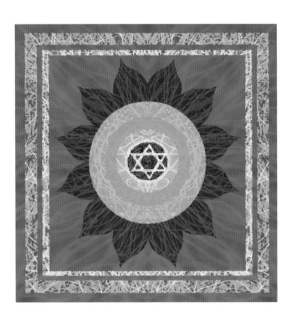

MANIPURA: SOLAR PLEXUS CHAKRA

This chakra governs such issues as personal power, fear, anxiety, opinion-formation, introversion and transition from simple or base emotions to complex.

Physically, this chakra governs digestion. Mentally, it governs personal power. Emotionally, it governs expansiveness, and spiritually, all matters of growth.

Element: Agni tatva (Fire)

Location: Naval and solar plexus

Function: Willpower

(The verb associated with this could be 'I AM CONFIDENT / I CAN'.)

Glands: Pancreas, digestive system, adrenal. Manipura is believed to correspond to the cells in the pancreas, as well as the outer adrenal glands. These play a vital role in digestion and the conversion of food matter into energy for the body.

Body parts it governs:

*   Upper abdomen
*   Stomach
*   Liver and spleen

Malfunction results: Acidity, stomach ulcers, diabetes

Food: Starch

Symbol: Lotus with 10 petals.

Colour: Yellow

Bija mantra / Seed mantra: 'Ram'

Yogic path: Asanas and mantra meditation

Asanas: Back-bending asanas e.g. Urdhva Dhanurasana, Chakrasana

SVADHISTHANA: SACRAL CHAKRA

This chakra governs the making of relationships, feeling of violence, addictions, basic emotional needs, and pleasure. Physically, this chakra governs reproduction. Mentally, it governs creativity. Emotionally, it governs joy, and spiritually, it governs enthusiasm.

Element: Apas tatva (Water)

Location: Sacrum, genitals and womb

Function: Procreation, sexual pleasure

(The verb associated with this could be 'I FEEL AFFECTION / DESIRE'.)

Glands: Adrenal, reproductive system – corresponding to the testes or ovaries that produce the sex hormones involved in the reproduction cycle.

Body parts it governs:

- Stomach
- Small Intestine
- Kidneys
- Reproductive organs

Malfunction results: Sex-related problems, problems in conceiving, kidney and bladder problems, serious imbalance in life like overindulgence and lack of control in emotions.

Food: Protein

Symbol: Lotus with 6 petals

Colour: Orange

Yogic path: Kriyas, bandhas and mudras

Bija mantra / Seed mantra: 'Vam'

Asanas: Bhujangasana, Salabasana, Dhanurasana, Makarasana

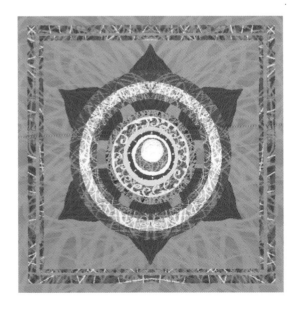

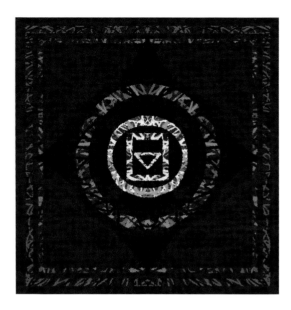

MULADHARA: BASE OR ROOT CHAKRA

This chakra is related to instinct, security, survival and also to basic human potentiality. Its centre is located in the region between the genitals and the anus. No endocrine organ is placed here. There is a muscle located in this region that controls ejaculation in the sexual act of the human male. A parallel is charted between the sperm cell and the ovum where the genetic code lies.

Physically, this chakra governs sexuality. Mentally, it governs stability. Emotionally, it governs sensuality, and spiritually, it governs a sense of security.

Element: Pritvi tatva (Earth)

Location: Pelvic floor

Function: Source of all energy

(The verb associated with it could be 'I FEEL CONTENT'.)

Glands: No gland is associated with this chakra.

Body parts it governs:

- Large intestine
- Colon
- Urethra and Anus

Malfunction results: Restlessness in various ways, depending on the situation the practitioner is in

Food: Bland food without salt or spice

Symbol: Lotus with 4 petals

Colour: Red

Yogic path: Asanas

Bija mantra / Seed mantra: 'Lam'

Asanas: Seated asanas lifted away from gravity e.g. Bakasana, Bhujapeedasana, Urdhva Dandasana, Tittibasana

NADIS

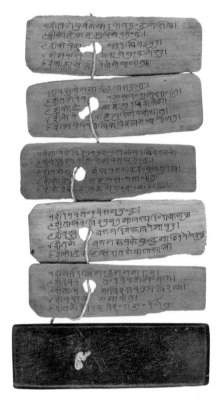

The Nadi Grantha *Manuscript*

The ancient texts on yoga mention subtle passages in the body which carry forth the vital force or pranic current, made up of subtle matter that cannot be seen by our physical eyes nor can it be captured to be tested by modern science. The body is filled with innumerable nadis that cannot be counted. Different texts state different numbers – from 72,000 to 3,50,000. These subtle passages of energy have a great influence on the physical functioning and operations of the body.

All nadis are believed to spring from the Kanda (junction where the Sushumna Nadi is connected to the Muladhara Chakra). Out of the innumerable nadis, 14 are recorded as significant. All these nadis are placed on the sides of the three most important nadis – Sushumna, Ida and Pingala – and proceed to various parts of the body, performing specific functions. Innumerable minor nadis spring from these.

SUSHUMNA
- Originates at the Muladhara Chakra and terminates at the Svadhisthana Chakra.
- Passes through the spinal column.
- Is activated only when the breath flows evenly and strongly from both nostrils simultaneously.
- Pranayama provides specific techniques to calm and activate this nadi, which is very helpful for meditation.

IDA
- Originates at the left of Sushumna and terminates in the left nostril.
- Criss-crosses the spinal column.
- Stimulates the right side of the brain.
- Carries pranic energy force to all the mental nadis.

PINGALA
- Originates at the right side of Sushumna and terminates at the right nostril.
- Is a powerful source of energy and carries solar energy.
- Builds in us vitality, strength (physical), and efficiency.
- Stimulates the left side of the brain.

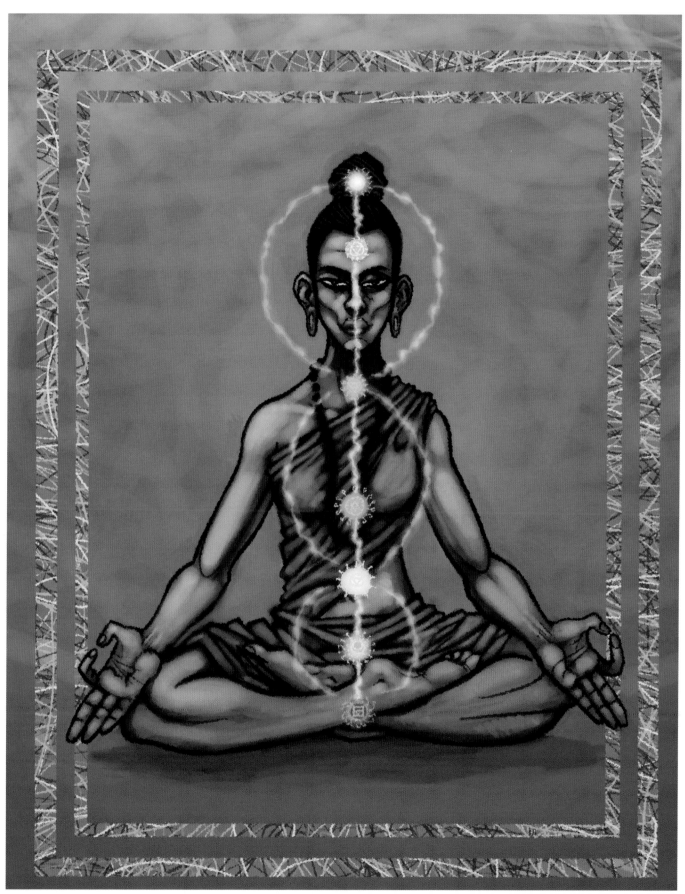

A picture from an 18th-century Nadi Grantha

MUDRAS AND BANDHAS

Bandhas and mudras help distribute energy and prevent its waste. The energy is directed to go up through the Sushumna channel to experience the state of deep relaxation, which will be helpful during the practice of meditation.

MUDRAS

'Mudra' means a seal or lock that closes the body apertures for a while. It is believed that prana flows in the body through various channels and energy points. Mudras help in diverting prana constantly back to the brain, otherwise it will flow into the atmosphere through the openings of the body and fingertips.

WARNING

All mudras are not practised as a routine. It is important for a practitioner to understand the purpose behind the practise of mudras. Proper guidance from a guru for the specific purpose either of yoga meditation or yoga asana, is imperative. The practice should progress slowly and steadily.

Some mudras can be practised before or after other yoga asanas or Pranayama. It appears that mudras were practised by ancient yogis to hear the internal sounds and to experience the most important energy of life force, the Kundalini.

Mudras are not as simple as they appear. No theory can explain their intricacies. The mudras specified here may sound different as there is no definitive method followed by all schools, and can be practised by Hatha Yoga practitioners. It is important to teach these mudras as a part of Kundalini..

KUNDALINI

The philosophy of yoga refers to spiritual energy as Kundalini. Located in the base of the spine, 'Kundalini', located at the base of the spine literally means that which is coiled. There are methods in yoga, which will enable a practitioner of the Kundalini form of yoga to uncoil and arouse energy through the spine upward, moving through the Ajna Chakra, then releasing from the Sahasrara Chakra. It is important to receive guidance from a guru to practise this. The practice of Kundalini benefits in many ways, from spiritual to physical and mental well-being. Studies have shown that the physical and physiological benefits cover a wide spectrum of ailments.

A. NABHO MUDRA
- Sit in a comfortable asana.
- Curl the tongue upward towards the palate of the mouth.
- The tongue should remain steady without movement.
- The lips are to be closed so that air does not enter into the mouth.
- Keep the eyes open and the gaze fixed to a point. Keep the thoughts steady and focus on the point of gaze all the time.
- Breathing has to be normal.
- Hold in this position for 2 minutes and release the tongue to rest. Repeat this mudra 5 times.
- Saliva gathered during this mudra has to be gently swallowed.

BENEFITS: This mudra causes the thymus gland to release beneficial hormones that release stress from the body.

B. BHUJANGINI MUDRA
- Relax on the ground with the chest facing the floor.
- Lift the chest up, and legs up similar to Salabasana and do a complete Adho Mukha Navasana.
- Look up towards the ceiling and fix the gaze at a point from the centre of the brow (Bhrumadhaya).
- Inhale deep and exhale with the a hissing soundlike that of a snake.
- Antara Kumbhaka (for 15 seconds) can be practised in this mudra before exhaling.
- Exhale completely and rest on the floor.
- Repeat again 3 times if you are doing it with Antara Kumbhaka or 5 times without Antara Kumbhaka.

BENEFITS: This mudra strengthens the abdomen and eliminates toxic gases from the abdominal region. It activates digestive juices and strengthens the digestive tract. It also subsides hunger.

C. KAKI MUDRA
- Sit in a comfortable asana.
- Inhale and exhale 5 times.
- Form an Uddiyana Bandha (p. 30) and a Jalandhara Bandha (p. 30)
- Point the mouth like you are trying to drink water from a straw.

- Keep the tongue inside the mouth stable and settled.
- Suck air into the mouth with pointed lips and swallow it, pushing the air into the area of the navel.
- Hold the breath for 10 seconds or till you are comfortable.
- The abdomen should not feel bloated.
- Lift the head up gently.
- Maintain a Samadrishti or close your eyes when you practise this mudra.
- Do not practise for more than 5 rounds.

BENEFITS: This mudra benefits the facial muscles, affects the thyroid and parathyroid glands and keeps the skin healthy and glowing.

D. MULA BANDHA MUDRA
- Place the left heel in the perineum.
- The heels should feel the contraction.
- Inhale and do Antara Kumbhaka before proceeding to do a Uddiyana Bandha.
- Fix the gaze at the Nasagrai (Nose centre).
- Do not repeat more than 5 times.

BENEFITS: Mula Bandha takes place in the centre of the body. It builds up core strength and establishes focus and concentration for higher spiritual practices.

E. SHANMUKHI MUDRA
- Sit in a comfortable asana.
- Spread your fingers above your eyes. Then close all your senses by the following steps:
  – Using your thumbs, close both the ears.
  – Using your index finger, close your eyes.
  – With the middle finger, block the nostrils.
  – Place the ring finger above the upper lip.
  – Place the little finger below the lower lip.
- Shape your lips into a gentle circle.
- Breathe in like you are sucking air. Hold the breath for a Antara Kumbhaka.
- Hold the Antara Kumbhaka for as long as possible and release through the nostrils at a slow, steady and comfortable pace.
- Relax for a while and repeat 5 more times.
- Do not exceed more than 10 times a day.

BENEFITS: This mudra calms the mind and relaxes disturbing thoughts. It also creates a balance in the thyroid that controls hormonal fluctuations.

F. TADAKA MUDRA
- Lie down on the floor with the chest upward in Supta Tadasana.
- Inhale as you raise your hands up towards the ceiling and exhale as you drop hands towards the ground behind the head.
- Observe the expansion of the chest as you breathe in and observe your navel dropping towards the ground as you breathe out.
- Set a breathing rhythm and get comfortable with it.
- The above points would be preparations for Tadaka Mudra.
- Keep the body in a completely stretched position.
- Breathe out completely and drop the navel towards the spine. Hold in that position for as long as you are comfortable.
- The hollow of your abdominal cavity will look like a pond.

BENEFITS: This mudra benefits the spine and hydrates it. It also benefits the circulatory system. Respiratory organs are strengthened to hold in the Kumbhaka which is important during spiritual practices.

G. MATANGI MUDRA
- Take a dip in the water until the head is completely inside
- Inhale through the nostril along with the water and fill the mouth with this water. Do not allow the water to enter into your lungs.
- After the mouth is full, stick the head out of the water and expel water from the mouth. (It should look like the water coming out of the tap.)

BENEFITS: This mudra removes restlessness from the mind and calms down excitement.

NOTE
Comfortable asanas recommended are Siddhasana, Padmasana, Swasthikasana, Veerasana, Vajrasana.

H. KECHARI MUDRA
- The tongue is pulled everyday till the tongue is able to touch the tip of the nose.
- Every week, the nerve below the tongue has to be cut further and pulled till it can be stretched into the nose.
- The tongue will then be swallowed and moved towards the throat till it reaches a point which is commonly known as second tongue.

- When the tongue touches this point, a juice is produced in the gland which yogis believe can conquer hunger and thirst.

BENEFITS: This mudra provides the body with youthful energy.

J. MAHA BANDHA MUDRA

- Press the anus carefully with the left heel.
- Place the right foot on the left thigh.
- Contract the anal muscles and pull the perineum upward.
- Draw air to do the Jalandhara Bandha.
- Then breathe out slowly.

BENEFITS: This mudra benefits the lower abdominal organs and increases energy in all the chakras.

K. MAHA VEDHA MUDRA

- Sit in Padmasana and do Jalandhara Bandha.
- Place the palms on the ground.
- With the support of the hands, palms pressed to the ground, lift the hip off the floor.
- The buttocks are to be hit to the ground gently several times by bouncing the hip up and down.

BENEFITS: This mudra aids in spiritual practices. The lifting and dropping in this mudra builds up cushioning in the sacral area which helps sit for long hours while practising meditation.

L. YOGA MUDRA

- Sit in Padmasana.
- Place the palms on the heels and bend forward.
- Exhale completely by the time you lean and touch the forehead to the ground.
- Deepen the pull of the navel towards the spine and stay there for as long as comfortable. Breathe normally.

BENEFITS: This mudra benefits the lower organs of the body by increasing circulation. It also helps expel toxic prana from the abdominal cavity, making the body light and comfortable.

M. VIPARITA KARANI MUDRA

- Lie on the ground with the chest facing up.
- Raise the legs to do the Sarvangasana with the palm supporting the hips, and elbows pressing to the ground.
- Keep your raised leg at an angle of 45°.
- Stay steady in this position.

- Gently pull in your neck and fix it into the collarbone to form a Jalandhara Bandha.
- Pull in the anal muscle and do a partial Mula Bandha (p. 29) and do not stress the muscle if it is tired.
- The position can be held for 2 to 3 minutes or more.

BENEFITS: This position increases blood supply to all areas of the body.

N. VAJROLI MUDRA

- Sit in the Padmasana with the palms placed on the thighs.
- Inhale through the nose and hold your breath.
- Pull up the sexual organs by contracting the lower abdominal muscles like you would to stop the flow of urine.
- Continue to hold the breath as you relax and contract these muscles ten times.
- On the tenth relaxation of the muscles, exhale completely.

BENEFITS: This mudra strongly influences the nadis that supply the sex organs with spiritual energy. This is practised before Kundalini meditation.

O. ASHWINI MUDRA

- Sit in a comfortable asana.
- Breathe normally.
- Gently contract the sphincter muscles and relax them.
- The action should be confined to the anus only.
- Repeat for 5 times and gradually increases the speed of the contraction.
- The contraction should be rhythmic.

BENEFITS: This mudra benefits the muscles of the rectum, colon and perineum. It builds up efficient functioning of the abdominal organs and keeps the body light and clean.

P. SHAKTI CHALANA MUDRA

This mudra is practised to reach the spiritual high of the Kundalini practice of yoga.

- Sit in the Padmasana on a wooden plank. Make sure the place of practice is quiet and secluded.
- Inhale air forcibly and hold a tight Mula Bandha.
- Close the right nostril with the right fingers (Shanka Mudra).
- Now swallow the air like you are swallowing food and push it towards the naval.
- Do this swallowing 4 to 5 times.

- Exhale gently and relax in the Shavasana.

BENEFITS: This mudra is practised to reach the spiritual high of the Kundalini Yoga practice. It improves the power of concentration and conquers lust, thus freeing the mind for higher spiritual practices.

Q. MANDUKA MUDRA

This mudra is usually conducted to control anger.

- Sit in a comfortable asana.
- Roll the tongue upward to touch the soft palate of the mouth called the Chandra Mandala.
- Move the tongue left to right in small movements until comfortable.
- A juice is produced when you do this. Swallow the juice. The juice is the nectar which helps control hunger.
- The mudra should be repeated of 4 or 5 times and not more.

BENEFITS: This mudra decreases the fluctuations of the mind and balances the energies of the Ida and Pingala.

R. SHAMBHAVI MUDRA

This mudra should be done only in sunlight, and can be done 2 to 3 times daily.

- Draw a circle of about 5-inches radius on a black paper.
- Mark a white spot in the centre of the circle.
- Sit in a comfortable position seven feet away from the circle.
- Stare into the white spot in a straight line without blinking.
- If you experience strain in the eyes, relax your eyes by blinking 10-15 times till you no longer feel the strain.
- Keep staring at the white point until tears form in the eyes.
- The eyes should be cleaned with a fresh handkerchief by dabbing them dry and not by rubbing.

BENEFITS: This mudra, while practised as a pre-meditation routine, improves the vision to see the self (self-assessment), which is an important step before meditation.

BANDHAS

In Sanskrit, 'Bandha' means binding. It refers to holding together in an asana certain organs or parts of the body. Bandhas are mainly performed to harmonise prana inside the body. This helps release blocked and repressed energy to replenishes the body with it. Initially bandhas are taught as a way of engaging specific muscle / muscle groups in physical movement. However, it is important to know that bandhas should never be viewed as muscular contraction as they are not physical locks but energy locks. When bandhas are practised with awareness, energy patterns underlying the physical body are noticeable.

The Classic Bandhas

a. Mula Bandha (Muladhara Chakra)
b. Uddiyana Bandha (Manipura Chakra)
c. Jalandhara Bandha (Vishuddha Chakra)
d. Traya Bandha (Maha Bandha holding all three Bandhas)

MULA BANDHA

In the Mula Bandha, the mula or root lock moves the earth energy from the Muladhara Chakra upward towards the water energy at the Svadhisthana Chakra.

Preparation

- The energy dynamics which occur in the perineal area require toning up of the nerves, glands and muscles of the area so that the energy point is recognised.
- It is important to learn to relax the perineum, to draw it upward rather than tighten and contract the muscles making it challenging to draw the perineum up.
- Body awareness and practice of concentration are very important to understand the movement of this subtle energy.

Procedure

- Focus on the sacrum / tailbone.
- Focus on the pubic bone in the front.
- Relax the area between the two points and practise to bring the two together, pulling them upward into the body.

Benefits

- Tones and purifies the pelvic and genital region.
- Forms a stable support to the entire torso and spine.
- Takes away the strain from the perineal and the lumbar region while sitting in meditation for long hours.
- Keeps the pranic energy circulating inside the body.
- Helps stabilise the other bandhas during the practice of Pranayama / asana.

Caution

- Imposing a practice instead of relaxing might result in constipation, tightness of the lower abdomen, hip, pelvis, legs and lower limbs. To avoid this, keep a check on the tailbone, which should be in a straight line with the spine and make sure it is relaxed and pointing towards the floor.
- Symptoms of depleted Mula energy could be in the form imbalanced physical tension in the initial stages. Try Nadi Shudha Pranayama to balance this effect.
- Avoid harsh, spicy, coarse and irritating foods, lustful and irritating thoughts.

UDDIYANA BANDHA

'Uddiyana' means upward-moving energy locks. Here the energy of the earth, water and fire chakras (Mula, Svadhisthana, Manipura) enters into the air chakra (Anahata).

Preparation

- Focus on your navel point. Feel the area around the navel and also feel the area exactly behind the navel near the lumbar curve.
- Align the asana to make sure that you do not have a curve in that area.
- Do not drop your shoulders into a curve, which results in the ribs dropping into the Manipura Chakra / Solar Plexus).
- Pull your navel inwards, moving it towards the spine, but make sure that the spine is not moving away in the process.
- Practise this a number of times till you start feeling comfortable to hold it for at least 1 minute.

Procedure

- Keep the knees slightly bent. Place the hands on the inside corner of the lower thighs (for better grip), with the heel of the palms resting on the top side of the thighs.
- Do not collapse the chest in the process and make sure the back and torso feel lengthened. While doing this, the chest area should feel lifted and relaxed.
- Make sure the pelvis is stable and pulled long in the Mula Bandha.
- Observe the curved vast space between the ribs and the hipbone area.
- The neck should be relaxed.

- Exhale all the air and maintain Bahya Kumbhaka (External Retention – Section B, Chapter 4).
- Try to maintain the Mula Bandha at all times to keep the energy flow moving upward.
- Relax the muscles of the diaphragm and start lifting the abdominal length into the diaphragm area. Keep the navel tucked in towards the spine. Observe the formation of a concave in the area right below the rib cage or the sternum – the region of the stomach, liver and pancreas.
- Hold the breath during the Uddiyana Bandha.
- Release the bandha just before you become uncomfortable or gasp for breath.

Benefits

- Tones the abdominal area.
- Increases gastric fire, thus stimulating the digestive organs.
- The back feels lengthened and relaxed after the Uddiyana Bandha.
- The Manipura Chakra feels charged and connected to the Svadhisthana Chakra from below and the Anahata Chakra from the top.

Caution

- Do not force the practice of the Uddiyana Bhandha. Instead keep practising until you feel confident.
- If you do not have the stamina to hold the bandha, practise the Preparation points for some more time.
- If you feel a strain around the throat area, release the diaphragm and the chest. It could be because you are pressing the diaphragm too much instead of emphasising on the length from the navel area.
- The Mula Bandha has to be maintained throughout the Uddiyana Bandha. Practise the Mula Bandha well before starting on the Uddiyana Bandha.

JALANDHARA BANDHA

The Jalandhara Bandha addresses the Throat Chakra or the Vishuddha Chakra. It connects the Anahata Chakra (Heart Chakra) to the Ajna Chakra. The Jalandhara Bandha is performed in many asanas.

Preparation and Procedure

- Make sure you relax the shoulders, throat, neck area, chin and face.

- The back of the neck should bend forward towards the collarbone without hunching the back or constricting the front of the throat.
- Practise lifting the chest up towards the descending chin.
- The jaws should feel relaxed and not clenched.
- Deep breathing could be practised in this position.

Benefits
- Tones the throat, shoulders and the neck area.
- Improves the voice quality and relaxes tension in the throat.
- Relieves pain and tension along the spine
- Makes the mind humble and mitigates arrogance.

Caution
- Make sure that you relax the bandha just before you gasp for breath.
- Make sure you practise this bandha well before you venture into the challenging Traya Bandha.
- Holding breath with the head down could make you feel giddy and tired. These symptoms are only during initial stages of the practice.

TRAYA (THREE-FOLD) BANDHA
When all the three bandhas (Mula, Uddiyana and Jalandhara) are engaged at the same time, it forms the Traya Bandha. The sequence while building the Traya Bandha is Mula Bandha, Uddiyana Bandha and Jalandhara Bandha. The sequence while releasing the Traya Bandha is exactly the opposite.

Preparation and Procedure
Same as explained in the above three bandhas.

Benefits
- Helps build concentration.
- The powerful energy flow to and fro, from the Muladhara Chakra can be felt in the Sushumna Nadi (Central Column).
- Helps prepare for advanced Pranayama practices and gives you a preview of the feeling of flow of energy. As the practice progresses, you will experience the pleasant feeling of the subtle energy flow, which will help the practice of meditation in the long run.

Caution
- Read any kind of discomfort as a warning to stop and if it settles, restart.
- The bandhas have to be practised with awareness, observation, patience and complete knowledge of the body.
- Do not be too anxious to feel the subtle energy flow as it requires calm and patient observation.

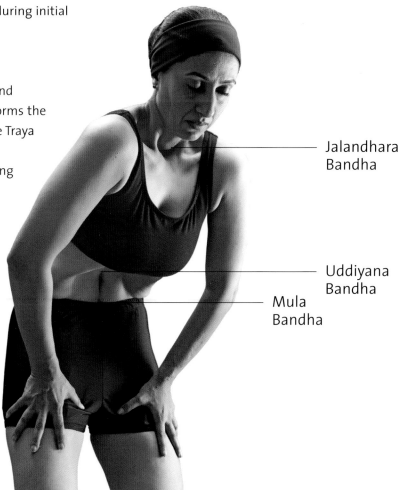

Jalandhara Bandha

Uddiyana Bandha

Mula Bandha

ASANAS

'Asana' literally means seat. In yoga, asana is defined as 'posture'. Asana deals with the physical aspects of the body. It is one of the eight limbs in the classical Ashtanga practice of yoga. Asanas helps strengthen and control the body and mind to progress towards higher aspects of yoga. This does not mean that asanas are just another exercise programme. The energy channels, chakras and psychic centre of the body are opened by performing various asanas, which in turn wake up the concerned energy centre.

BENEFITS OF YOGA ASANAS

The physical benefits of asanas are many. They give the practitioner an opportunity to improve awareness, to get to know the body well with all its limitations. Asanas involve voluntary exercises, which help channelise awareness of all dimensions of the body, including bone density, muscular flexibility and structure, tissue strength, glandular function and internal organs, thus improving health at a higher level.

IMPORTANT

It is very important to note a few things while practising yoga asanas. Asanas are to be approached gently and cautiously. The progress of asanas is generally slow and needs to be monitored. It is important to learn about the points of resistance in the body and the pain which is experienced while meeting these points. A momentary lapse of attention, misjudgment about preparedness for a particular asana, or a basic slip-up is sometimes all it takes to get injured and injuries can set us back. Mistakes can also help our practice evolve by teaching us how we should or shouldn't practice. Almost any asana, if performed incorrectly can cause problems.

The awareness a yoga asana practice helps achieve maximum flow of vital energy to the entire body, thus benefiting the physical body which is relieved of all discomfort so that the mind reaches the state of concentration which is the actual purpose of the practice.

CATEGORIES OF YOGA ASANAS

A. PARSVA OR LATERAL STRETCHES

Lateral-bending or asymmetric asanas aim at stretching the body intensely, from toe to fingertip. Stretching improves lung capacity by expanding the chest and tones the muscles of the heart. Stretches form an important part of the practice as they free all muscles in the body, which helps to progress in the practice.

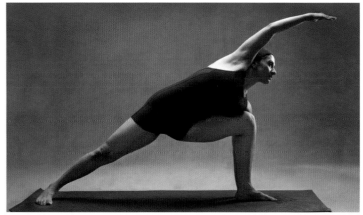

PARSVAKONASANA

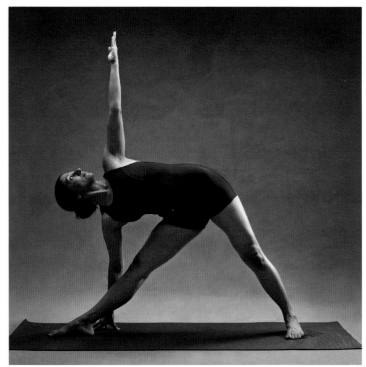

TRIKONASANA

B. PURVATTANA OR BACKWARD STRETCHES

Back-bending asanas are particularly useful when there are conditions of tightness in the front torso, or when there is a need to increase the thoracic mobility or to expand the chest. They improve blood circulation to all the organs of the body. They tone the muscles of the back and remove stiffness from the shoulders. They also enhance the capacity for inhalation and energise the entire system.

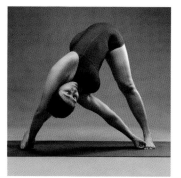
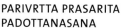
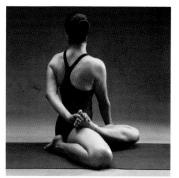

PARIVRTTA PRASARITA PADOTTANASANA

BHARADWAJASANA

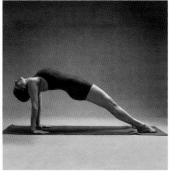
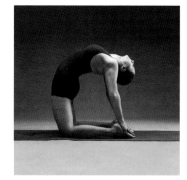

PURVOTTANASANA

USHTRASANA

C. PASCHIMOTTANA OR FORWARD STRETCHES

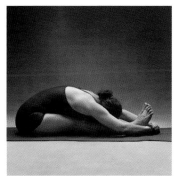
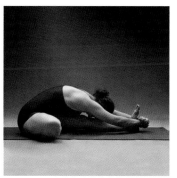

PASCHIMOTTANASANA

JANU SHIRSASANA

Forward-bending asanas are particularly useful when there are conditions of increasing lumbar curve or tightness in the back or when there is a need to enhance digestion. These relieve mental and physical exhaustion and tone the abdominal organs including the liver, spleen, kidneys, intestines etc. They help relieve stomach aches, ease stiffness in the shoulders and legs, and help stabilise blood pressure.

D. PARIVRTTA OR TWISTS

Twisting asanas help particularly when there are conditions of scoliosis, asymmetries in the body, tightness in the shoulders and neck or the pelvic girdle, and when digestion and absorption need to be stimulated. These relieve discomfort in the shoulder and spinal areas, increase their flexibility and ease pain or strain from stiff lumbar spine.

E. VIPARITA OR INVERTED ASANAS

These asanas reverse the effects of gravity on our system. They are useful in strengthening the neck, spine, muscles of the back and the respiratory system. They build stamina and reduce palpitations while strengthening the lungs and improving the functions of the nervous system.

F. VISHESHA OR EXTREME ASANAS

Unusual or extreme asanas that challenge the body, these should be attempted only when the body is ready for them. They are particularly useful in building a sense of confidence, strengthening the body, flexibility of the spine and increasing

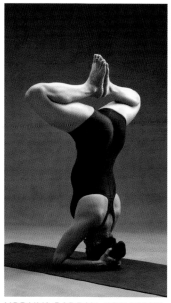
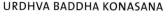
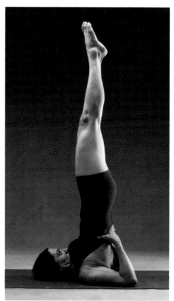

URDHVA BADDHA KONASANA

SARVANGASANA

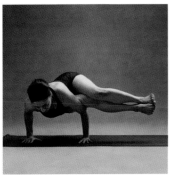

DWI PADA KOUNDINYASANA

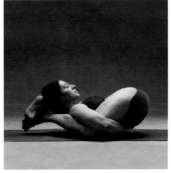

YOGA NIDRASANA

concentration. Often, these advanced variations are natural progressions from the easier ones.

BEFORE ASANA PRACTICE

Mentioned below are a few points to be followed for asana practice:

- Drink a glass of fresh lukewarm water 45 minutes before practice.
- The stomach should be clean and empty.
- Food timings should be adjusted according to your practice timings.
  - 4 hours after a vegetarian meal.
  - 5 hours after a non-vegetarian meal, though it is best to avoid all forms of meat during practice days.
  - 2 hours after a light snack or beverages.
- Avoid rich food, very dry food, very spicy / hot food, left-overs, refrigerated / frozen food and very importantly avoid overeating.
- Keep the body warm at least for half an hour after practice.
- Practise a steady rhythm of breathing throughout the yoga session.
- Move the body steadily and observe every movement. This helps avoid injury.
- Asanas should be ideally practised early in the morning. If this is not possible, the next best time is evening, around dusk.
- Ensure Ujjayee breathing to follow a rhythmic pattern of deep, diaphragm breathing, during asana practice.
- Stop when the body is stressed. Relax tensed muscles, wait till the breathing and the heart rate settle.
- Asanas should be performed in a well-ventilated, peaceful and calm room.
- Light physical exercises as warm-up are essential before practising Pranayama.

ASANA / POSTURE PRACTICE POINTS

It is important to conduct the asanas systematically. Each asana is an experience. Take time to explore each of them. The journey throughout your practice will be that of pleasure and awakening rather than mere difficult physical movements. The student should focus on experiencing the asana rather than forcing the body to achieve the final pose.

Patience is the key. Be aware of every movement of the body as each day the body rhythms are different due to a lot of circumstances. During a particular day if you find certain asanas too challenging, revert to asanas which the body is more comfortable with.

Yield yourself to the flow of the body and surrender to the force of gravity. Release tension from the muscles after achieving the final position of the asana. Try to hold the asana at least for 30 seconds.

- Always practise bare foot and on a clean mat.
- Warm-up is very important.
- Freeing and loosening up limbs will help avoid injuries.
- Start all the asanas from the Samasthiti (Start pose).
- Keep the feet firm on the ground and keep the spine elongated and firm with the tailbone tucked inside the body.
- The power of yoga is only felt with proper rhythmic breathing. Observe the breath. Any discomfort whilst breathing could be an indication that you are pushing yourself too much. Focus on steady deep diaphragm breathing, before you progress from one asana to another.
- Do not rush through the practice. Excessive sweating indicates this in a tense body and an agitated mind.

PLEASE NOTE

This practice manual suggests (a) moderated sequence of practice (b) shortened sequence of practice (c) specific target practice. Lifestyle-based sequence of practice has also been suggested. It is important to become familiar with all the asanas and then pick a practice sequence according to what suits you best.

Study the asanas. Develop a mental and visual understanding of each. If while practising any of these asanas, you feel uncomfortable, consult a qualified yoga teacher.

PRANAYAMA

INTRODUCTION

'Prana' is the life force or the subtle form of energy carried by air, food, water and sunlight. 'Ayama' means to exercise, to stretch, to expand, to control, to restrain, to energise. This process of self-energising the body by utilising the existing prana is known as Pranayama. It is believed that our prana is exercised through controlled breathing techniques, which draw in more oxygen into the body thus invigorating it.

> **NOTE**
> Pranayama needs training from an expert. Theoretical study is good but, practical learning and corrections are vital.

Pranayama, a form of perfect breathing, is fifth amongst the eight basic principles of yoga (Ashtanga). Before the practice of Pranayama, it is important to note a few points on the mechanics of breathing.

Observe the stages of breathing
A. Inhalation – taking air inside the body.
B. Pause before exhalation.
C. Exhalation – pushing air out of the body.
D. Now again pause before inhaling.

This is the normal breathing / respiration procedure, where the inhalation and exhalation are at a ratio of 1:2. In Pranayama, this normal respiration procedure is practised in various methods. Each variation has its target point in the body and the nervous system, which can be gradually experienced when practised consistently with focus and observation.

Observe the breathing patterns

A. CHEST-LEVEL BREATHING

In this kind of respiration, only the upper part of the lungs is activated. It makes the ribs, collarbone and shoulders rise, which can be stressful. This is the least advisable breathing as the upper part of the lungs has small air capacity and the ribs are rigid in the upper region of the chest, which makes expansion of the lungs difficult. People suffering from asthma, an obese person and people wearing tight clothes get into this kind of breathing habit.

B. LOW BREATHING

This breathing primarily takes place in the lower region of the chest and lungs. It is the most effective form of breathing with a slight movement of the abdomen (in and out) and also of the diaphragm. It is a relaxing form of breathing and can be seen and observed when a person is fast asleep. It can also be observed in an active person, while walking, running, lifting weights. While low breathing, the stomach is slightly pushed forward at the time of inhalation, and the stomach gets back into position during exhalation.

Benefits
- More air, hence more oxygen, is taken in while inhaling.
- Expands the diaphragm, drawing more venous blood and thus improving the body's general circulation.
- The abdominal organs are gently massaged by the up-and-down movement of the diaphragm.

C. MIDDLE-LEVEL BREATHING

This type of breathing involves primarily the middle part of the lungs. This is also shallow breathing which means though it expands the chest, it does not move the diaphragm up and down. The ribs expand sideways, which is not a very helpful breathing habit.

D. COMPLETE BREATHING

This involves breathing into all the three parts of the lungs – upper, middle and lower – thus engaging the entire respiratory system. In this kind of breathing, maximum air is inhaled, expanding the lungs to its full capacity. It opens up the areas of the shoulders, collarbones, ribs and the diaphragm, creating a power house of energy.

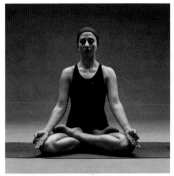

PADMASANA

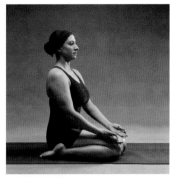

VEERASANA

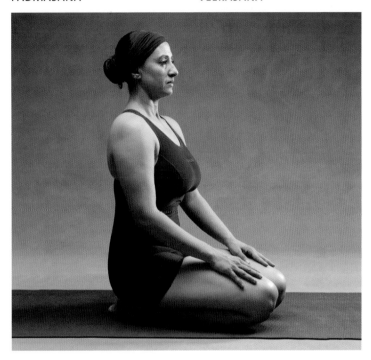

VAJRASANA

PRANAYAMA (PRACTICE OF BREATHING)

Note the following before and during practice of Pranayama:

- Establish a comfortable posture. It need not necessarily be on the floor. However, the back should be straight and knees relaxed.
- Normal respiration should fall into a steady and rhythmic pace.
- Kumbhakas (holding of breath) are traditionally performed 4 times a day (early morning, noon, evening and midnight) until the number of Kumbhakas in one sitting is 80.

DOS AND DON'TS

- When Pranayama is performed properly, it eradicates all diseases, but done improperly may even generate disease.
- Please follow all the instructions carefully as it is necessary not to omit any instruction.

- In the enthusiasm to master Pranayama at the earliest, practitioners may use too much force during inhalation, holding or expelling the air. This may cause undue pressure on the eyes, ears, etc. and can cause pain.
- There should be a gap of eight hours between each Pranayama session.

INTRODUCING SOME PRANAYAMA TECHNIQUES

(Practise it first with a yoga guru)

UJJAYEE

'Ujjayee' means victorious. This breathing can be done standing, sitting or even lying down.

Steps

- Face the incoming air, while performing Ujjayee.
- First exhale air with force, throwing out all air through the mouth. When completely exhaled, the stomach should be pulled inside, squeezing out all the stale air.
- Inhale steadily with both nostrils, making 'ssss' sound from the epiglottis. Keep the body relaxed and at ease while inhaling.
- The air is inhaled through the back of the nostrils.
- After inhalation, observe that the chest has expanded while the stomach is rolled inward. Slowly tighten the abdominal muscles and hold the breath inside for as long as you are comfortable.

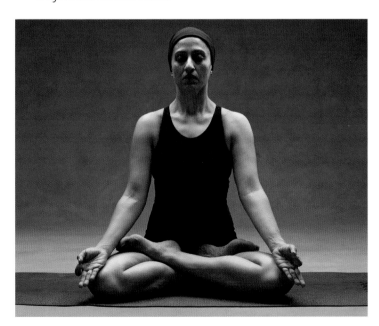

PADMASANA

- Exhale slowly, relaxing and easing tension. It is important to synchronise the relaxation with the exhalation.
- Rest for ten seconds, breathing normally.

Sitting

Try the following asanas: Padmasana, Siddhasana, Vajrasana or Veerasana. However, make sure a comfortable posture is adopted. The seat bones should be firmly anchored. You can sit on a chair too, with a straight back. The breathing process remains the same as while standing.

Lying Down

This position is recommended for weak or disabled people, who could feel dizzy standing.

Posture

- Lie straight on the floor with palms close to the body.
- The heels together should point towards the ceiling.
- The process of breathing remains the same as already explained above.

Restrictions

- Start with 5 rounds and gradually increase to eight rounds in one session.
- Make sure you do not stress your breath or feel out of breath at any point in time.
- Retain the breath only for as long as you are comfortable.

Benefits

- Helps in energising the body.
- Helps internal purification and conditions the body.
- Increases oxygen supply to the haemoglobin.
- Calms down the heart rate and benefits the central nervous system.
- Helps maintain vibrant health, nourishing the physical body.

SHITAKARI PRANAYAMA

This Pranayama cools the body and hence the name. It can be practised anytime at any place.

Steps

- Sit comfortably on the floor.
- Place the tongue closer to the lines of the teeth, with the lips slightly apart.
- Inhale fresh air steadily through and in between teeth at a medium speed.
- Air should be inhaled in a manner that it touches the tongue all the way from the tip to the very base.
- After inhaling sufficient air, exhale through the nostrils at medium speed.
- Repeat at least 5 times.

Caution

- Do not practise for more than ten rounds.
- There are chances of getting a cold or sore throat during the initial stages of practice. Take a break for a few days and restart the practice.

Benefits

- Cools the whole body and the nervous system.
- Activates the liver and spleen and also improves digestion.
- Helps relieve thirst.
- Recommended as a remedy for nervousness.

SHITALI PRANAYAMA

This Pranayama is similar to the previous one. The only change would be, instead of clenching the teeth while

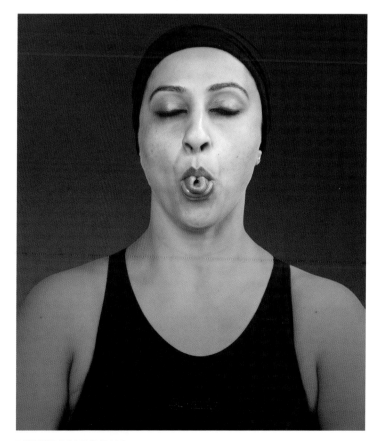

SHITALI PRANAYAMA

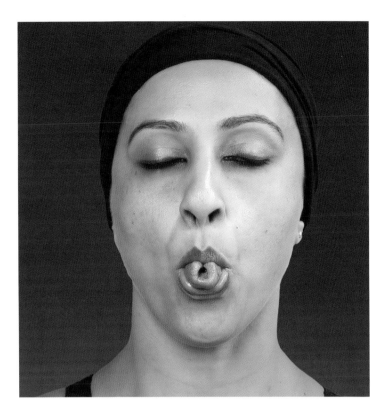

Steps
- Relax in a comfortable position.
- Exhale completely until all air in the lungs is expelled.
- Inhale for 5 seconds, pause and hold the breath for 5 seconds.
- Exhale for 5 seconds, pause and hold the breath for 5 seconds.
- Gradually release the tension around the abdomen which was established while the breath was held.

Benefits
- Brings lightness and a feeling of ease in the body.
- A good warm-up for the respiratory system.

NADI SHUDDHI PRANAYAMA
This is similar to Anuloma Viloma Pranayama, the only difference being that the breath is not held. Inhalation and exhalation are a continuous process through alternate nostrils.

breathing in through the mouth, with the tongue slightly touching the gap between the teeth as in Sitakari, in Shitali the tongue is rolled out of the lips and air is breathed through the tongue like breathing in through a straw. The advantage is that more air can be sucked which adds to the benefit mentioned in the Sitakari Pranayama. Beginners can start with 5:10 breathing and progress to 6:12 depending on their comfort. This Pranayama should be stopped if the practitioner feels a little dizzy or nauseous.

The cooling sensation inside the body, around the lips and in the throat is normal. If the throat starts itching, the Pranayama has to be stopped. People with a cold should not practise this Pranayama.

Caution
People with low blood pressure should not practise this Pranayama as it might further lower the BP, but can do Sitakari Pranayama.

ANULOMA VILOMA
- 'Anuloma' means aligned with the natural order and 'Viloma' means against the natural order. In this Pranayama, inhalation and exhalation is a continuous process, but interrupted by several pauses.
- Can be done in the sitting or lying-down positions.

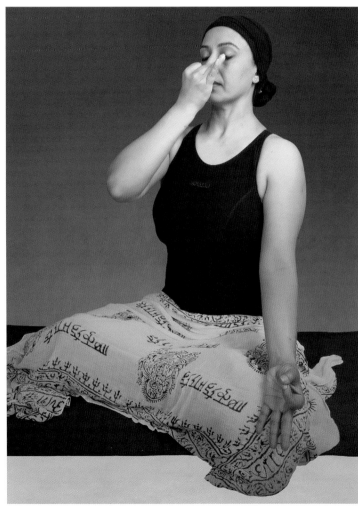

NADI SHUDDHI PRANAYAMA

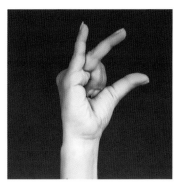 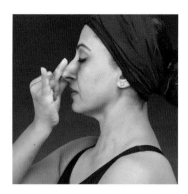

VISHNU MUDRA

KAPALABHATI

'Kapala' means skull and 'Bhati' means lustre / shine

- Always done sitting. Select any asana you are comfortable with: Padmasana, Siddhasana, Vajrasana, Sukhasana or Veerasana.

Steps

- First exhale air from the lungs.
- Inhale slowly, relaxing the abdomen, allowing the air to fill in the lungs gently. Try not to do Ujjayee.
- Exhale short blasts of air by contracting and releasing the abdomen quickly, thus raising the diaphragm upward.
- Start with slow blasts of air (about 20 per exhale) and relax to observe.
- You can repeat the cycles till whenever comfortable.

Caution

- Stop the practice if you experience cramps, or a pull in any muscle. This indicates that you are not gentle with the muscle contraction.
- Begin with 3 to 5 cycles and gradually increase.
- People with poor lung capacity, high / low blood pressure, backaches, or suffering from eye / ear disorder must not attempt this Pranayama.

Benefits

- Helps the body eliminate large quantities of carbon-dioxide and toxins / impurities.
- Purifies the nasal passages and lungs.
- Activates pancreas, spleen and abdominal muscles, and improves digestion.
- Asthma patients, those suffering from sinusitis and air pollution (traffic, industry, cigarette, etc.) will benefit from this asana.

SURYA BHEDANA PRANAYAMA

This refers to a breathing technique in which you inhale through the right nostril, hold the inhaled breath for as long as comfortable and exhale through the left.

'Surya' means Sun, referring to the right nostril which is the path of the Pingala Nadi (Section B, Chapter 4).

Steps

- Hold a mudra by pressing the index finger and the middle finger of the right hand on the mound of the palm below the thumb, (see left for illustration of the Vishnu Mudra)
- Whenever needed, use the thumb to close the right nostril. The ring finger and the little finger are used to close the left nostril.

Benefits

- Daily practice keeps air passages clean and free from blockages in the length of the Pingala Nadi.

CHANDRA BHEDANA PRANAYAMA

This refers to breathing exercises in which you inhale through the left nostril, hold the inhaled breath for as long as it is comfortable to do so, and exhale through the right nostril.

'Chandra' means moon, referring to the left nostril which is the path of the Ida Nadi (Section B, Chapter 6).

Steps

- Hold a mudra by pressing the index finger and the middle finger of the left hand on the mound of the palm below the thumb.
- Use the thumb close the left nostril and ring, and the little finger to close the right nostril.

Benefits

- Daily practice keeps air passages clean and free from blockages at the Ida and keeps the mind alert and awake.
- Beneficial for children who feel stressed out, especially during exams.

BHASTRIKA

'Bhastrika' means bellows. In the Bhastrika Pranayama, the air is inhaled and exhaled rapidly and forcefully. This creates a sound similar to bellows when they are used.

Procedure

- Relax in a comfortable seated position.
- Inhale rapidly and forcefully. Then exhale rapidly, making the sound of a sneeze from the nostril.
- The sound should be like that of a bellow.
- Do around 5 cycles of about 20 each and relax into breathing Ujjayee. Try Antara Kumbhaka between Ujjayee.
- Then move back to Bhastrika.

KUMBHAKA

'Kumbhaka' means holding of breath. The two important Kumbhakas are:
A. Bhahya: External retention of breath after exhalation.
B. Antara: Internal retention of breath after inhalation.

BRAHMARI

The word 'Brahmari' means bee. The characteristic of this Pranayama is to create a sound like a humming bee.

Steps

- Sit in a comfortable position.
- Inhale quickly with both nostrils.
- During exhalation, bring out the sound of the bee. For this, the soft palate gets naturally lifted towards the pharynx sufficiently (while imitating a bee's buzzing sound) to produce a controlled vibrating sound.
- Become one with the sound of the vibrations and let them fill your whole head and gradually the whole body.

Duration

- Start by practising about 5 times and then slowly increase to 11 and then 21, which would take around 20 minutes.

Benefits

- Delights the mind.
- Useful in elevating mood, relieving anxiety, tension and depression.
- Helpful for people suffering from thyroid disorders.
- Helps lower blood pressure and regulate blood circulation.
- Helps control asthma and other respiratory diseases.

NOTE: Combine the practice of Brahmari along with Anuloma Viloma, which is of great benefit.
Caution

- If there is a feeling of dizziness, take a break.
- Do not hold the breath during the course of Brahmari.
- Keep the mouth dry to avoid discomfort or choking while swallowing the saliva.

OMKARA SADHANA

Getting into a state of tranquility and peace is an important purpose behind the practice of yoga. There are various methods of practice which lead a practitioner into this state of mind known as dhyana or meditation. Practitioners understand dhyana in different ways. For some, it is a way of self-observation; for others, it is breath awareness, thinking, or reflecting. Omkara Sadhana is a very powerful traditional practice where the mind is filled with the sound of AUM'.

The sound of 'AUM' is traditionally referred to as Omkara Sadhana. Omkara acts as a centering sound. It offers the mind a place to rest. The sound of Omkara is believed to absorb all distracting energies and induce spiritual insight, making the mind calm. With regular practice, focus and concentration on the sound will increase. Eventually, the sound will seem to be at the back of the mind all the time.

Practice Tips

- Rest your body into a comfortable position (Padmasana).
- Adjust and tune the voice into a comfortable pitch.
- Visualise the formation of the bell curve with a gentle sound of A – U – M.
- Centre your vision to the heart centre and focus your mind to the sound.
- If distracting thoughts disturb the focus, pause for a while, then gently direct attention to the sound again.
- The time, place and right hour are very important to the sadhana of Omkara. It is ideal after asana practice because the body will be in total balance of the three doshas: Vata, Pitta and Kapha.

Sunrise and sunset are traditional timings. Never practise Omkara immediately after meals in the afternoon.

DRISHTI

Drishti — point of focus or gaze — helps to concentrate and mentally focus on the positioning and balance of an asana. Drishti is said to direct oxygen to the brain which further releases tension from the brain. Drishti facilitates avoid distractions and helps attain a higher awareness of an asana. A steady point of focus provides orientation and balance to an asana when it is to be held for a long time. A proper positioning of drishti helps relax the neck by positioning the head properly, making breathing comfortable.

Angushtagrai	Tip of the thumb
Bhoomigrai	Ground
Bhrumadhya	Centre of the brows
Dhyana	Inward-looking
Hastagrai	Hand / Palm
Nabi	Centre of the navel
Nasagrai	Tip of the nose
Padayoragrai	Tip of the toes
Parsva	Side (Left / Right)
Purva	Backward
Sama	Straight
Urdhva	Upward

The drishti positions are different in each asana. The prescribed drishti in the asana allows the eyes to fix at one point. This ensures mental focus, balance and a comfortable neck position, all essential for steady and easy breathing. Drishti also improves the muscles of the eyes.

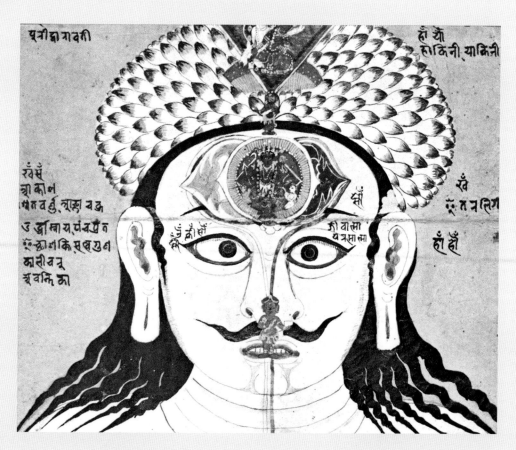

CHAPTER 5
SURYA NAMASKARA (SUN SALUTATION)

SURYA NAMASKARA A

Surya Namaskara is the most important foundation routine in yoga asana practice. It sets a certain rhythm and pace to the practice. It helps focus and concentrate, preparing the practitioner by warming up the body and establishing stability – both in the body and mind. The series of asanas prescribed by the yogis intend to awaken the energy of the sun that normally lies dormant inside our body in the Svadhisthana Chakra. The asanas in the Surya Namaskara allow us to reach deep into the chakras of the body and stimulate them to produce the radiant energy which has healing powers.

It helps:
- Calm the mind
- Balance the pranic flow
- Balance the heating and cooling system in the body (Ida and Pingala Nadis)
- Energise the body's nervous system

Surya Namaskara can be practised by anyone, as it is not the property of any caste, creed or religion, just like sunlight that is showered upon everyone on earth. According to ancient scriptures, Surya or the sun is considered to be the one who bestows health (both physical and mental) upon all life form. Venerating his stature is best achieved by Surya Namaskara.

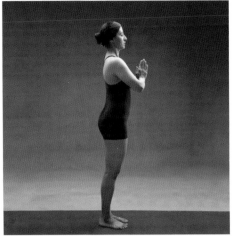

0. SAMASTHITI

1. URDHVA MUKHA TADASANA

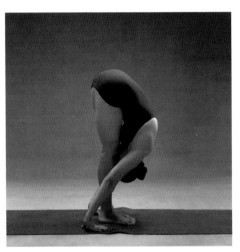

2. UTTANASANA

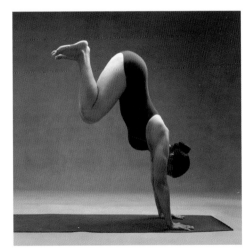

3. JUMP BACK

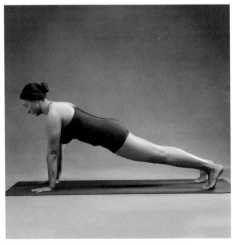

4A. CHADURANGA DANDASANA 1

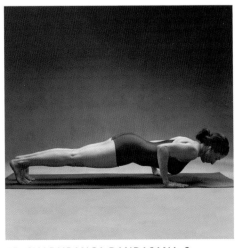

4B. CHADURANGA DANDASANA 2

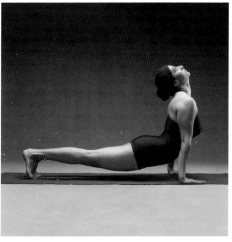

5. URDHVA MUKHA SVANASANA

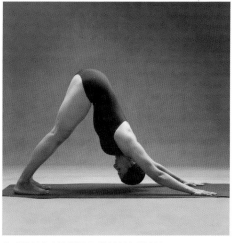

6. ADHO MUKHA SVANASANA

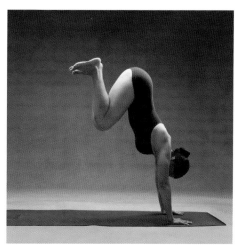

7. JUMP FORWARD

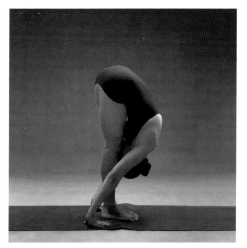

8. UTTANASANA

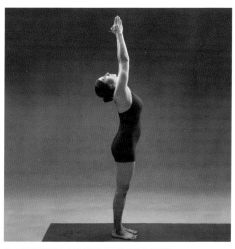

9. URDHVA MUKHA TADASANA

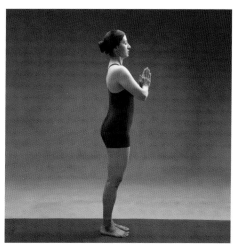

0. SAMASTHITI

SURYA NAMASKARA B

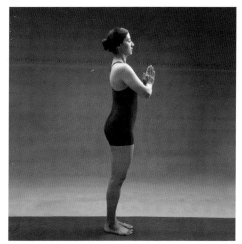

0 SAMASTHITI

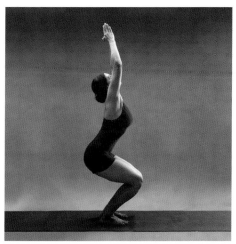

1. UTKATASANA

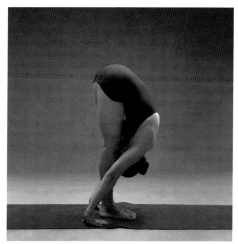

2. UTTANASANA

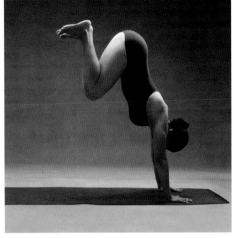

3. JUMP BACK

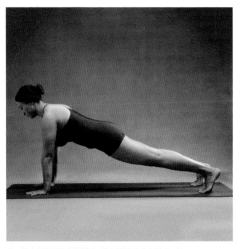

4. CHADURANGA DANDASANA 1

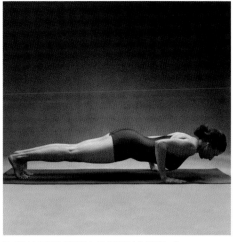

5. CHADURANGA DANDASANA 2

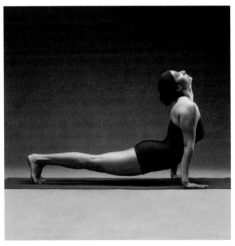

6. URDHVA MUKHA SVANASANA 1

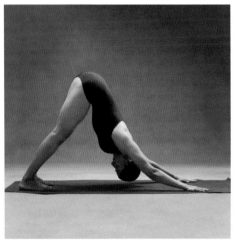

7. ADHO MUKHA SVANASANA

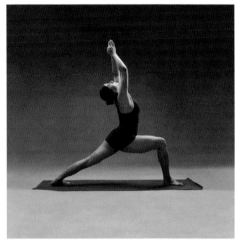

8. VEERABHADRASANA RIGHT LEG

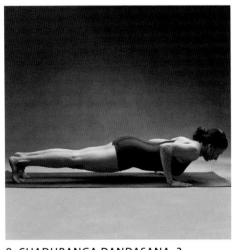

9. CHADURANGA DANDASANA 2

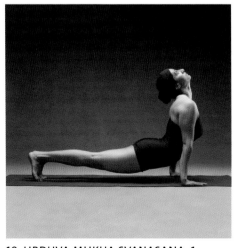

10. URDHVA MUKHA SVANASANA 1

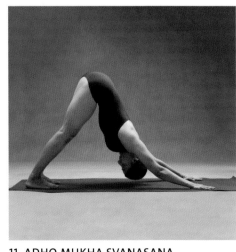

11. ADHO MUKHA SVANASANA

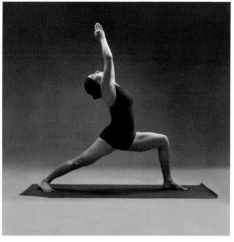

12. VEERABHADRASANA LEFT LEG

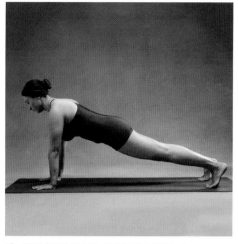

13. CHADURANGA DANDASANA 1

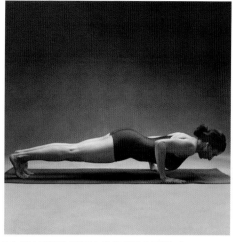

14. CHADURANGA DANDASANA 2

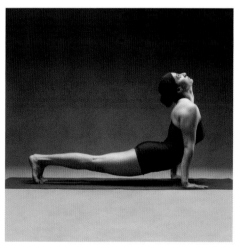

15. URDHVA MUKHA SVANASANA 1

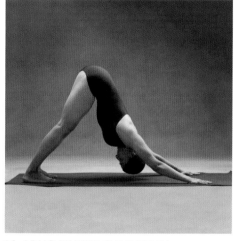

16. ADHO MUKHA SVANASANA

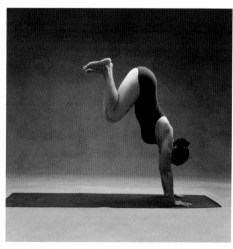

17. JUMP FORWARD

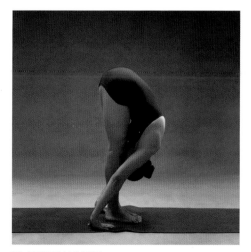

18. UTTANASANA

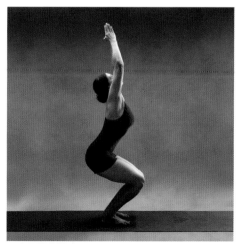

19. UTKATASANA

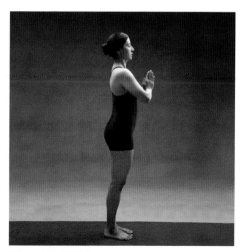

20. SAMASTHITI

CHAPTER 6
PRE-SEQUENCE

Except for the cooling down routine, the below routines should be done by all practitioners before following any specified sequences in the following chapters. However, depending on the practitioner's health condition, specific asanas have either been added or deleted from this routine. Please study SectionC, The Sequence Manual, for details of any such change in the order of the asanas. It is good practice to hold an asana for a minimum of 5 deep breaths or 30 seconds.

A cooling down routine should be followed at the end of any sequence, and is detailed in each of the specific sequences that follow.

I. WARM UP

- Perform soft rhythmic jumps 50 times.
- Swing the arms forward and backward powerfully 10 times.
- Circle the shoulders forward and backward 10 times.
- Twist the waist with arms open and stretched 5 times each side.
- Gently circle the knees, left & right sides, 5 times each.
- Circle ankles clockwise and anti-clockwise, with front sole pressed to the ground and heel raised – 5 times each.

II. PRANAYAMA

Sit in a comfortable, relaxed position. Calm your mind and observe your thoughts.

- Perform Ujjayee for 5 minutes.
- Ujjayee with Antara Kumbhaka (holding breath after inhaling) – 5 min.
- Perform Anuloma Viloma for 10 minutes.

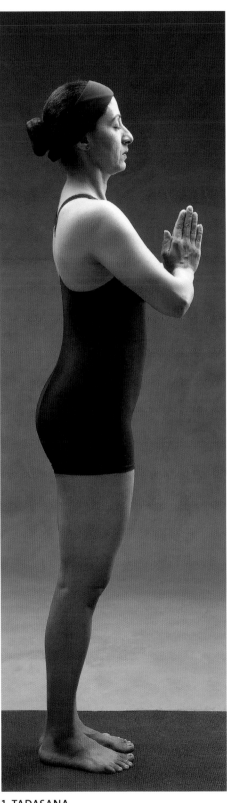

1. TADASANA

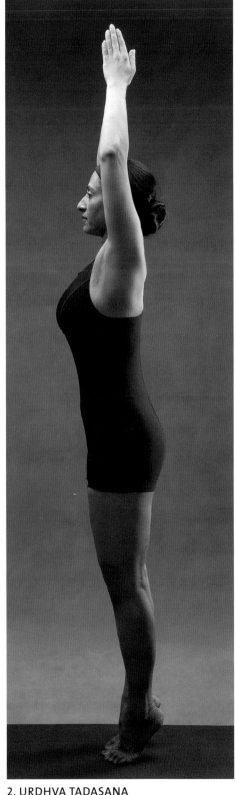

2. URDHVA TADASANA

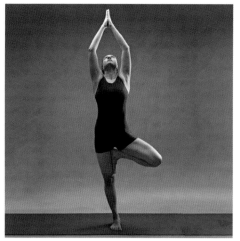

3. VRIKSHASANA

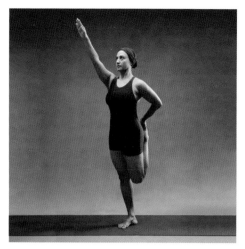

4. SANTULANASANA

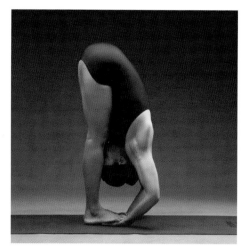

5. PADANGUSTASANA

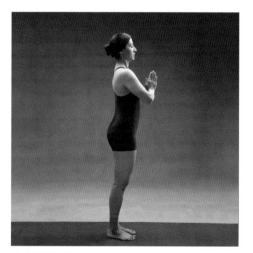

6. SURYA NAMASKARA
Alternate between A & B – 5 times each.

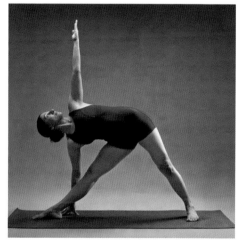

7. TRIKONASANA

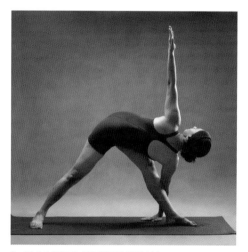

8. PARIVRTTA TRIKONASANA

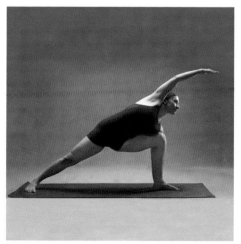

9. PARSVAKONASANA

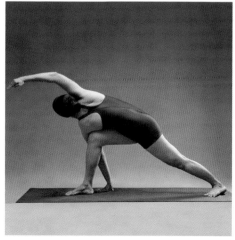

10. PARIVRTTA PARSVAKONASANA

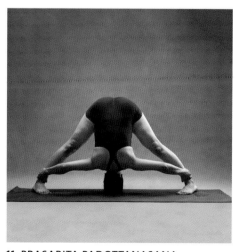

11. PRASARITA PADOTTANASANA

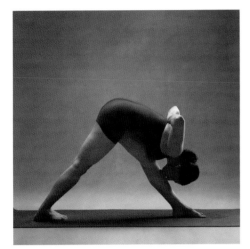

12. PARSVOTTANASANA

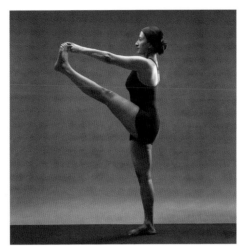

13. UTTHITA HASTA PADANGUSTASANA
Featured asana

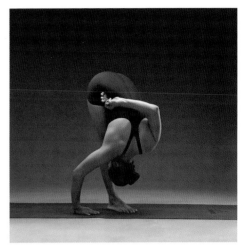

14. ARDHA BADDHA PADMOTTANASANA

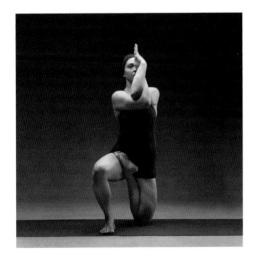

15. VATAYANASANA

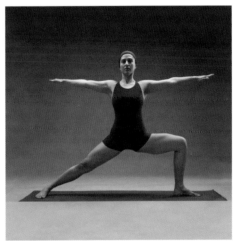

16. VEERABHADRASANA 3

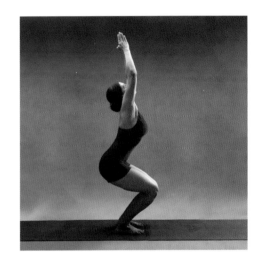

17. UTKATASANA

FLOOR ASANA SEQUENCE

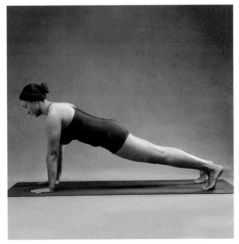

1. CHADURANGA DANDASANA 1

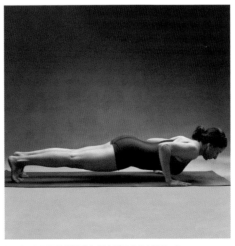

2. CHADURANGA DANDASANA 2

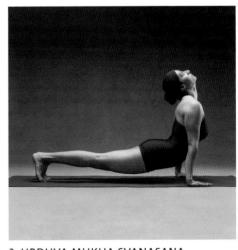

3. URDHVA MUKHA SVANASANA

COOLING DOWN

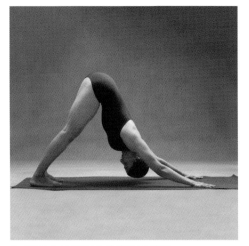

4. ADHO MUKHA SVANASANA

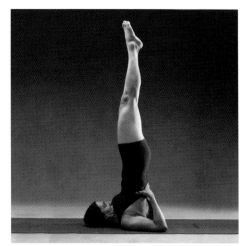

1. SARVANGASANA

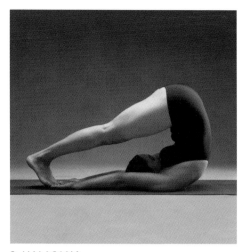

2. HALASANA

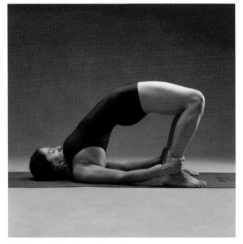

3. SETU BANDHASANA

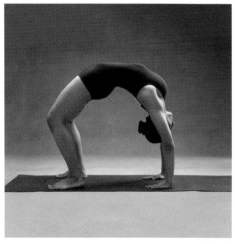

4. URDHVA DHANURASANA

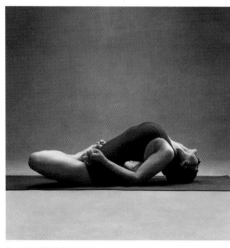

5. MATSYASANA

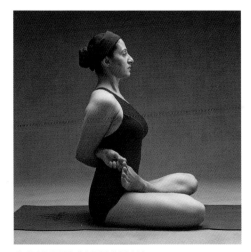

6. BADDHA PADMASANA

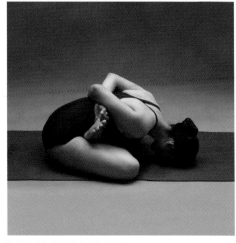

7. YOGA MUDRASANA

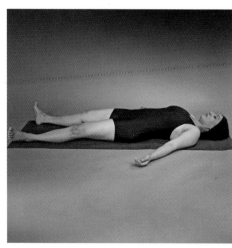

8. SHAVASANA
5 minutes

Sit in Padmasana for a count of 5 breaths before leaving the mat.

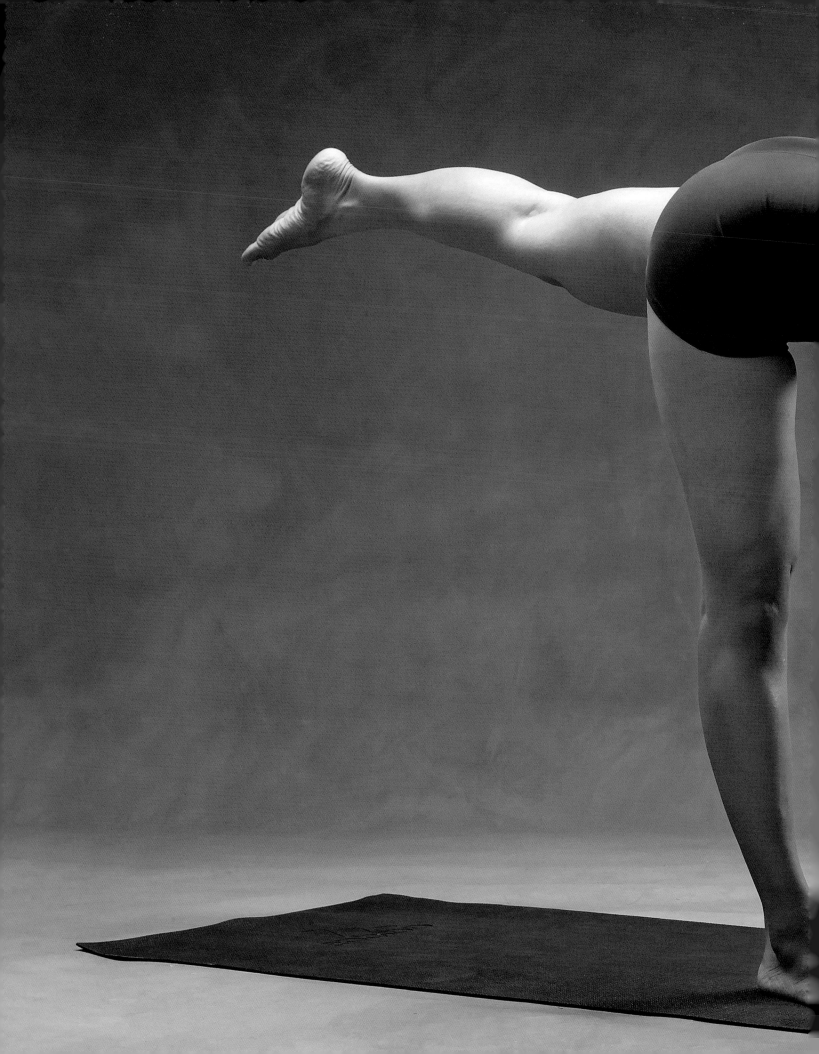

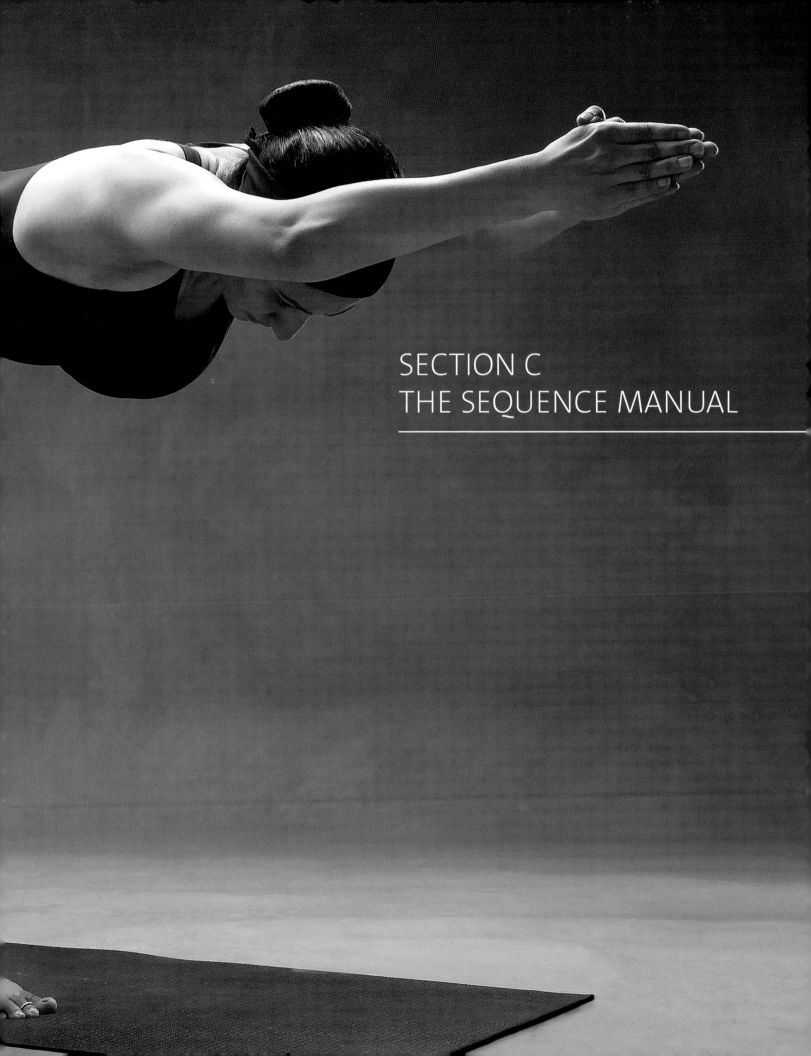

SECTION C
THE SEQUENCE MANUAL

CHAPTER 7

SEQUENCE TO OVERCOME ADDICTION AND DETOX THE BODY

WARM-UP ROUTINE
Perform soft rhythmic jumps 50 times.
Swing the arms forward and backward powerfully 10 times.
Circle the shoulders forward and backward 10 times.
Twist the waist with arms open and stretched 5 times each side.
Gently circle the knees, left & right sides, 5 times each.
Circle the ankles clockwise and anti-clockwise with the front sole pressed to the ground and heel raised, 5 times each.

PRANAYAMA ROUTINE
Sit in a comfortable, relaxed position. Calm your mind and observe your thoughts.
Perform Ujjayee for 5 minutes.
Perform Ujjayee with Antara Kumbhaka (holding breath after inhaling) for 5 minutes.
Perform Anuloma Viloma for 10 minutes.

STANDING-ASANAS ROUTINE
1. Surya Namaskara: Alternate between A & B – 5 times each.
2. Trikonasana
3. Parivrtta Trikonasana
4. Parsvakonasana
5. Parivrtta Parsvakonasana
6. Ardha Chandrasana
7. Parivrtta Ardha Chandrasana – Featured Asana
8. Parsvottanasana
9. Trianga Mukhottasana
10. Utthita Hasta Padangustasana
11. Ardha Baddha Padmottanasana
12. Vatayanasana
13. Veerabhadrasana 3
14. Utkatasana

FLOOR-ASANAS ROUTINE
15. Chaduranga Dandasana
16. Urdhva Mukha Svanasana
17. Adho Mukha Svanasana
18. Adho Mukha Shavasana
19. Paschimottanasana
20. Purvottanasana
21. Bhardwajasana
22. Marichyasana 1
23. Marichyasana 2
24. Baddha Konasana
25. Navasana
26. Upavishtakonasana
27. Ubhaya Upavishtakonasana
28. Urdhva Mukha Upavishtakonasana

COOLING-DOWN ROUTINE
29. Supta Padangustasana 1
30. Sarvangasana
31. Halasana
32. Setu Bandhasana
33. Urdhva Dhanurasana
34. Matsyasana
35. Shavasana – 5 min
Sit in Padmasana for a count of 5 breaths, before leaving the mat.

The sequence prescribed is based on self-study and years of experience teaching various categories of students. The feedback from students who have benefited from these sequences inspired the author to document them. The symptoms of any discomfort have been observed, studied and discussed with friends who are doctors and psychotherapists.

IMPORTANT

Please make sure that all the asanas and Pranayama techniques have been taught to you by your yoga guru. A doctor's permission could be essential in some cases. Before starting on this sequence, it is imperative that the practitioner follows the Warm-up Exercises, Surya Namaskara (A&B) (Section B, Chapter 5) and Asanas (Section B, Chapters 3 & 4; Section C, Chapter 9).

However, a few asanas like Tadasana, Urdhva Tadasana, Vrikshasana, Santulanasana, could be avoided as the body may be difficult to balance when it needs to detox. Even forward-bending asanas like Padangustasana and Prasarita Padottanasana should be avoided.

It is recommended that the Pranayama Routine in Section B, Chapter 4, be practised after the Cooling-down Routine prescribed in this chapter, but before Shavasana.

ABOUT ADDICTION

- Addiction starts as a habit by choice. You seem still in control and enjoying the habit. Subsequently, if this habit gets beyond a stage where it is difficult to stop, it becomes an addiction.
- An addiction could be behavioural, substance-related or even to a simple game.
- The chemical balance in the body will get temporarily altered, especially if it involves substances like alcohol, tobacco and drugs.
- Though the chemical reactions are different, people with an addiction for gambling, work, exercising, internet, sex etc. exhibit similar psychological dependence.
- Addictions can lead to feelings of guilt, shame, hopelessness, despair, failure, rejection, anxiety and humiliation, which cause serious problems in life, be it at home, work or during other social interactions.
- An addiction could be the result of a combination of physical, mental, circumstantial and emotional factors.
- Often a person suffering from an addiction is completely unaware that there is a problem and even when realisation occurs, there could be denial.
- The practice of asanas will break the thought pattern to cultivate bodily awareness in a kind and nurturing way. It allows the practitioner to bring steadiness to the mind and help detoxify.

DEPLETED CHAKRAS

Visudha, Manipura and Muladhara

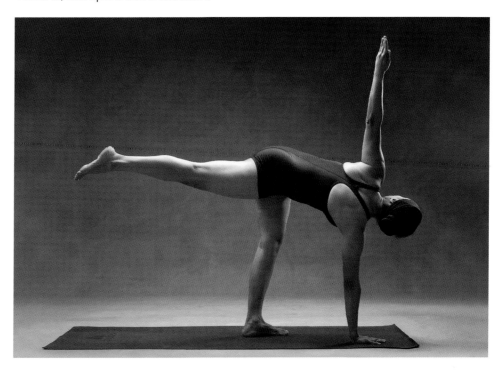

Standing Asana Sequence Start with pre-sequence asanas 1-5, then follow sequence below.

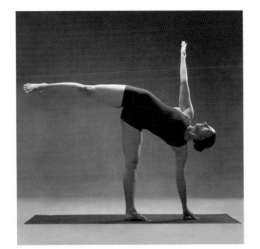

6. ARDHA CHANDRASANA

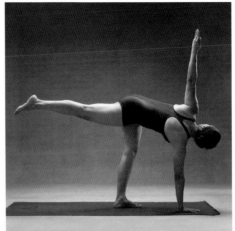

7. PARIVRTTA ARDHA CHANDRASANA
Featured asana

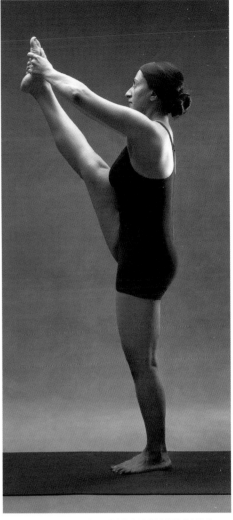

10. UTTHITA HASTA PADANGUSTASANA

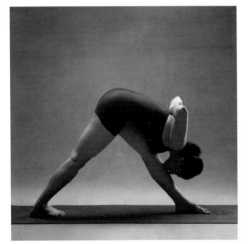

8. PARSVOTTANASANA

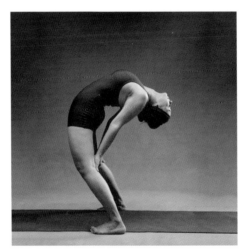

9. TRIANGA MUKHOTTASANA

FLOOR ASANA SEQUENCE *Continue with Pre-sequence floor asanas 15-18, then follow sequence below.*

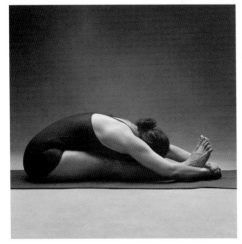

19. PASCHIMOTTANASANA

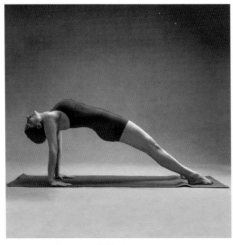

20. PURVOTTANASANA

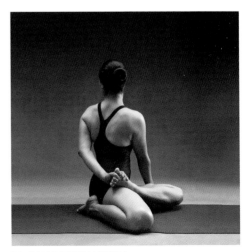

21. BHARDWAJASANA

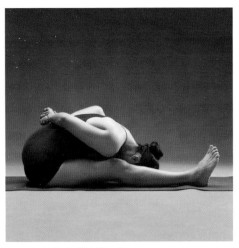

22. MARICHYASANA 1

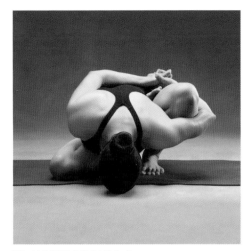

23. MARICHYASANA 2

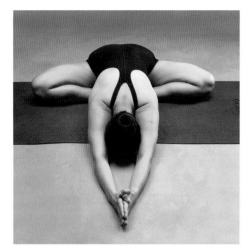

24. BADDHA KONASANA

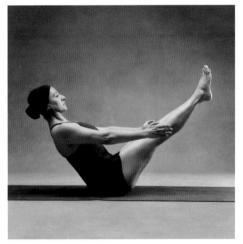

25. NAVASANA

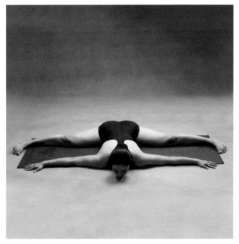

26. UPAVISHTAKONASANA

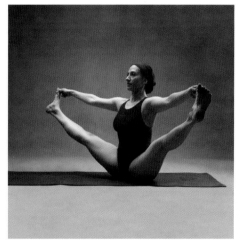

27. UBHAYA UPAVISHTAKONASANA

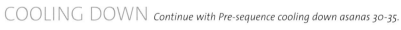

COOLING DOWN *Continue with Pre-sequence cooling down asanas 30-35.*

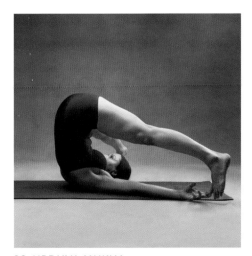

28. URDHVA MUKHA
UPAVISHTAKONASANA

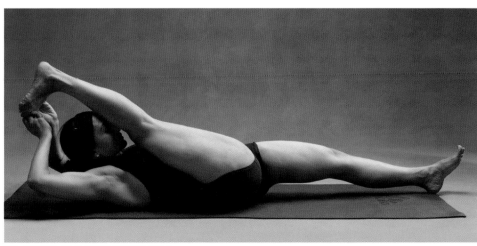

29. SUPTA PADANGUSTASANA 1

SEQUENCE TO SUPPRESS AGITATION IN THE MIND AND THE BODY

WARM-UP ROUTINE

Perform soft rhythmic jumps 50 times.

Swing the arms forward and backward powerfully 10 times.

Circle the shoulders forward and backward 10 times.

Twist the waist with arms open and stretched 5 times each side.

Gently circle the knees, left & right sides, 5 times each.

Circle the ankles clockwise and anti-clockwise with the front sole pressed to the ground and heel raised 5 times each.

PRANAYAMA ROUTINE

Sit in a comfortable, relaxed position. Calm your mind and observe your thoughts.

Perform Ujjayee for 5 minutes.

Perform Ujjayee with Antara Kumbhaka (holding breath after inhaling) for 5 minutes.

Perform Anuloma Viloma for 10 minutes.

STANDING-ASANAS ROUTINE

1. Tadasana
2. Urdhva Tadasana
3. Vrikshasana
4. Santulanasana
5. Padangustasana
6. Surya Namaskara: Alternate between A & B – 5 times each.
7. Trikonasana
8. Parivrtta Trikonasana
9. Parsvottanasana
10. Veerabhadrasana 6
11. Utthita Hasta Padangustasana
12. Ardha Baddha Padmottanasana
13. Vatayanasana
14. Natarajasana
15. Veerabhadrasana 3
16. Utkatasana

FLOOR-ASANAS ROUTINE

1. Chaduranga Dandasana
2. Urdhva Mukha Svanasana
3. Adho Mukha Svanasana
4. Adho Mukha Shavasana
5. Vajrasana
6. Paryankasana – Featured Asana
7. Ushtrasana
8. Bharadwajasana
9. Janu Shirsasana
10. Parivrtta Janu Shirsasana
11. Baddha Konasana
12. Navasana
13. Ubhaya Upavishtakonasana
14. Purvottanasana

COOLING-DOWN ROUTINE

1. Sarvangasana
2. Halasana
3. Setu Bandhasana
4. Urdhva Dhanurasana
5. Matsyasana
6. Shavasana – 5 min

Sit in Padmasana for a count of 5 breaths before leaving the mat.

IMPORTANT

Please make sure that all the asanas and Pranayama techniques have been taught to you by your yoga guru. A doctor's permission could be essential in some cases. Before starting on this sequence, it is imperative that the practitioner follows the Warm-up Exercises, Surya Namaskara (A&B) (Section B, Chapter 5) and Asanas (Section B, Chapters 3 & 4; Section C, Chapter 9).

However, if you are battling chronic agitation, please avoid asanas like Parsvakonasana, Parivrtta Parsvakonasana and Prasarita Padottanasana that require extreme stretching or twisting.

The sequence prescribed is based on self-study and years of experience teaching various categories of students. The feedback from students who have benefited from these sequences inspired the author to document them. The symptoms of any discomfort have been observed, studied and discussed with friends who are doctors and psychotherapists.

UNDERSTANDING AGITATION

- Agitation in mind and body could be a form of depression.
- The symptoms shown are usually restlessness and irritability. This could be due to intense inner tension with racing thoughts, continuous talking, verbal outbursts, over-reacting, etc.
- Frequently getting into agitated situations could lead a person to mental restlessness as a habit would be set in the mind due to repeated reinforcement.
- For an outsider, a person suffering from an agitated mind would seem obnoxious, angry, irritable and unwilling.
- Agitated depression is most commonly seen in middle-aged people and older adults. They have outbursts of agitated behaviour which leave them tired, sad and hopeless, and affect their quality of life.
- Agitated depression is due to the predominance of the Rajas.
- Yoga asana and Pranayama techniques will help to come out of this situation.
- However, agitated practitioners would have difficulty in exhaling fully. Hence, all the asanas prescribed in this sequence would aim at challenging the body. Also, rigorous asana practice is an advantage, which could help burn off some energy and also bring drifting attention back to focus.
- Regular yoga practice would ensure steady improvement. However, the progress has to be monitored.
- In extreme cases of agitation, it is recommended to seek medical advice.

DEPLETED CHAKRAS

Almost all the chakras are disturbed in the state of agitation.

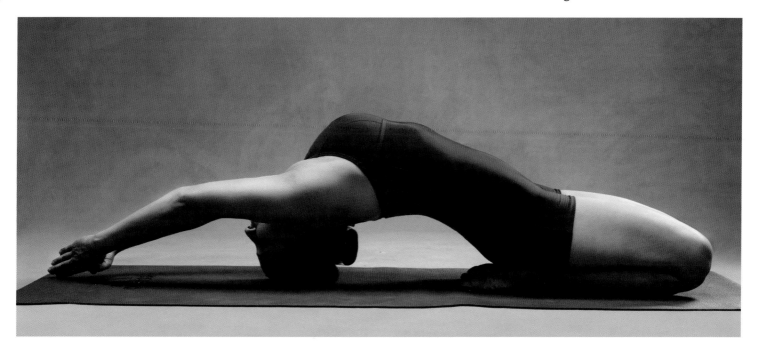

STANDING ASANA SEQUENCE

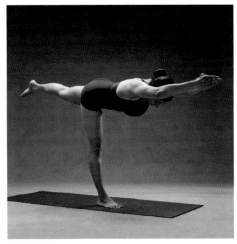

10. VEERABHADRASANA 6

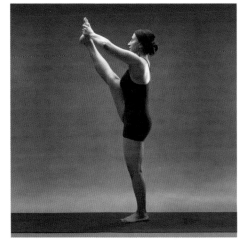

11. UTTHITA HASTA PADANGUSTASANA

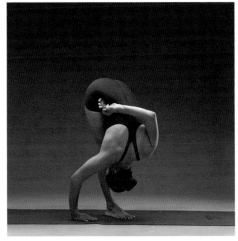

12. ARDHA BADDHA PADMOTTANASANA

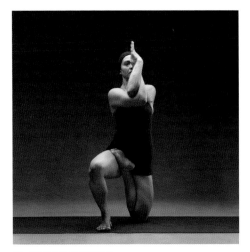

13. VATAYANASANA

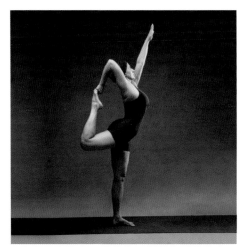

14. NATARAJASANA

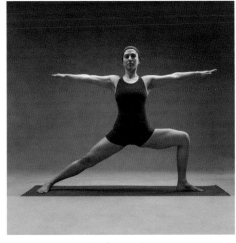

15. VEERABHADRASANA 3

FLOOR ASANA SEQUENCE

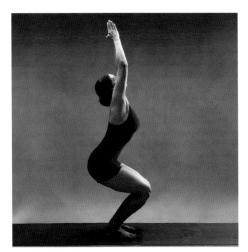

16. UTKATASANA

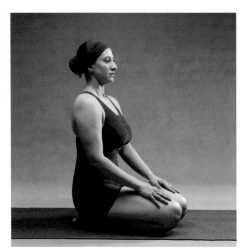

5. VAJRASANA

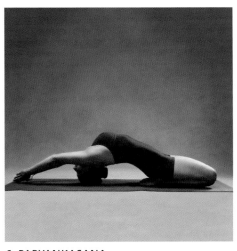

6. PARYANKASANA
Featured asana

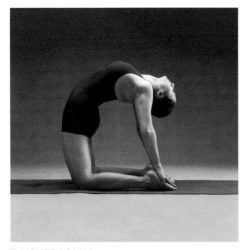

7. USHTRASANA

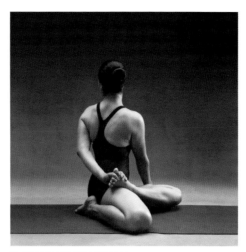

8. BHARADWAJASANA

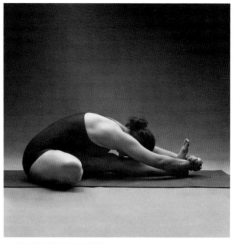

9. JANU SHIRSASANA

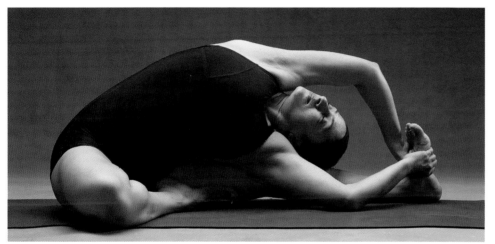

10. PARIVRTTA JANU SHIRSASANA

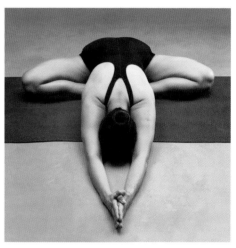

11. BADDHA KONASANA

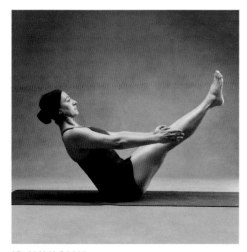

12. NAVASANA

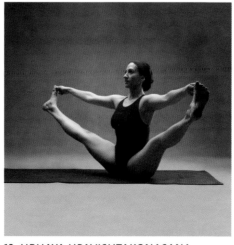

13. UBHAYA UPAVISHTAKONASANA

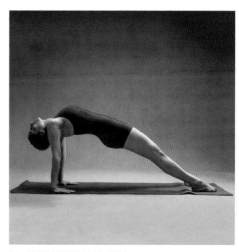

14. PURVOTTANASANA

SEQUENCE TO MANAGE ANGER

WARM-UP ROUTINE

Perform soft rhythmic jumps 50 times.

Swing the arms forward and backward powerfully 10 times.

Circle the shoulders forward and backward 10 times.

Twist the waist with arms open and stretched 5 times each side.

Gently circle the knees, left & right sides, 5 times each.

Circle the ankles clockwise and anti-clockwise with the front sole pressed to the ground and heel raised 5 times each.

PRANAYAMA ROUTINE

Sit in a comfortable, relaxed position. Calm your mind and observe your thoughts.

Perform Ujjayee for 5 minutes.

Perform Ujjayee with Antara Kumbhaka (holding breath after inhaling) for 5 minutes.

Perform Anuloma Viloma for 10 minutes.

STANDING-ASANAS ROUTINE

1. Tadasana
2. Urdhva Tadasana
3. Vrikshasana
4. Santulanasana
5. Surya Namaskara: Alternate between A & B – 5 times each.
6. Trikonasana
7. Parivrtta Trikonasana
8. Parsvakonasana
9. Parivrtta Parsvakonasana
10. Ardha Chandrasana
11. Parsvottanasana
12. Utthita Hasta Padangustasana
13. Vatayanasana
14. Veerabhadrasana 3
15. Utkatasana
16. Veerabhadrasana 6
17. Natarajasana – Featured Asana

FLOOR-ASANAS ROUTINE

1. Chaduranga Dandasana
2. Urdhva Mukha Svanasana
3. Adho Mukha Svanasana
4. Adho Mukha Shavasana
5. Dhanurasana: Follow with relaxing the back. Lie with chest down and move feet up and down with bent knees.
6. Ushtrasana
7. Veerasana
8. Supta Veerasana
9. Baddha Konasana
10. Kurmasana
11. Shayanasana
12. Ananta Shayanasana

COOLING-DOWN ROUTINE

1. Sarvangasana
2. Halasana
3. Setu Bandhasana
4. Urdhva Dhanurasana
5. Matsyasana
6. Shavasana – 5 min

Sit in Padmasana for a count of 5 breaths before leaving the mat.

The sequence prescribed is based on self-study and years of experience teaching various categories of students. The feedback from students who have benefited from these sequences inspired the author to document them. The symptoms of any discomfort have been observed, studied and discussed with friends who are doctors and psychotherapists.

UNDERSTANDING ANGER

- Anger is basically a response to an unhappy feeling.
- Anger is circumstantial and can happen anytime, anywhere.
- Anger can make the mind go out of control.
- An unpleasant situation releases stress hormones which releases adrenal to the blood, creating a violent feeling in the mind.
- Anger results in complete loss of control in the chakra levels. It disrupts the entire body mechanism.
- A chronically angry person is prone to a variety of chronic diseases like high blood pressure, migraine, fatigue, indigestion etc. as the adrenaline gland gets exhausted.
- Yoga asanas recommended in this sequence aim at calming and stilling the mind.
- While there is medication for a chronically angry person, it is best to aim at a long-time cure which would work on gently easing away from situations that cause anger.

DEPLETED CHAKRAS

Manipura and Ajna

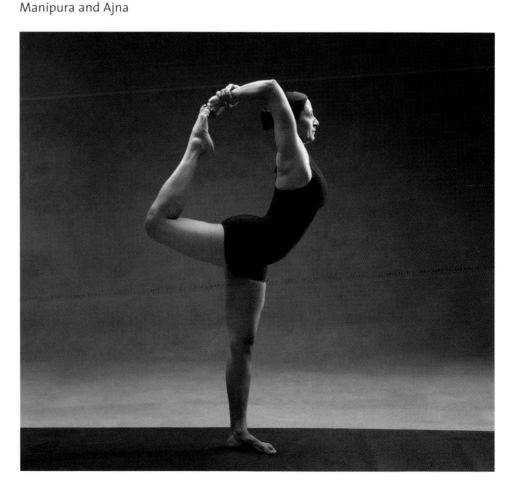

STANDING ASANA SEQUENCE

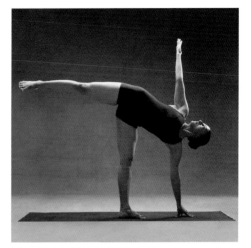

10. ARDHA CHANDRASANA

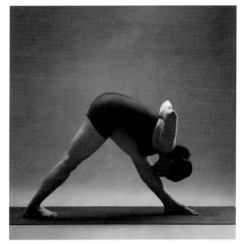

11. PARSVOTTANASANA

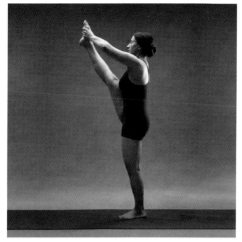

12. UTTHITA HASTA PADANGUSTASANA

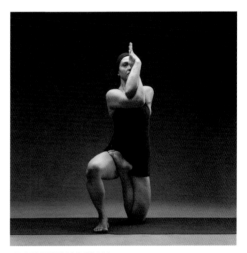

13. VATAYANASANA

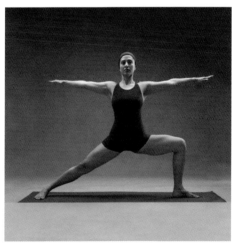

14. VEERABHADRASANA 3

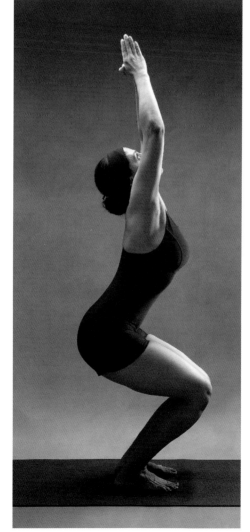

15. UTKATASANA

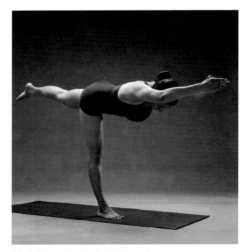

16. VEERABHADRASANA 6

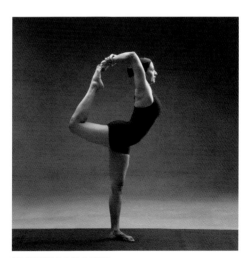

17. NATARAJASANA
Featured asana

FLOOR ASANA SEQUENCE

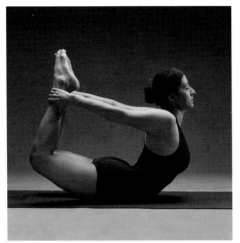

5. DHANURASANA
Follow with relaxing the back. Lie with chest down and move feet up and down with bent knees.

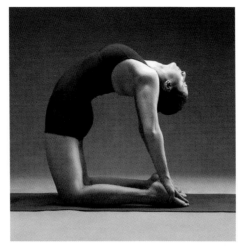

6. USHTRASANA

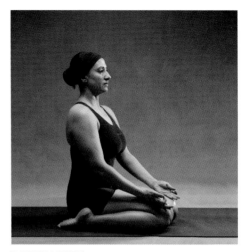

7. VEERASANA

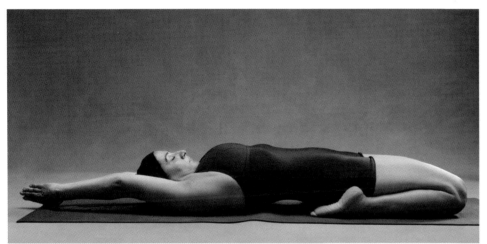

8. SUPTA VEERASANA

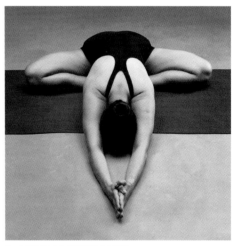

9. BADDHA KONASANA

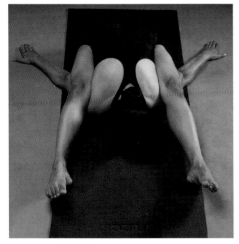

10. KURMASANA

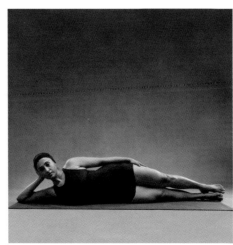

11. SHAYANASANA

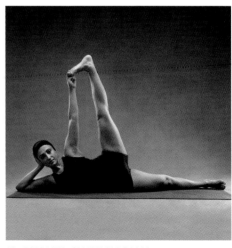

12. ANANTA SHAYANASANA

SEQUENCE TO OVERCOME ANXIETY DUE TO STRESS

WARM-UP ROUTINE

Perform soft rhythmic jumps 50 times.

Swing the arms forward and backward powerfully 10 times.

Circle the shoulders forward and backward 10 times.

Twist the waist with arms open and stretched 5 times each side.

Gently circle the knees, left & right sides, 5 times each.

Circle the ankles clockwise and anti-clockwise with the front sole pressed to the ground and heel raised 5 times each.

PRANAYAMA ROUTINE

Sit in a comfortable, relaxed position. Calm your mind and observe your thoughts.

Perform Ujjayee for 5 minutes.

Perform Ujjayee with Antara Kumbhaka (holding breath after inhaling) for 5 minutes.

Perform Anuloma Viloma for 10 minutes.

STANDING-ASANAS ROUTINE

1. Tadasana
2. Urdhva Tadasana
3. Vrikshasana
4. Santulanasana
5. Padangustasana
6. Surya Namaskara: Alternate between A & B – 5 times each.
7. Trikonasana
8. Trianga Mukhottasana – Featured Asana
9. Prasarita Padottanasana
10. Parivrtta Prasarita Padottanasana
11. Ardha Chandrasana
12. Utthita Hasta Padangustasana
13. Ardha Baddha Padmottanasana
14. Vatayanasana
15. Veerabhadrasana C
16. Utkatasana

FLOOR-ASANAS ROUTINE

1. Chaduranga Dandasana
2. Urdhva Mukha Svanasana
3. Adho Mukha Svanasana
4. Adho Mukha Shavasana
5. Shalabhasana
6. Dhanurasana: Follow with relaxing the back. Lie with chest down and move feet up and down with bent knees.
7. Vajrasana
8. Ushtrasana
9. Veerasana
10. Ardha Padma Paschimottanasana
11. Baddha Konasana
12. Kurmasana
13. Shayanasana
14. Ananta Shayanasana

COOLING-DOWN ROUTINE

1. Sarvangasana
2. Halasana
3. Setu Bandhasana
4. Urdhva Dhanurasana
5. Matsyasana
6. Shavasana – 5 min

Sit in Padmasana for a count of 5 breaths before leaving the mat.

IMPORTANT

Please make sure that all the asanas and Pranayama techniques have been taught to you by your yoga guru. A doctor's permission could be essential in some cases. Before starting on this sequence, it is imperative that the practitioner follows the Warm-up Exercises, Surya Namaskara (A&B) (Section B, Chapter 5) and Asanas (Section B, Chapters 3 & 4; Section C, Chapter 9).

However, if you are battling severe anxiety issues, please remove asanas like Parivrtta Trikonasana, Parsvakonasana, Parivrtta Parsvakonasana, Parsvottanasana from the Standing Asanas Sequence, as the focus of this sequence should be to ensure that the energy flow is directed backward than forward.

The sequence prescribed is based on self-study and years of experience teaching various categories of students. The feedback from students who have benefited from these sequences inspired the author to document them. The symptoms of any discomfort have been observed, studied and discussed with friends who are doctors and psychotherapists.

UNDERSTANDING ANXIETY

- The daily routine of a modern-day lifestyle is sufficient to lead to an anxiety disorder. A relaxing holiday would prove to be a good therapy.
- There are emotional symptoms and physical symptoms which could lead to an anxiety attack.
- Few emotional symptoms could be irritability, lack of concentration, feeling tense all the time, restlessness, and anticipating the worst.
- Some physical symptoms could include being lethargic and sluggish all the time, muscular tightness, stomach upsets, dizziness, frequent urination, loose motions, excessive sweating.
- If you notice such symptoms, please check for thyroid disorder, hypoglycaemia and for asthma.

DEPLETED CHAKRAS

Manipura and Anahata

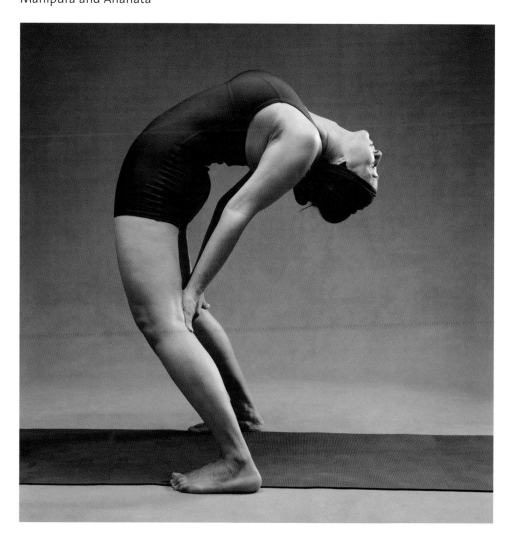

STANDING ASANA SEQUENCE

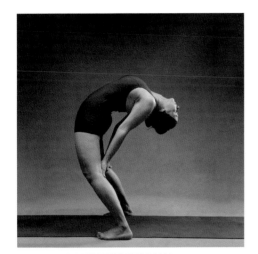

8. TRIANGA MUKHOTTASANA
Featured asana

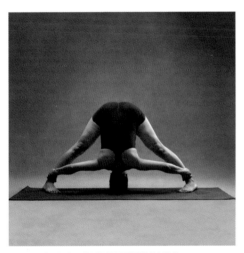

9. PRASARITA PADOTTANASANA

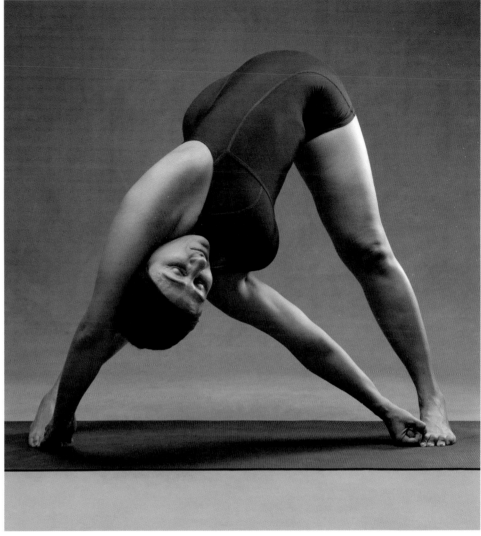

10. PARIVRTTA PRASARITA PADOTTANASANA

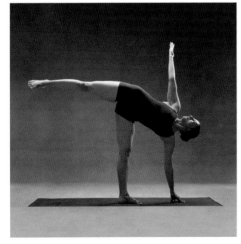

11. ARDHA CHANDRASANA

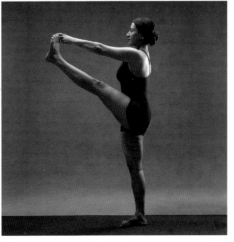

12. UTTHITA HASTA PADANGUSTASANA

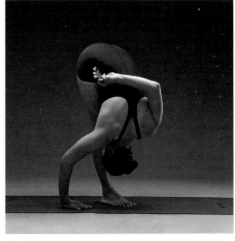

13. ARDHA BADDHA PADMOTTANASANA

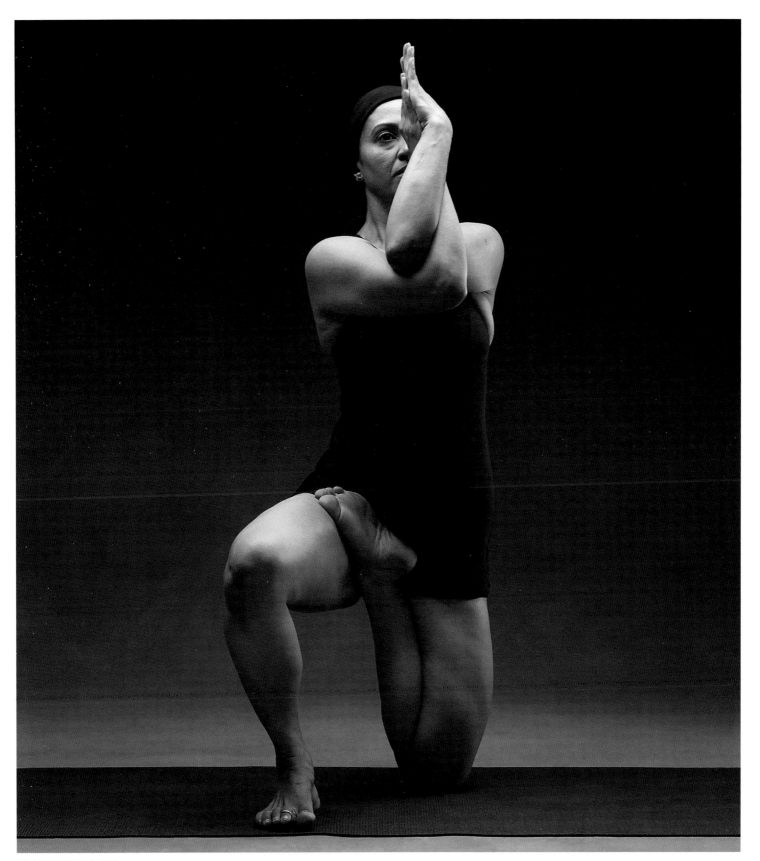

14. VATAYANASANA

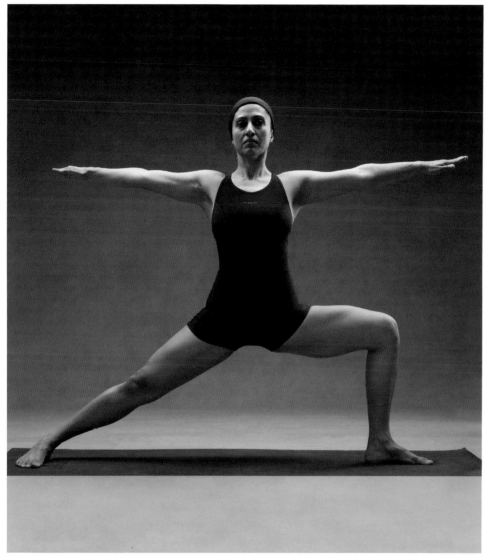

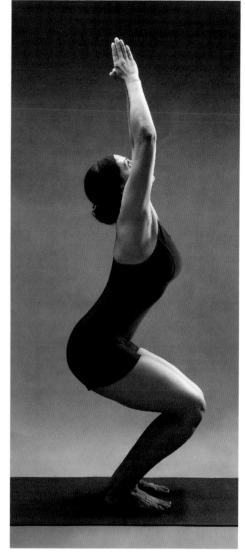

15. VEERABHADRASANA C

16. UTKATASANA

FLOOR ASANA SEQUENCE

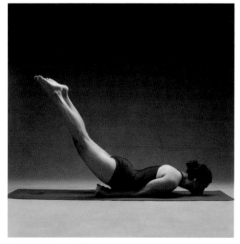

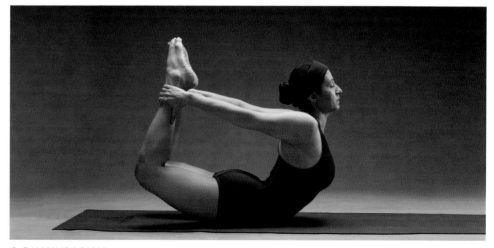

5. SHALABHASANA

6. DHANURASANA
Follow with relaxing the back. Lie with chest down and move feet up and down with bent knees.

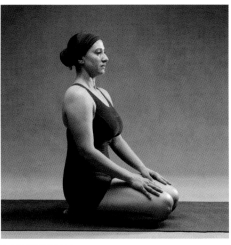

7. VAJRASANA

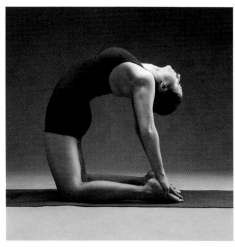

8. USHTRASANA

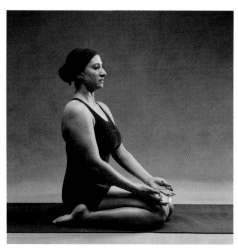

9. VEERASANA

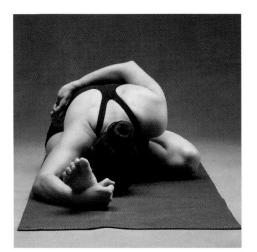

10. ARDHA PADMA PASCHIMOTTANASANA

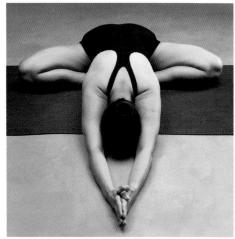

11. BADDHA KONASANA

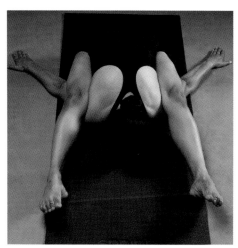

12. KURMASANA

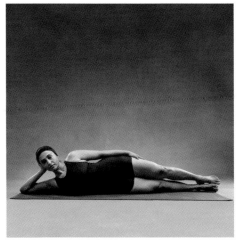

13. SHAYANASANA

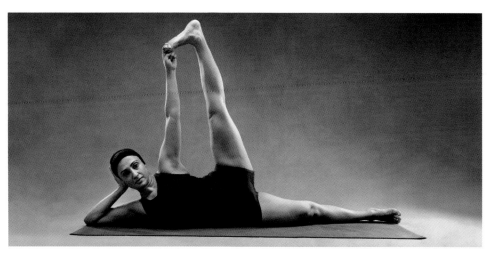

14. ANANTA SHAYANASANA

SEQUENCE TO INCREASE FOCUS AND CONCENTRATION

WARM-UP ROUTINE

Perform soft rhythmic jumps 50 times.

Swing the arms forward and backward powerfully 10 times.

Circle the shoulders forward and backward 10 times.

Twist the waist with arms open and stretched 5 times each side.

Gently circle the knees, left & right sides, 5 times each.

Circle the ankles clockwise and anti-clockwise with the front sole pressed to the ground and heel raised 5 times each.

PRANAYAMA ROUTINE

Sit in a comfortable relaxed position. Calm your mind and observe your thoughts.

Perform Ujjayee for 5 minutes.

Perform Ujjayee with Antara Kumbhaka (holding breath after inhaling) for 5 minutes.

Perform Surya Bedhana Pranayama for 10 minutes.

Perform Kapalabhati – 300 blows – with adequate rest in between.

STANDING-ASANAS ROUTINE

1. Tadasana
2. Urdhva Tadasana
3. Vrikshasana
4. Santulanasana
5. Padangustasana
6. Surya Namaskara: Alternate between A & B – 5 times each.
7. Trikonasana
8. Parivrtta Trikonasana
9. Parsvakonasana
10. Parivrtta Parsvakonasana
11. Ardha Chandrasana
12. Parivrtta Ardha Chandrasana
13. Parsvottanasana
14. Prasarita Padottanasana
15. Utthita Hasta Padangustasana
16. Ardha Baddha Padmottanasana
17. Vatayanasana
18. Veerabhadrasana 6
19. Utkatasana
20. Vashistasana

FLOOR-ASANAS ROUTINE

1. Chaduranga Dandasana
2. Urdhva Mukha Svanasana
3. Adho Mukha Svanasana
4. Adho Mukha Shavasana
5. Dhanurasana: Follow with relaxing the back. Lie with chest down and move feet up and down with bent knees.
6. Bekasana
7. Ushtrasana
8. Vajrasana
9. Shirsasana (Featured Asana)
10. Marichyasana 1
11. Marichyasana 2
12. Baddha Konasana
13. Gomukhasana
14. Navasana
15. Purvottanasana

COOLING-DOWN ROUTINE

1. Sarvangasana
2. Halasana
3. Setu Bandhasana
4. Urdhva Dhanurasana
5. Matsyasana
6. Shavasana – 5 min (with Brahmari Pranayama)

Sit in Padmasana for a count of 5 breaths before leaving the mat.

The sequence prescribed is based on self-study and years of
experience teaching various categories of students. The
feedback from students who have benefited from these
sequences inspired the author to document them. The
symptoms of any discomfort have been observed, studied
and discussed with friends who are doctors and
psychotherapists.

UNDERSTANDING LACK OF CONCENTRATION

- Stress, lack of sleep, nutritional deficiency, lack of exercise, depression, attention-deficit disorder are some of the reasons for lack of concentration.
- Medical reasons like thyroid imbalance, pituitary gland disorder, hypoglycaemia, and certain kinds of hormonal fluctuations could also result in lack of focus.
- Research shows that protein and iron deficiencies lead to lack of concentration.
- Situational depression may bring about lack of concentration.

DEPLETED CHAKRAS

Vishuddha and Sahasrara

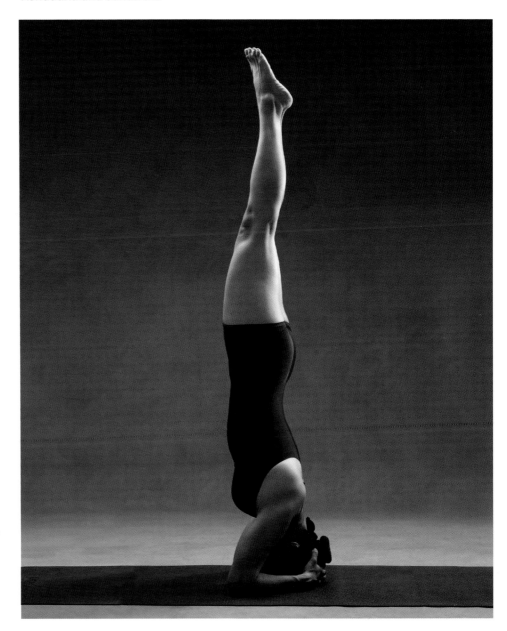

STANDING ASANA SEQUENCE

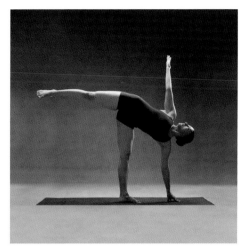

11. ARDHA CHANDRASANA

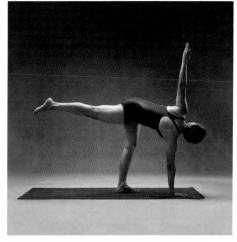

12. PARIVRTTA ARDHA CHANDRASANA

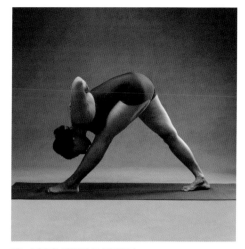

13. PARSVOTTANASANA

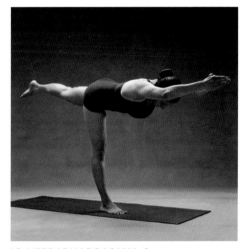

18. VEERABHADRASANA 6

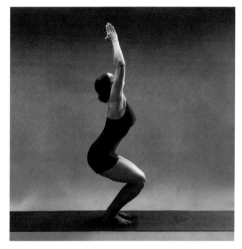

19. UTKATASANA

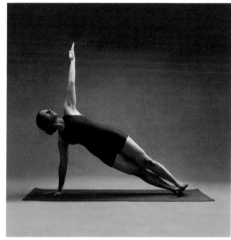

20. VASHISTASANA

FLOOR ASANA SEQUENCE

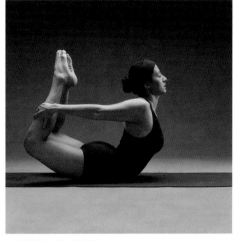

5. DHANURASANA
*Follow with relaxing the back. Lie with chest down
and move feet up and down with bent knees.*

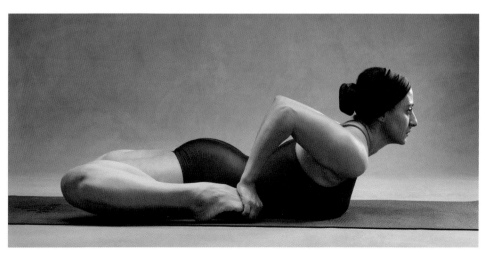

6. BEKASANA

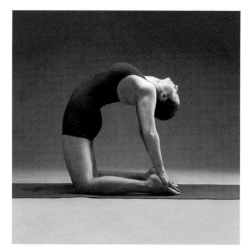

7. USHTRASANA

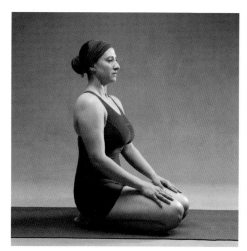

8. VAJRASANA

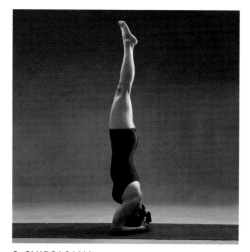

9. SHIRSASANA
Featured asana

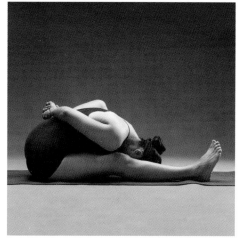

10. MARICHYASANA 1

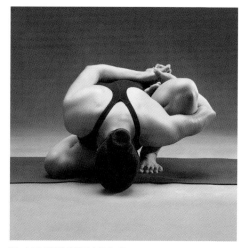

11. MARICHYASANA 2

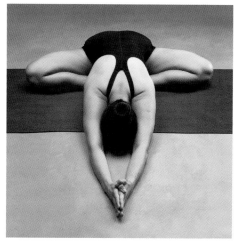

12. BADDHA KONASANA

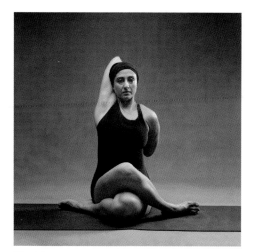

13. GOMUKHASANA

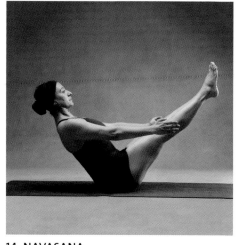

14. NAVASANA

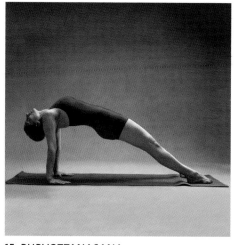

15. PURVOTTANASANA

SEQUENCE TO HANDLE DEPRESSION

WARM-UP ROUTINE

Perform soft rhythmic jumps 50 times.

Swing the arms forward and backward powerfully 10 times.

Circle the shoulders front and backward – 10 times.

Twist the waist with arms open and stretched 5 times each side.

Gently circle the knees, left & right sides, 5 times each.

Circle the ankles clockwise and anti-clockwise with the front sole pressed to the ground and heel raised 5 times each.

PRANAYAMA ROUTINE

Sit in a comfortable, relaxed position. Calm your mind and observe your thoughts.

Perform Ujjayee for 5 minutes.

Perform Ujjayee with Antara Kumbhaka (holding breath after inhaling) for 5 minutes.

Perform Anuloma Viloma for 10 minutes.

Perform Surya Bedhana Pranayama for 5 minutes (inhale and exhale through right nostril only).
OR
21 counts of Omkara (Om chanting).

STANDING-ASANAS ROUTINE

1. Tadasana
2. Urdhva Tadasana
3. Vrikshasana
4. Santulanasana
5. Padangustasana
6. Surya Namaskara: Alternate between A & B – 5 times each.
7. Trikonasana
8. Parivrtta Trikonasana
9. Parsvakonasana
10. Parivrtta Parsvakonasana
11. Parsvottanasana
12. Prasarita Padottanasana
13. Veerabhadrasana 3
14. Utkatasana
15. Urdhva Dhanurasana
16. Upadasana – Featured Asana
17. Eka Pada Kapotasana

FLOOR-ASANAS ROUTINE

1. Chaduranga Dandasana
2. Urdhva Mukha Svanasana
3. Adho Mukha Svanasana
4. Adho Mukha Shavasana
5. Dhanurasana
6. Shalabhasana: Follow with relaxing the back. Lie with chest down and move feet up and down with bent knees.
7. Ushtrasana
8. Vajrasana
9. Supta Veerasana
10. Marichyasana 1
11. Marichyasana 2
12. Matsyendrasana
13. Navasana
14. Purvottanasana
15. Simhasana (Get into position and inhale deep and breathe out with a roar like that of a lion, keeping the mouth open and tongue out.)

COOLING-DOWN ROUTINE

1. Sarvangasana
2. Halasana
3. Setu Bandhasana
4. Urdhva Dhanurasana
5. Matsyasana
6. Shavasana – 5 min

Sit in Padmasana for a count of 5 breaths before leaving the mat.

UNDERSTANDING DEPRESSION

- Depression could be a form of anxiety.
- The symptoms are sadness and lack of ability to take rational decisions.
- Mental distress, restlessness and loneliness are features of depression.
- A person suffering from a depressed mind would be sluggish and unwilling to do anything.
- Agitated depression is most commonly seen in middle-aged people and older adults.
- Outbursts of depression make people tired, sad and hopeless which negatively affect the quality of their lives.
- Medical advice is necessary in extreme cases.
- Regular yoga practice would ensure steady improvement. However, the progress has to be monitored.

DEPLETED CHAKRAS

Manipura, Anahata and Vishuddha

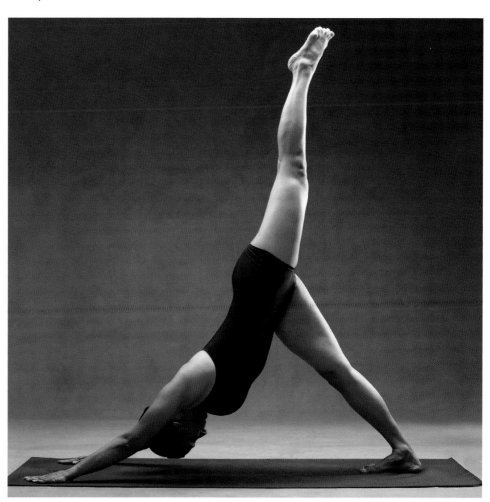

The sequence prescribed is based on self-study and years of experience teaching various categories of students. The feedback from students who have benefited from these sequences inspired the author to document them. The symptoms of any discomfort have been observed, studied and discussed with friends who are doctors and psychotherapists.

STANDING ASANA SEQUENCE

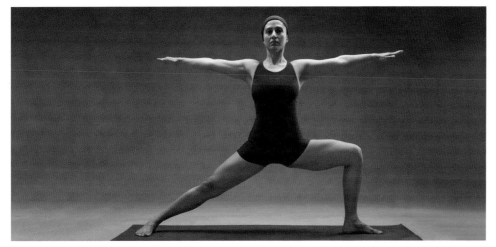

13. VEERABHADRASANA 3

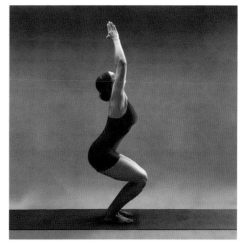

14. UTKATASANA

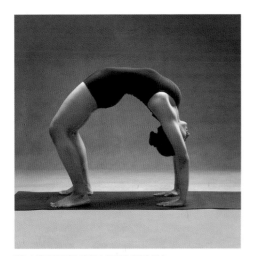

15. URDHVA DHANURASANA

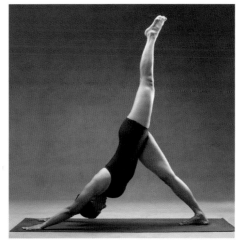

16. UPADASANA
Featured asana

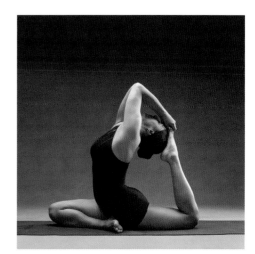

17. EKA PADA KAPOTASANA

FLOOR ASANA SEQUENCE

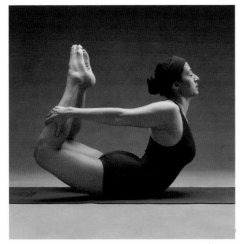

5. DHANURASANA

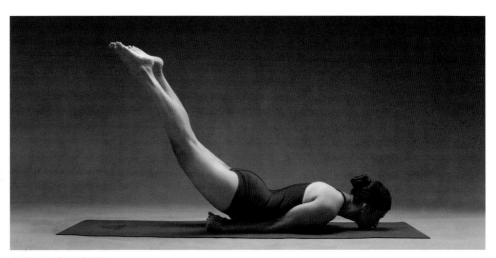

6. SHALABHASANA
Follow with relaxing the back. Lie with chest down and move feet up and down with bent knees.

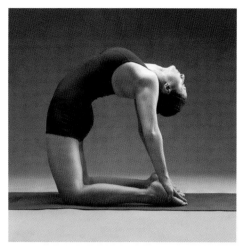

7. USHTRASANA

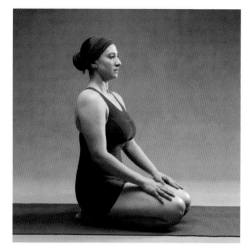

8. VAJRASANA

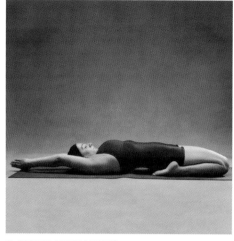

9. SUPTA VEERASANA

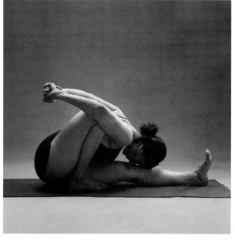

10. MARICHYASANA 1

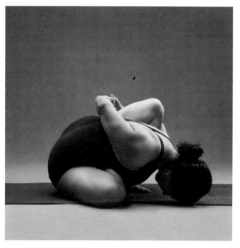

11. MARICHYASANA 2

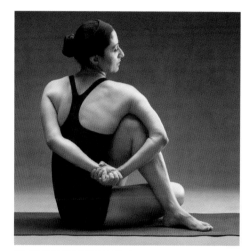

12. MATSYENDRASANA

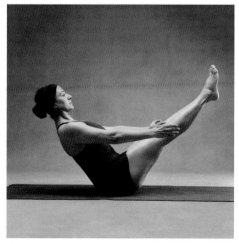

13. NAVASANA

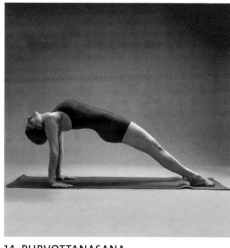

14. PURVOTTANASANA

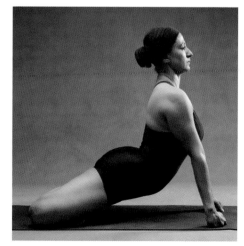

15. SIMHASANA
(Get into position and inhale deep and breathe out with a roar like that of a lion, keeping mouth open and tongue out.)

SEQUENCE TO IMPROVE DIGESTION AND ASSIMILATION

WARM-UP ROUTINE

Perform soft rhythmic jumps 50 times.

Swing the arms forward and backward powerfully 10 times.

Circle the shoulders forward and backward 10 times.

Twist the waist with arms open and stretched 5 times each side.

Gently circle the knees, left & right sides, 5 times each.

Circle the ankles clockwise and anti-clockwise with the front sole pressed to the ground and heel raised 5 times each.

PRANAYAMA ROUTINE

Sit in a comfortable relaxed position. Calm your mind and observe your thoughts.

Perform Ujjayee in Vajrasana for 5 minutes (sit in Vajrasana).

Perform Ujjayee with Antara Kumbhaka (holding breath after inhaling) for 5 minutes.

Perform Anuloma Viloma for 10 minutes.

STANDING-ASANAS ROUTINE

1. Tadasana
2. Urdhva Tadasana
3. Vrikshasana
4. Santulanasana
5. Padangustasana
6. Surya Namaskara: Alternate between A & B – 5 times each.
7. Trikonasana
8. Parivrtta Trikonasana
9. Parsvakonasana
10. Parivrtta Parsvakonasana
11. Parsvottanasana
12. Prasarita Padottanasana
13. Utthita Hasta Padangustasana
14. Ardha Baddha Padmottanasana
15. Vatayanasana
16. Veerabhadrasana 3
17. Utkatasana

FLOOR-ASANAS ROUTINE

1. Chaduranga Dandasana
2. Urdhva Mukha Svanasana
3. Adho Mukha Svanasana
4. Adho Mukha Shavasana
5. Shalabhasana
6. Dwi Pada Kapotasana
7. Vajrasana – Featured Asana
8. Paryankasana
9. Veerasana
10. Supta Veerasana
11. Ushtrasana
12. Baddha Konasana
13. Gomukhasana

COOLING-DOWN ROUTINE

1. Sarvangasana
2. Halasana
3. Setu Bandhasana
4. Urdhva Dhanurasana
5. Matsyasana
6. Shavasana – 5 min

Sit in Padmasana for a count of 5 breaths before leaving the mat.

NEED FOR GOOD DIGESTION AND ASSIMILATION

- Stress of all kinds – physical, emotional and mental – may be the cause for poor digestion.
- Infection, trauma from injuries, surgery and environmental toxins could affect digestion.
- Symptoms of indigestion could be in the form of abdominal discomfort like gas, feeling of bloating, heartburn, diarrhoea, heartburn, constipation, food allergies, nausea and vomiting.

DEPLETED CHAKRAS

Muladhara and Svadhisthana

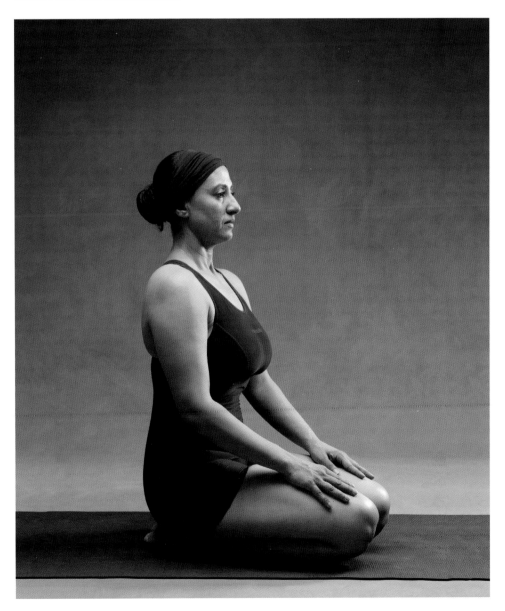

The sequence prescribed is based on self-study and years of experience teaching various categories of students. The feedback from students who have benefited from these sequences inspired the author to document them. The symptoms of any discomfort have been observed, studied and discussed with friends who are doctors and psychotherapists.

FLOOR ASANA SEQUENCE

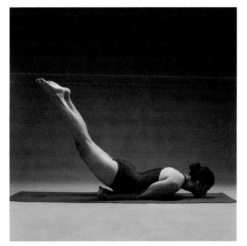

5. SHALABHASANA

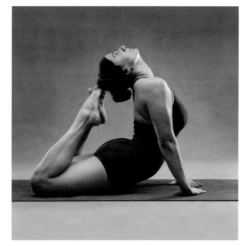

6. DWI PADA KAPOTASANA

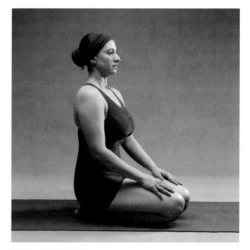

7. VAJRASANA
Featured asana

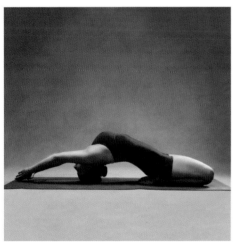

8. PARYANKASANA

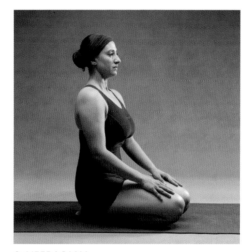

9. VEERASANA

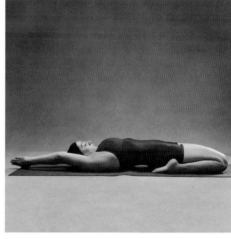

10. SUPTA VEERASANA

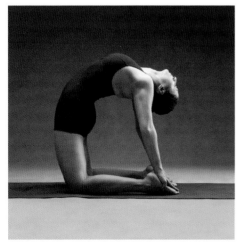

11. USHTRASANA

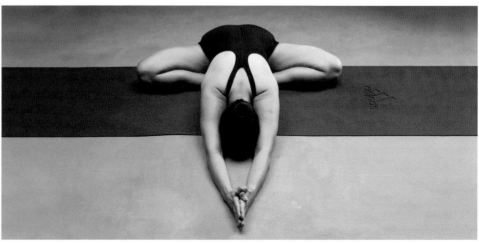

12. BADDHA KONASANA

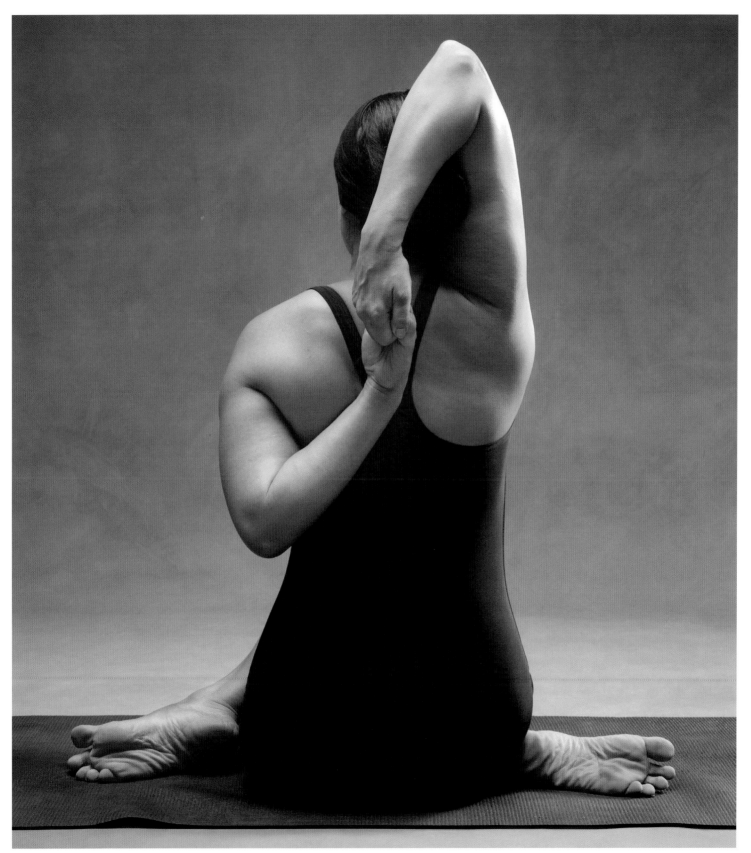

13. GOMUKHASANA

SEQUENCE TO INCREASE ENERGY

WARM-UP ROUTINE

Perform soft rhythmic jumps 50 times.

Swing the arms forward and backward powerfully 10 times.

Circle the shoulders forward and backward 10 times.

Twist the waist with arms open and stretched 5 times each side.

Gently circle the knees, left & right sides, 5 times each.

Circle the ankles clockwise and anti-clockwise with the front sole pressed to the ground and heel raised 5 times each.

PRANAYAMA ROUTINE

Sit in a comfortable relaxed position. Calm your mind and observe your thoughts.

Perform Ujjayee for 5 minutes.

Perform Ujjayee with Antara Kumbhaka (holding breath after inhaling) for 5 minutes.

Perform Anuloma Viloma for 10 minutes.

Perform Kapalabhati – 300 blows – with adequate rest in between.

STANDING-ASANAS ROUTINE

1. Tadasana
2. Urdhva Tadasana
3. Vrikshasana
4. Santulanasana
5. Padangustasana
6. Surya Namaskara: Alternate between A & B – 5 times each.
7. Trikonasana
8. Parivrtta Trikonasana
9. Parsvakonasana
10. Ardha Chandrasana
11. Trianga Mukhottasana
12. Prasarita Padottanasana
13. Utthita Hasta Padangustasana
14. Ardha Baddha Padmottanasana
15. Vatayanasana
16. Veerabhadrasana 3
17. Utkatasana

FLOOR-ASANAS ROUTINE

1. Chaduranga Dandasana
2. Urdhva Mukha Svanasana
3. Adho Mukha Svanasana
4. Adho Mukha Shavasana
5. Shalabhasana
6. Dhanurasana: Follow with relaxing the back. Lie with chest down and move feet up and down with bent knees.
7. Ushtrasana
8. Vajrasana
9. Paryankasana
10. Paschimottanasana – Featured Asana
11. Navasana
12. Purvottanasana

COOLING-DOWN ROUTINE

1. Sarvangasana
2. Halasana
3. Setu Bandhasana
4. Urdhva Dhanurasana
5. Matsyasana
6. Shavasana – 5 min (with Brahmari)

Sit in Padmasana for a count of 5 breaths before leaving the mat.

IMPORTANT

Please make sure that all the asanas and Pranayama techniques have been taught to you by your yoga guru. A doctor's permission could be essential in some cases. Before starting on this sequence, it is imperative that the practitioner follows the Warm-up Exercises, Surya Namaskara (A&B) (Section B, Chapter 5) and Asanas (Section B, Chapters 3 & 4; Section C, Chapter 9).

Add Ardha Chandrasana and Trianga Mukhottasana to the Standing- Asanas Routine instead of Parivrtta Parsvakonasana and Parsvottanasana.

It would help if Kapalabhati is added to the Pranayama Routine. Also, include Brahmari at the end of the entire sequence while lying down in Shavasana for 5 minutes.

UNDERSTANDING LACK OF ENERGY

- Lifestyle factors could be poor eating habits, use of caffeine and alcohol, sleep deprivation and a sedentary lifestyle.
- Physical factors are allergies, persistent muscular pains, diabetes, overactive or underactive thyroid, obesity, nutritional deficiencies, etc.
- Psychological conditions can make the body weak and tired when dealing with depression or grief. Boredom with the current state of affairs could add to the lack of energy.

DEPLETED CHAKRAS

Anahata and Ajna

The sequence prescribed is based on self-study and years of experience teaching various categories of students. The feedback from students who have benefited from these sequences inspired the author to document them. The symptoms of any discomfort have been observed, studied and discussed with friends who are doctors and psychotherapists.

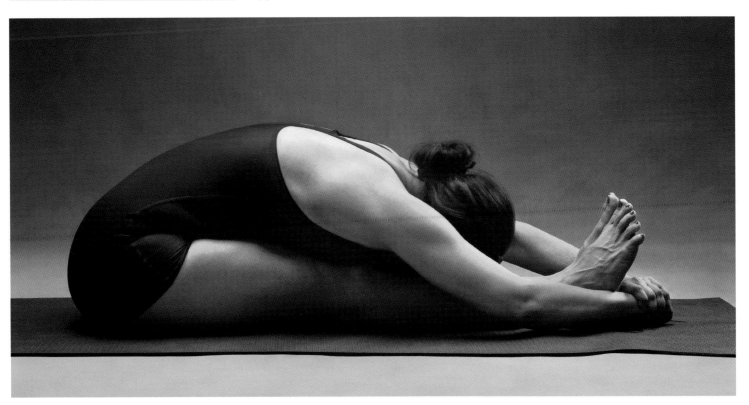

STANDING ASANA SEQUENCE

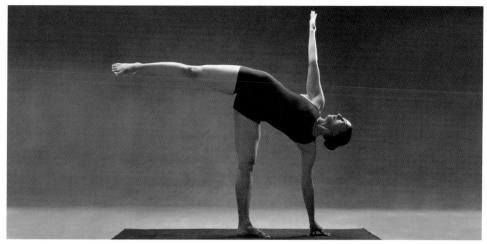

10. ARDHA CHANDRASANA

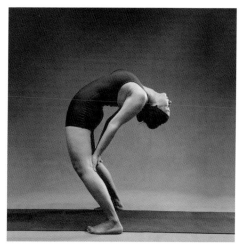

11. TRIANGA MUKHOTTASANA

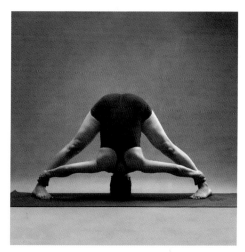

12. PRASARITA PADOTTANASANA

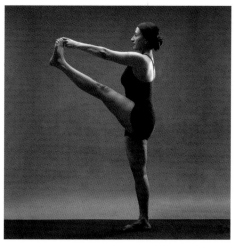

13. UTTHITA HASTA PADANGUSTASANA

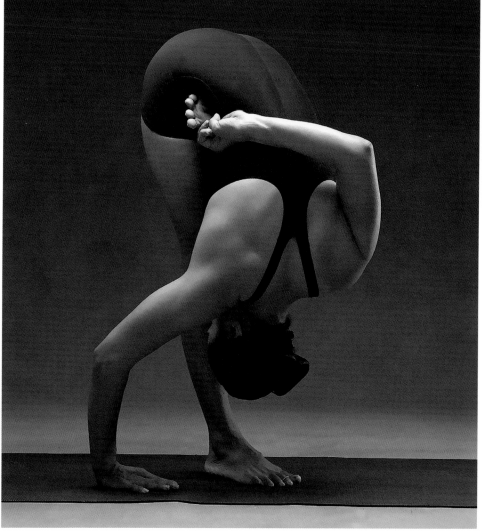

14. ARDHA BADDHA PADMOTTANASANA

FLOOR ASANA SEQUENCE

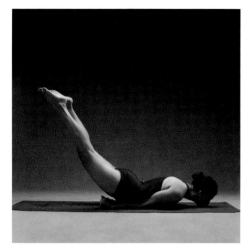

5. SHALABHASANA

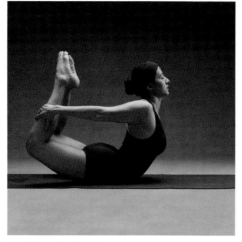

6. DHANURASANA
Follow with relaxing the back. Lie with chest down and move feet up and down with bent knees.

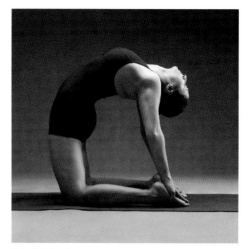

7. USHTRASANA

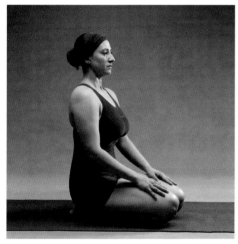

8. VAJRASANA

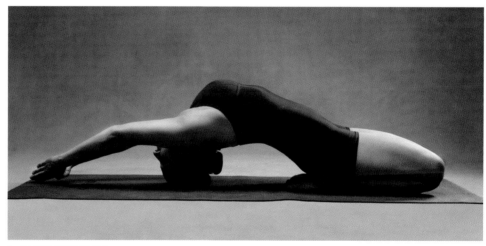

9. PARYANKASANA

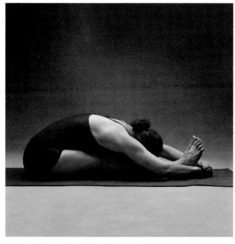

10. PASCHIMOTTANASANA
Featured asana

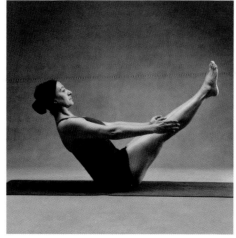

11. NAVASANA

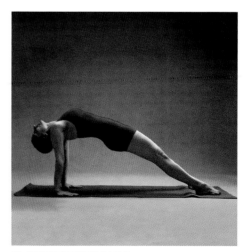

12. PURVOTTANASANA

SEQUENCE TO IMPROVE FLEXIBILITY

WARM-UP ROUTINE

Perform soft rhythmic jumps 50 times.
Swing the arms forward and backward powerfully 10 times.
Circle the shoulders forward and backward 10 times.
Twist the waist with arms open and stretched 5 times each side.
Gently circle the knees, left & right sides, 5 times each.
Circle ankles clockwise and anti-clockwise with front sole pressed to the ground and heel raised – 5 times each

PRANAYAMA ROUTINE

Sit in a comfortable relaxed position. Calm your mind and observe your thoughts.
Perform Ujjayee for 5 minutes.
Perform Ujjayee with Antara Kumbhaka (holding breath after inhaling) for 5 minutes.
Perform Anuloma Viloma for 10 minutes.

STANDING-ASANAS ROUTINE

1.	Tadasana
2.	Urdhva Tadasana
3.	Vrikshasana
4.	Santulanasana
5.	Padangustasana
6.	Surya Namaskara: Alternate between A & B – 5 times each.
7.	Trikonasana
8.	Parivrtta Trikonasana
9.	Parsvakonasana
10.	Parivrtta Parsvakonasana
11.	Ardha Chandrasana
12.	Parivrtta Ardha Chandrasana
13.	Utthita Hasta Padangustasana
14.	Ardha Baddha Padmottanasana
15.	Vatayanasana
16.	Chakrasana 1
17.	Chakrasana 2
18.	Uttanasana
19.	Utkatasana
20.	Updasana

FLOOR-ASANAS ROUTINE

1.	Chaduranga Dandasana
2.	Urdhva Mukha Svanasana
3.	Adho Mukha Svanasana
4.	Adho Mukha Shavasana
5.	Pashasana
6.	Malasana – Featured Asana
7.	Paschimottanasana
8.	Purvottanasana
9.	Baddha Konasana
10.	Veerasana
11.	Supta Veerasana
12.	Bharadwajasana
13.	Gomukhasana

COOLING-DOWN ROUTINE

1.	Supta Padangustasana 1
2.	Supta Padangustasana 2
3.	Supta Padangustasana 3
4.	Sarvangasana
5.	Halasana
6.	Setu Bandhasana
7.	Urdhva Dhanurasana
8.	Matsyasana
9.	Shavasana – 5 min
Sit in Padmasana for a count of 5 breaths, before leaving the mat.

IMPORTANT
Please make sure that all the asanas and Pranayama techniques have been taught to you by your yoga guru. A doctor's permission could be essential in some cases. Before starting on this sequence, it is imperative that the practitioner follows the Warm-up Exercises, Surya Namaskara (A&B) (Section B, Chapter 5) and Asanas (Section B, Chapters 3 & 4; Section C, Chapter 9).

The sequence prescribed is based on self-study and years of experience teaching various categories of students. The feedback from students who have benefited from these sequences inspired the author to document them. The symptoms of any discomfort have been observed, studied and discussed with friends who are doctors and psychotherapists.

UNDERSTANDING FLEXIBILITY

- Flexibility depends on the genetic composition of the body-like bone structure, muscle mass, excess fatty tissue, connective tissue, physical injury, etc.
- Age is another important factor which impacts flexibility.
- Excessive muscle mass (heavily built muscle) and excessive fatty tissue restricts flexibility as these interfere with a complete range of movement.
- Flexibility in one area does not mean flexibility in all areas of the body. There are internal and external factors governing flexibility. A few are mentioned below
- Internal factors:
  - Elasticity of muscle tissue
  - Ability of the muscle to relax
  - Temperature in the joint (this mainly depends on atmospheric temperature)
- External factors:
  - Climate
  - Injuries (injured areas of the body take a long time to get back flexibility due to tissue damage)
  - Limited flexibility due to insufficient water in the body

DEPLETED CHAKRAS

While almost all the chakras are depleted, the actual impact is on the nadis, which are less energised.

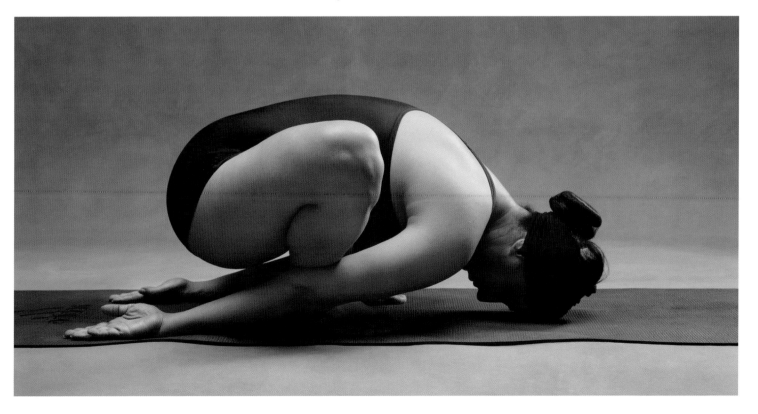

STANDING ASANA SEQUENCE

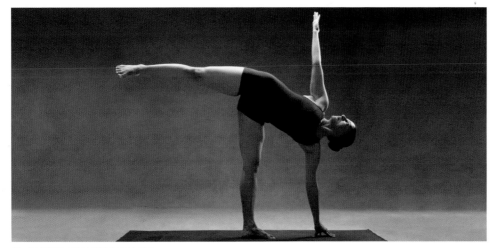

11. ARDHA CHANDRASANA

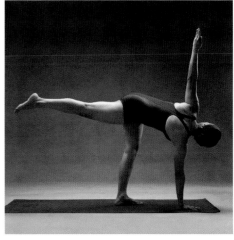

12. PARIVRTTA ARDHA CHANDRASANA

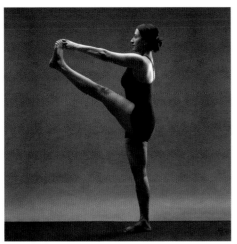

13. UTTHITA HASTA PADANGUSTASANA

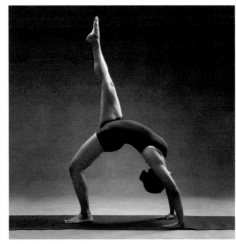

16. CHAKRASANA 1

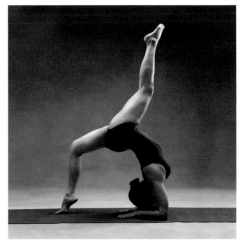

17. CHAKRASANA 2

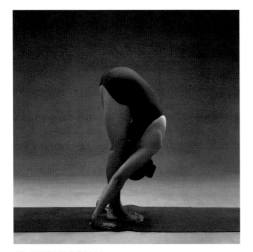

18. UTTANASANA

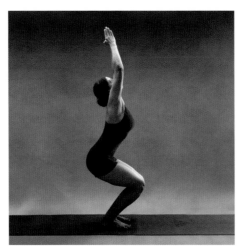

19. UTKATASANA

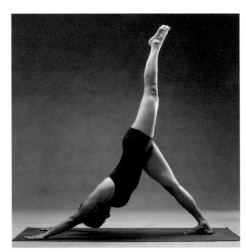

20. UPDASANA

FLOOR ASANA SEQUENCE

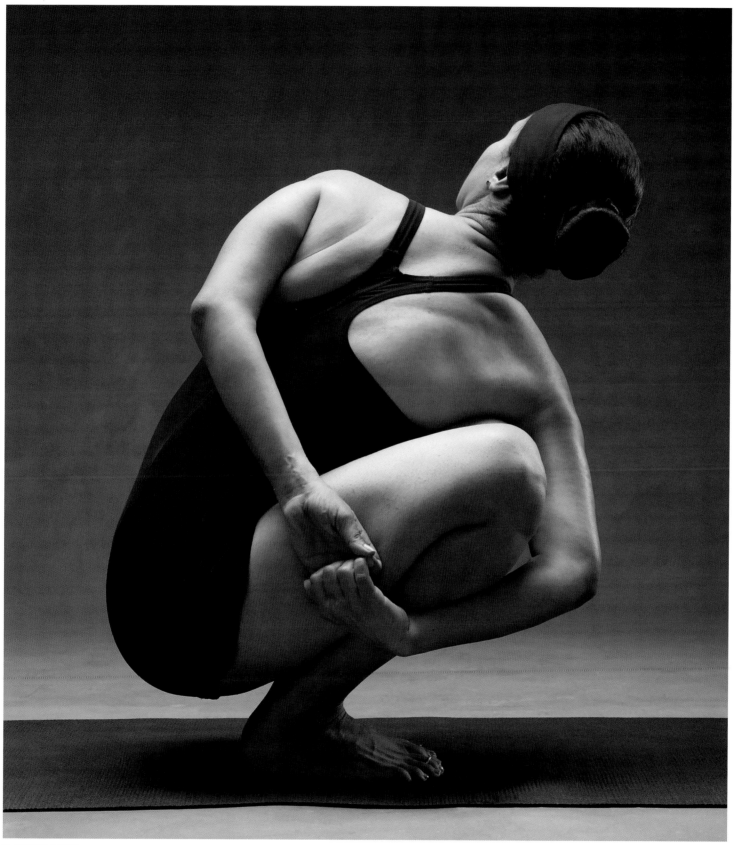

5. PASHASANA

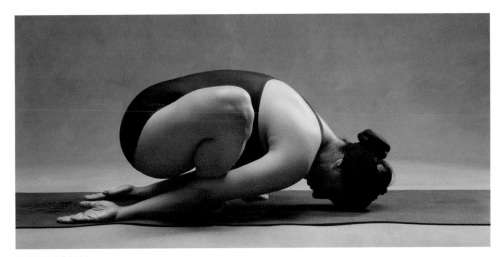

6. MALASANA
Featured asana

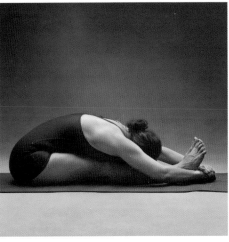

7. PASCHIMOTTANASANA

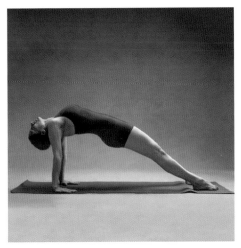

8. PURVOTTANASANA

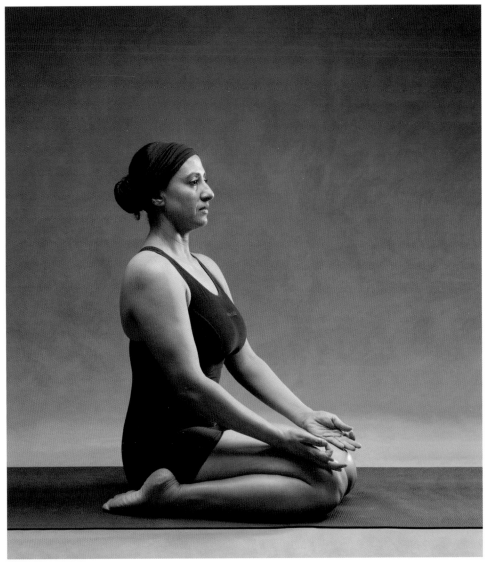

10. VEERASANA

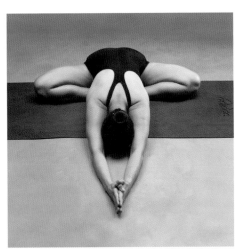

9. BADDHA KONASANA

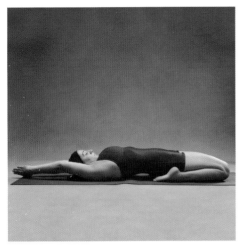

11. SUPTA VEERASANA

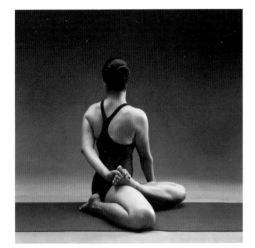

12. BHARADWAJASANA

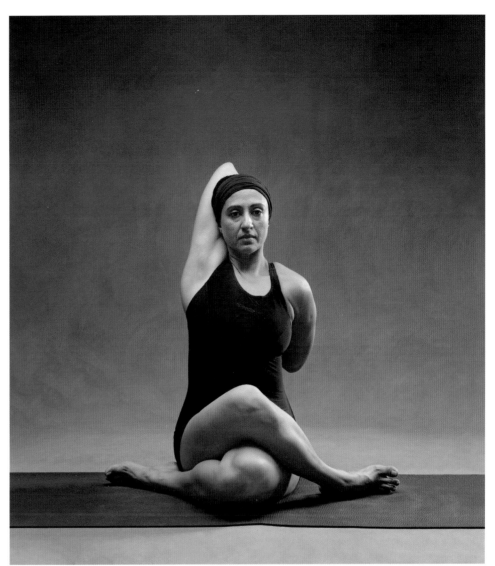

13. GOMUKHASANA

COOLING DOWN

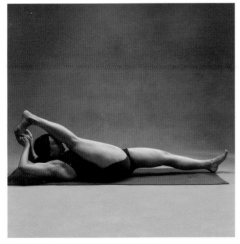

1. SUPTA PADANGUSTASANA 1

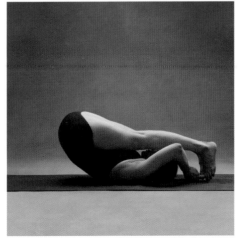

2. SUPTA PADANGUSTASANA 2

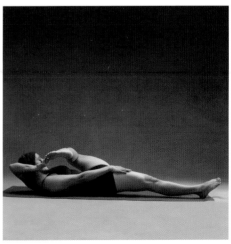

3. SUPTA PADANGUSTASANA 3

SEQUENCE TO MAINTAIN HORMONAL BALANCE

WARM-UP ROUTINE

Perform soft rhythmic jumps 50 times.

Swing the arms forward and backward powerfully 10 times.

Circle the shoulders forward and backward 10 times.

Twist the waist with arms open and stretched 5 times each side.

Gently circle the knees, left & right sides, 5 times each.

Circle the ankles clockwise and anti-clockwise with the front sole pressed to the ground and heel raised 5 times each.

PRANAYAMA ROUTINE

Sit in a comfortable relaxed position. Calm your mind and observe your thoughts.

Perform Ujjayee for 5 minutes.

Perform Ujjayee with Antara Kumbhaka (holding breath after inhaling) for 5 minutes.

Perform Anuloma Viloma for 10 minutes.

Perform Brahmari 5 times.

STANDING-ASANAS ROUTINE

1. Tadasana
2. Urdhva Tadasana
3. Vrikshasana
4. Santulanasana
5. Padangustasana
6. Surya Namaskara: Alternate between A & B – 5 times each.
7. Trikonasana
8. Parivrtta Trikonasana
9. Parsvakonasana
10. Parivrtta Parsvakonasana
11. Parsvottanasana
12. Prasarita Padottanasana
13. Utthita Hasta Padangustasana
14. Ardha Chandrasana
15. Ardha Baddha Padmottanasana
16. Vatayanasana
17. Veerabhadrasana 3
18. Utkatasana

FLOOR-ASANAS ROUTINE

1. Chaduranga Dandasana
2. Urdhva Mukha Svanasana
3. Adho Mukha Svanasana
4. Adho Mukha Shavasana
5. Shalabhasana
6. Dhanurasana: Follow with relaxing the back. Lie with chest down and move feet up and down with bent knees.
7. Ushtrasana
8. Kapotasana – Featured Asana
9. Janu Shirsasana
10. Parivrtta Janu Shirsasana
11. Trianga Mukhapeeda Paschimottanasana
12. Baddha Konasana
13. Upavishtakonasana
14. Bharadwajasana
15. Gomukhasana

COOLING-DOWN ROUTINE

1. Sarvangasana
2. Halasana
3. Setu Bandhasana
4. Urdhva Dhanurasana
5. Viparita Dandasana
6. Matsyasana
7. Shavasana – 5 min

Sit in Padmasana for a count of 5 breaths before leaving the mat.

UNDERSTANDING HORMONAL IMBALANCE

- Hormones are secreted from the pituitary gland and the adrenal glands. They essentially balance the vital functions of the body to keep it fit and healthy.
- Several reasons can disrupt the hormonal balance in the body – age, pollution, stress, change in lifestyle, etc.
- Environmental pollution increases toxins in the body which affects hormonal secretion and the overall function of the glands.
- Symptoms of hormonal malfunction can be detected when one suddenly gains weight, is irritable and tired, has frequent mood swings, heart disease, etc.
- In women, hormonal imbalance leads to energy loss, migraines, dizziness, fatigue, hair loss, anxiety, urinary tract infections, obesity, wrinkles, water retention and a feeling of bloatedness.
- Hormonal imbalance can be handled by adjusting lifestyle, acquiring good eating habits and through proper exercise, especially yoga.

DEPLETED CHAKRAS
Manipura and Vishuddha

The sequence prescribed is based on self-study and years of experience teaching various categories of students. The feedback from students who have benefited from these sequences inspired the author to document them. The symptoms of any discomfort have been observed, studied and discussed with friends who are doctors and psychotherapists.

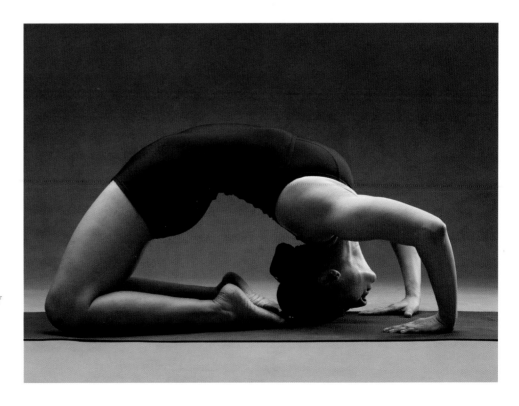

STANDING ASANA SEQUENCE

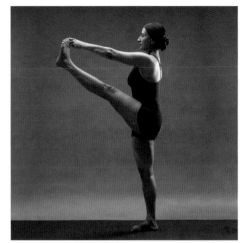

13. UTTHITA HASTA PADANGUSTASANA

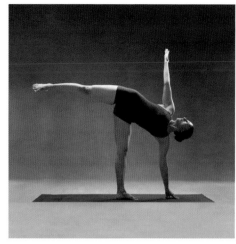

14. ARDHA CHANDRASANA

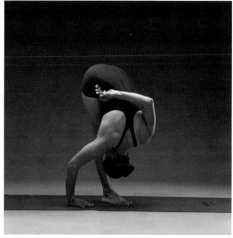

15. ARDHA BADDHA PADMOTTANASANA

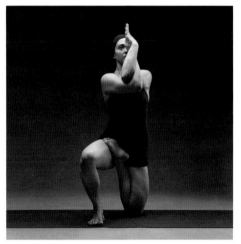

16. VATAYANASANA

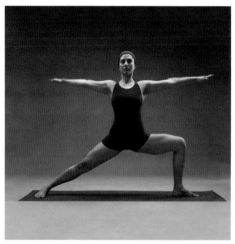

17. VEERABHADRASANA 3

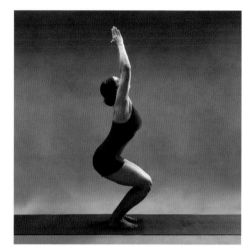

18. UTKATASANA

FLOOR ASANA SEQUENCE

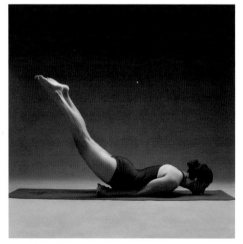

5. SHALABHASANA

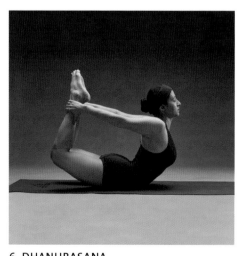

6. DHANURASANA

*Follow with relaxing the back. Lie with chest down
and move feet up and down with bent knees.*

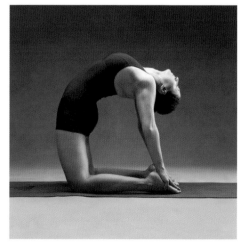

7. USHTRASANA

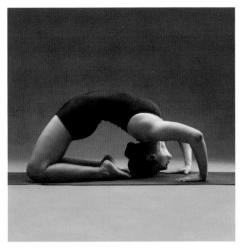

8. KAPOTASANA
Featured asana

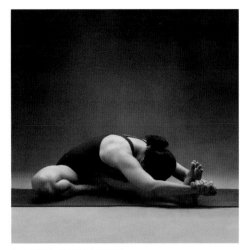

9. JANU SHIRSASANA

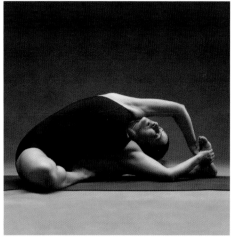

10. PARIVRTTA JANU SHIRSASANA

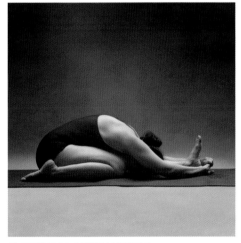

**11. TRIANGA MUKHAPEEDA
PASCHIMOTTANASANA**

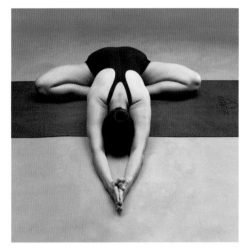

12. BADDHA KONASANA

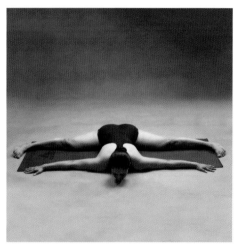

13. UPAVISHTAKONASANA

COOLING DOWN

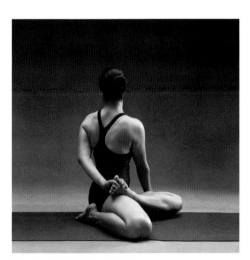

14. BHARADWAJASANA

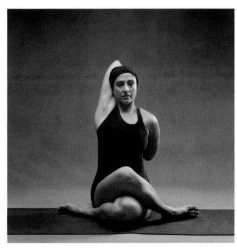

15. GOMUKHASANA

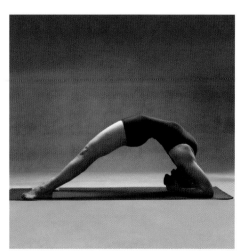

5. VIPARITA DANDASANA

SEQUENCE TO BALANCE THE IMMUNE SYSTEM

WARM-UP ROUTINE

Perform soft rhythmic jumps 50 times.

Swing the arms forward and backward powerfully 10 times.

Circle the shoulders forward and backward 10 times.

Twist the waist with arms open and stretched 5 times each side.

Gently circle the knees, left & right sides, 5 times each.

Circle the ankles clockwise and anti-clockwise with the front sole pressed to the ground and heel raised 5 times each.

PRANAYAMA ROUTINE

Sit in a comfortable, relaxed position. Calm your mind and observe your thoughts.

Perform Ujjayee for 5 minutes.

Perform Ujjayee with Antara Kumbhaka (holding breath after inhaling) for 5 minutes.

Perform Anuloma Viloma for 10 minutes.

Perform Kapalabhati – 150 blows – with adequate rest in between.

STANDING-ASANAS ROUTINE

1. Tadasana
2. Urdhva Tadasana
3. Vrikshasana
4. Santulanasana
5. Padangustasana
6. Surya Namaskara: Alternate between A & B – 5 times each.
7. Trikonasana
8. Parivrtta Trikonasana
9. Parsvakonasana
10. Parivrtta Parsvakonasana
11. Parsvottanasana
12. Prasarita Padottanasana
13. Utthita Hasta Padangustasana
14. Ardha Baddha Padmottanasana
15. Garudasana / Vatayanasana
16. Veerabhadrasana 3
17. Utkatasana
18. Uttanasana
19. Upadasana
20. Eka Pada Kapotasana

FLOOR-ASANAS ROUTINE

1. Chaduranga Dandasana
2. Urdhva Mukha Svanasana
3. Adho Mukha Svanasana
4. Adho Mukha Shavasana
5. Shalabhasana
6. Dhanurasana: Follow with relaxing the back. Lie with chest down and move feet up and down with bent knees.
7. Vajrasana
8. Ushtrasana
9. Baddha Konasana
10. Gomukhasana – Featured Asana
11. Navasana
12. Purvottanasanana

COOLING-DOWN ROUTINE

1. Supta Padangustasana 1
2. Supta Padangustasana 2
3. Sarvangasana
4. Halasana
5. Setu Bandhasana
6. Shirsasana
7. Matsyasana
8. Shavasana – 5 min

Sit in Padmasana for a count of 5 breaths before leaving the mat.

IMPORTANT

Please make sure that all the asanas and Pranayama techniques have been taught to you by your yoga guru. A doctor's permission could be essential in some cases. Before starting on this sequence, it is imperative that the practitioner follows the Warm-up Exercises, Surya Namaskara (A&B) (Section B, Chapter 5) and Asanas (Section B, Chapters 3 & 4; Section C, Chapter 9).

To increase immunity, asanas that increase energy flow to the neck region should be practised.

It would help if Kapalabhati is added to the Pranayama Routine. Including Uttanasana, Upadasana and Eka Pada Kapotasana to the end of the Standing-Asanas Routine in Section B, Chapters 3 & 4, would strengthen immunity in the body.

The sequence prescribed is based on self-study and years of experience teaching various categories of students. The feedback from students who have benefited from these sequences inspired the author to document them. The symptoms of any discomfort have been observed, studied and discussed with friends who are doctors and psychotherapists.

UNDERSTANDING LOW-IMMUNITY SYMPTOMS

- Seasonal allergies indicate imbalance in the immune system.
- Symptoms would be stuffy nose, ears and sinuses, inflamed eyes, headaches, sore throat and difficulty in breathing, caused by the mucus-producing process of the immune system. Mucus is released from the body to prevent foreign bacteria from entering it.
- Emotional stress can also cause low immunity.
- The thymus gland would be the focus in the asanas.
- People with low immunity should practise asanas at a slow and a gentle pace, paying a lot of attention to breathing.

DEPLETED CHAKRAS
Anahata and Vishuddha

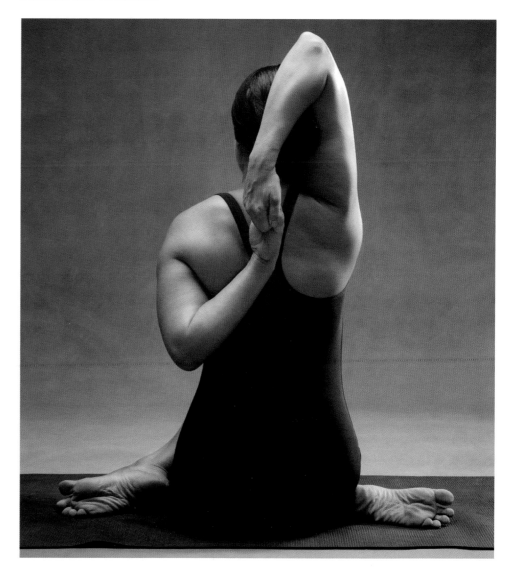

STANDING ASANA SEQUENCE

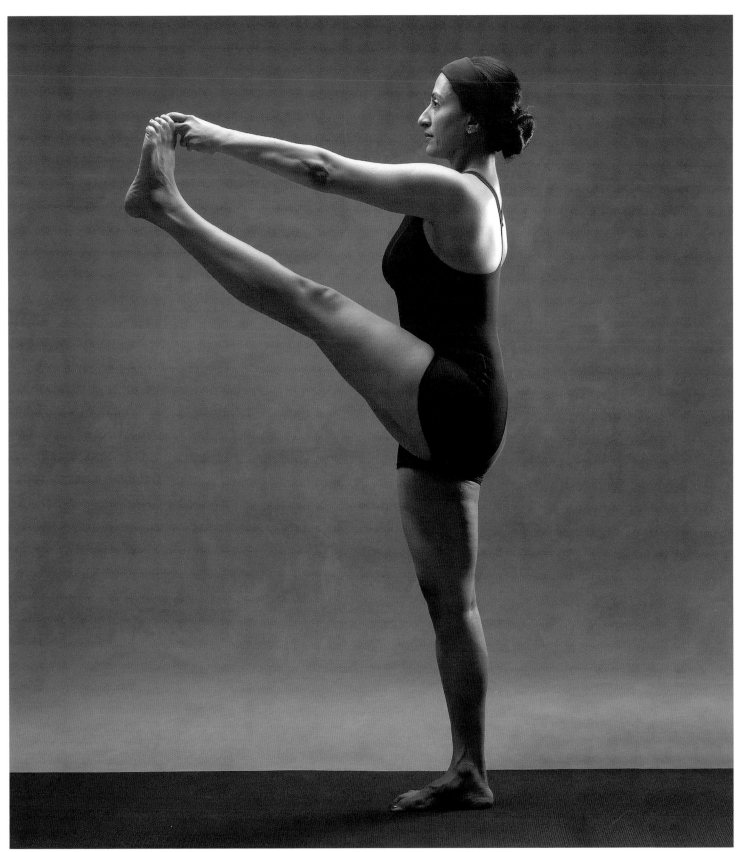

13. UTTHITA HASTA PADANGUSTASANA

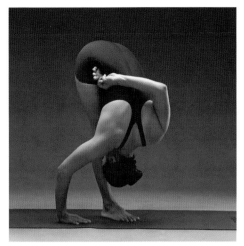

14. ARDHA BADDHA PADMOTTANASANA

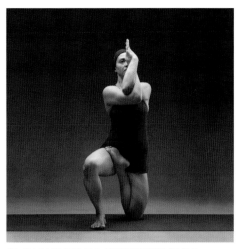

15. GARUDASANA / VATAYANASANA

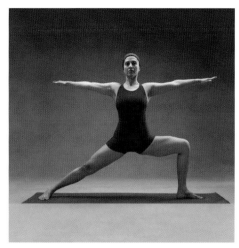

16. VEERABHADRASANA 3

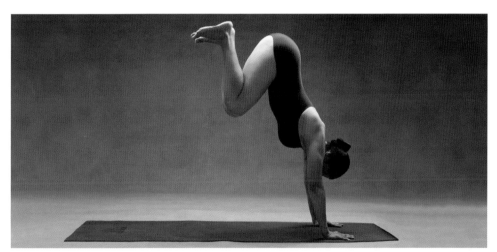

17. UTKATASANA

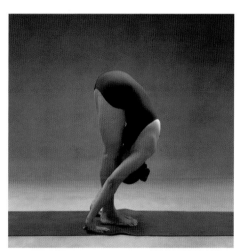

18. UTTANASANA

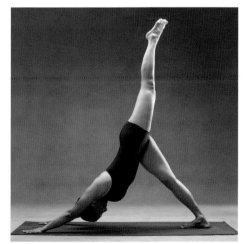

19. UPADASANA

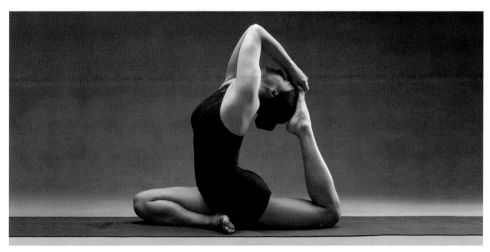

20. EKA PADA KAPOTASANA

FLOOR ASANA SEQUENCE

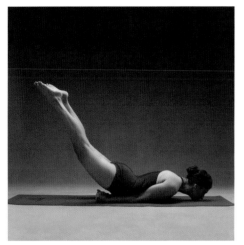

5. SHALABHASANA

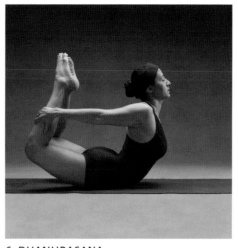

6. DHANURASANA
Follow with relaxing the back. Lie with chest down and move feet up and down with bent knees.

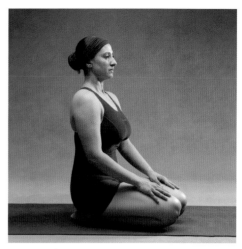

7. VAJRASANA

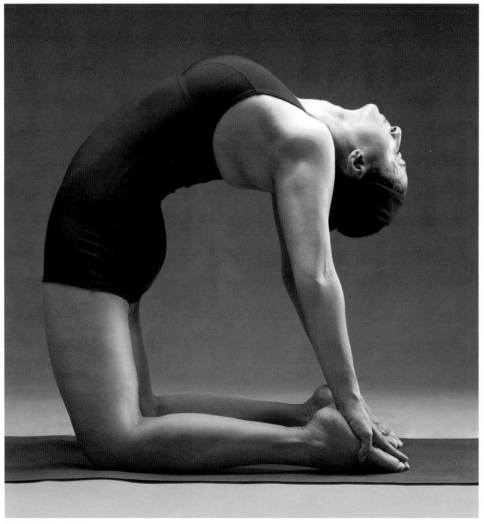

8. USHTRASANA

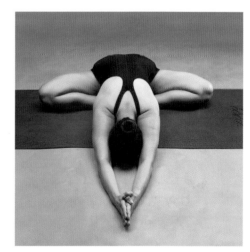

9. BADDHA KONASANA

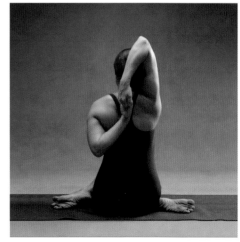

10. GOMUKHASANA
Featured asana

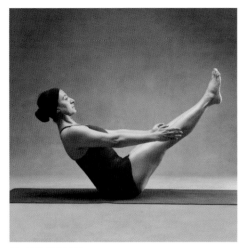

11. NAVASANA

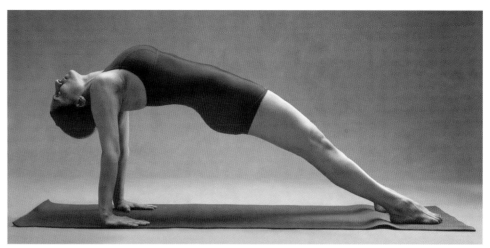

12. PURVOTTANASANA

COOLING DOWN

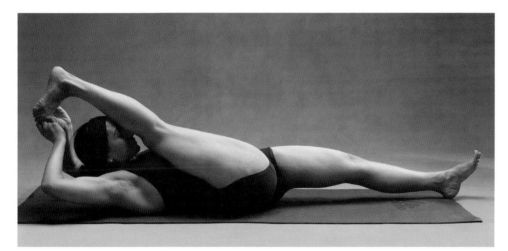

1. SUPTA PADANGUSTASANA 1

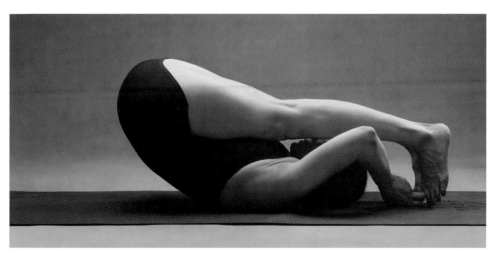

2. SUPTA PADANGUSTASANA 2

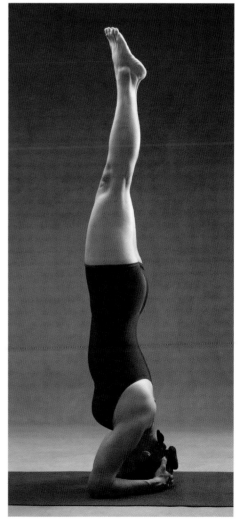

6. SHIRSASANA

SEQUENCE TO OVERCOME INSECURITY

WARM-UP ROUTINE
Perform soft rhythmic jumps 50 times.
Swing the arms forward and backward powerfully 10 times.
Circle the shoulders forward and backward 10 times.
Twist the waist with arms open and stretched 5 times each side.
Gently circle the knees, left & right sides, 5 times each.
Circle the ankles clockwise and anti-clockwise with the front sole pressed to the ground and heel raised 5 times each.

PRANAYAMA ROUTINE
Sit in a comfortable, relaxed position. Calm your mind and observe your thoughts.
Perform Ujjayee for 5 minutes.
Perform Ujjayee with Antara Kumbhaka (holding breath after inhaling) for 5 minutes.
Perform Anuloma Viloma for 10 minutes.
Perform Shitali 5 times.

STANDING-ASANAS ROUTINE
1. Tadasana
2. Urdhva Tadasana
3. Vrikshasana
4. Santulanasana
5. Padangustasana
6. Surya Namaskara: Alternate between A & B – 5 times each.
7. Trikonasana
8. Parivrtta Trikonasana
9. Parsvakonasana
10. Parivrtta Parsvakonasana
11. Parsvottanasana
12. Prasarita Padottanasana
13. Utthita Hasta Padangustasana
14. Ardha Baddha Padmottanasana
15. Vatayanasana
16. Veerabhadrasana 3
17. Vashistasana 1
18. Vashistasana 2
19. Chaduranga Dandasana
20. Upadasana
21. Eka Pada Kapotasana

FLOOR-ASANAS ROUTINE
1. Chaduranga Dandasana
2. Urdhva Mukha Svanasana
3. Adho Mukha Svanasana
4. Adho Mukha Shavasana
5. Dhanurasana
6. Shalabhasana: Follow with relaxing the back. Lie with chest down and move feet up and down with bent knees.
7. Veerasana
8. Supta Veerasana
9. Baddha Konasana
10. Kurmasana – Featured Asana
11. Marichyasana 2
12. Marichyasana 4
13. Navasana
14. Purvottanasana
15. Tolasana

COOLING DOWN ROUTINE
1. Supta Padangustasana 1
2. Supta Padangustasana 2
3. Sarvangasana
4. Halasana
5. Setu Bandhasana
6. Urdhva Dhanurasana
7. Matsyasana
8. Shavasana – 5 min
Sit in Padmasana for a count of 5 breaths before leaving the mat.

IMPORTANT
Please make sure that all the asanas and Pranayama techniques have been taught to you by your yoga guru. A doctor's permission could be essential in some cases. Before starting on this sequence, it is imperative that the practitioner follows the Warm-up Exercises, Surya Namaskara (A&B) (Section B, Chapter 5) and Asanas (Section B, Chapters 3 & 4; Section C, Chapter 9).

Add Shitali (not more than 5 repetitions) to the Pranayama Routine, which would help cool the body down and release tension. Adding Vashistasana, Upadasana and Eka Pada Kapotasana to the Standing-Asanas Routine would go a long way in helping the body.

UNDERSTANDING INSECURITY

- Insecurity could be physical or emotional. It makes a person nervous and suffer from low self-esteem. This can be overcome by understanding the circumstances calmly and working on facing it confidently.

- If the feeling of insecurity becomes persistent, there are substantial changes in the personality. The person would be over-talkative, untimely joking, always defensive, always talking about themselves, a workaholic, materialistic, spendthrift, abusive etc.

- The feeling of insecurity can grow to such an extent that it starts affecting the overall health. The signs would start with muscle tension, palpitation, dry mouth, sweating, lack of concentration, sleeplessness and gasping, with a feeling that some great disaster would strike any moment, though there are no real external threats.

- Insecure people tend to have regular gastrointestinal problems, abdominal pain, along with insomnia, irritation, sweaty hands, shortness of breath and a choking sensation.

- Medical causes like seizures, strokes, thyroid or hormonal imbalance could also lead to this dreaded feeling of insecurity.

DEPLETED CHAKRAS
Muladhara, Manipura, Anahata and Vishuddha

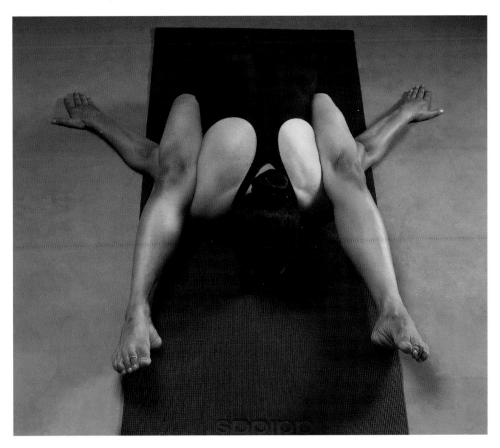

The sequence prescribed is based on self-study and years of experience teaching various categories of students. The feedback from students who have benefited from these sequences inspired the author to document them. The symptoms of any discomfort have been observed, studied and discussed with friends who are doctors and psychotherapists.

STANDING ASANA SEQUENCE

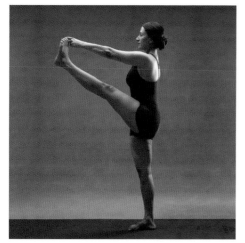

13. UTTHITA HASTA PADANGUSTASANA

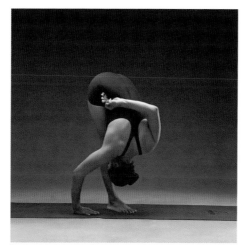

14. ARDHA BADDHA PADMOTTANASANA

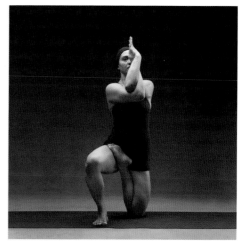

15. VATAYANASANA

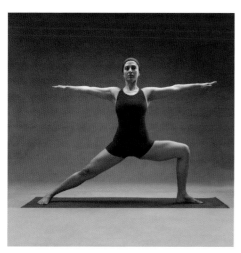

16. VEERABHADRASANA 3

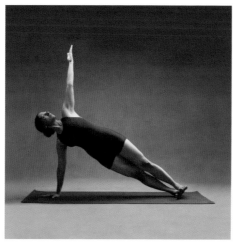

17. VASHISTASANA 1

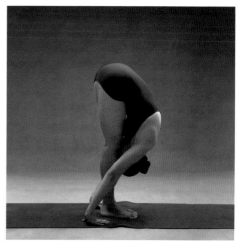

18. VASHISTASANA 2

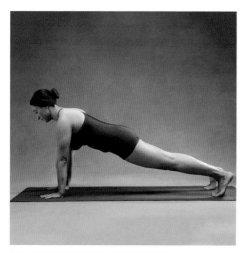

19. CHADURANGA DANDASANA

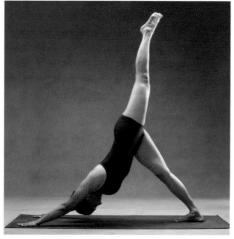

20. UPADASANA

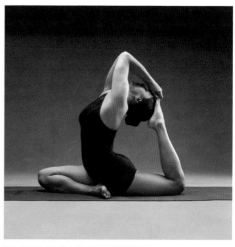

21. EKA PADA KAPOTASANA

FLOOR ASANA SEQUENCE

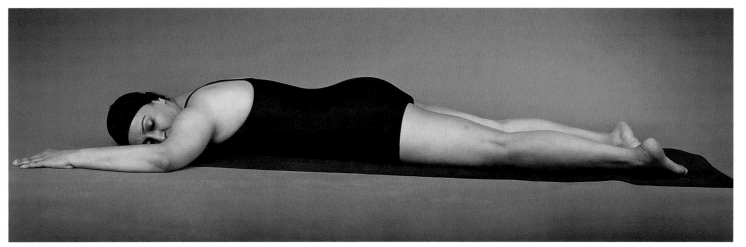

4. ADHO MUKHA SHAVASANA

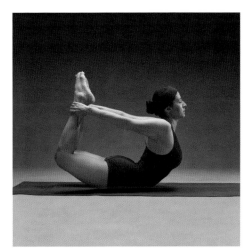

5. DHANURASANA

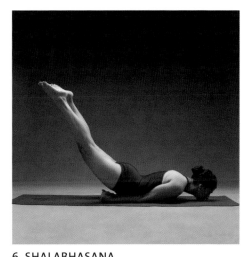

6. SHALABHASANA
Follow with relaxing the back. Lie with chest down and move feet up and down with bent knees.

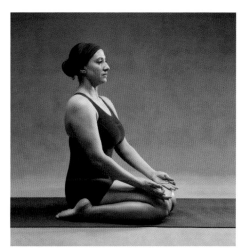

7. VEERASANA

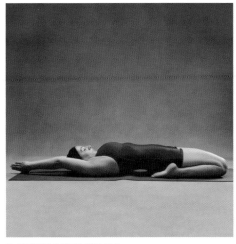

8. SUPTA VEERASANA

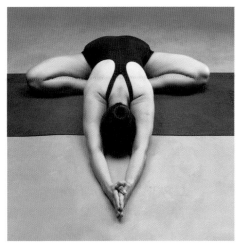

9. BADDHA KONASANA

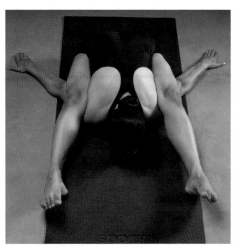

10. KURMASANA
Featured asana

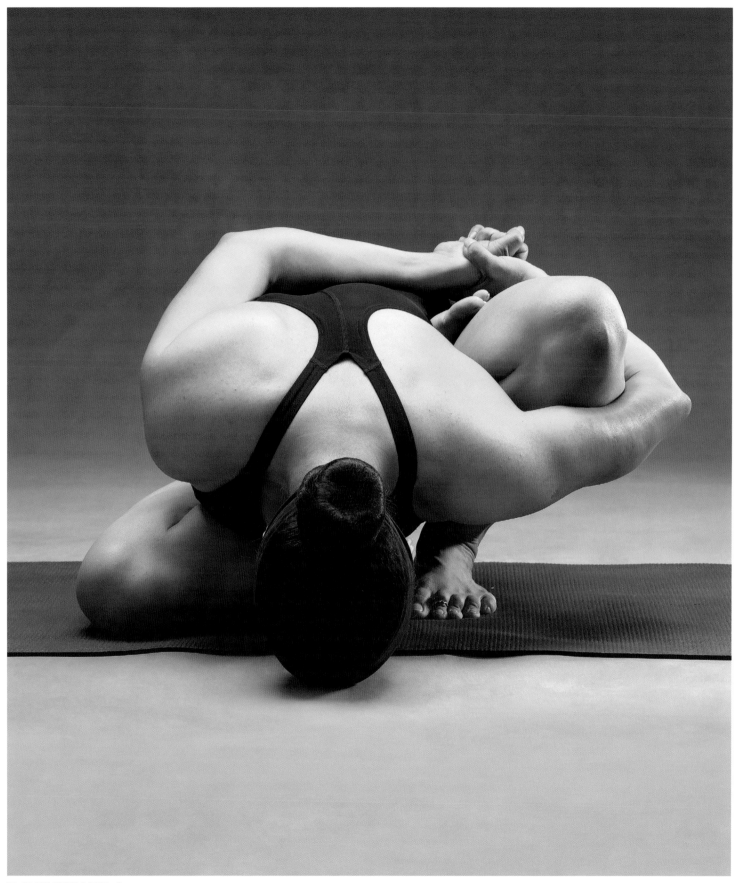

11. MARICHYASANA 2

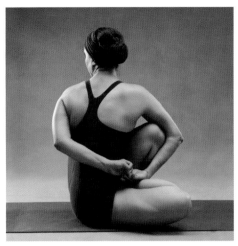

12. MARICHYASANA 4

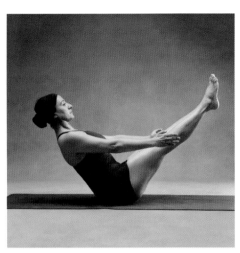

13. NAVASANA

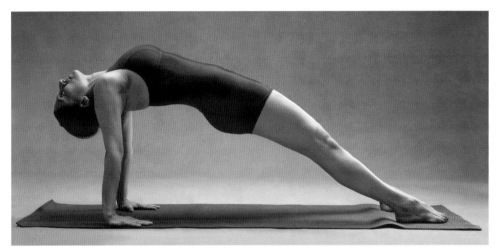

14. PURVOTTANASANA

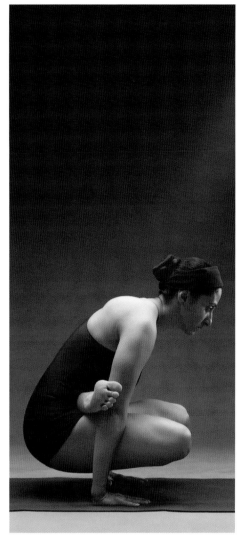

15. TOLASANA

COOLING DOWN

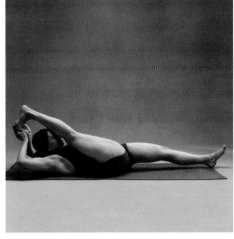

1. SUPTA PADANGUSTASANA 1

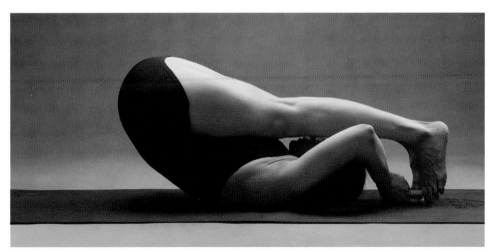

2. SUPTA PADANGUSTASANA 2

SEQUENCE TO INCREASE METABOLISM

WARM-UP ROUTINE

Perform soft rhythmic jumps 50 times.
Swing the arms forward and backward powerfully 10 times.
Circle the shoulders forward and backward 10 times.
Twist the waist with arms open and stretched 5 times each side.
Gently circle the knees, left & right sides, 5 times each.
Circle the ankles clockwise and anti-clockwise with the front sole pressed to the ground and heel raised 5 times each.

PRANAYAMA ROUTINE

Sit in a comfortable, relaxed position. Calm your mind and observe your thoughts.
Perform Ujjayee for 5 minutes.
Perform Ujjayee with Antara Kumbhaka (holding breath after inhaling) for 5 minutes.
Perform Anuloma Viloma for 10 minutes.
Perform Bhastrika – 50 blows – with adequate rest in between.

STANDING-ASANAS ROUTINE

1.	Tadasana
2.	Urdhva Tadasana
3.	Vrikshasana
4.	Santulanasana
5.	Padangustasana
6.	Surya Namaskara: Alternate between A & B – 5 times each.
7.	Trikonasana
8.	Parivrtta Trikonasana
9.	Parsvakonasana
10.	Parivrtta Parsvakonasana
11.	Parsvottanasana
12.	Prasarita Padottanasana
13.	Trianga Mukhottasana
14.	Utthita Hasta Padangustasana
15.	Ardha Baddha Padmottanasana
16.	Garudasana / Vatayanasana
17.	Veerabhadrasana 3
18.	Utkatasana
19.	Bakasana
20.	Tittibasana – Featured Asana

FLOOR-ASANAS ROUTINE

1.	Chaduranga Dandasana
2.	Urdhva Mukha Svanasana
3.	Adho Mukha Svanasana
4.	Adho Mukha Shavasana
5.	Dhanurasana: Follow with relaxing the back. Lie with chest down and move feet up and down with bent knees.
6.	Ushtrasana
7.	Janu Shirsasana
8.	Parivrtta Janu Shirsasana
9.	Baddha Konasana
10.	Navasana
11.	Purvottanasanana
12.	Gomukhasana
13.	Padmasana
14.	Tolasana

COOLING-DOWN ROUTINE

1.	Supta Padangustasana 2
2.	Supta Padangustasana 3
3.	Sarvangasana
4.	Halasana
5.	Setu Bandhasana
6.	Urdhva Dhanurasana
7.	Matsyasana
8.	Shavasana – 5 min
Sit in Padmasana for a count of 5 breaths before leaving the mat.	

IMPORTANT

Please make sure that all the asanas and Pranayama techniques have been taught to you by your yoga guru. A doctor's permission could be essential in some cases. Before starting on this sequence, it is imperative that the practitioner follows the Warm-up Exercises, Surya Namaskara (A&B) (Section B, Chapter 5) and Asanas (Section B, Chapters 3 & 4; Section C, Chapter 9).

Adding the vigorous Bastrika to the Pranayama Routine would help increase the body's metabolic rate.

The sequence prescribed is based on self-study and years of experience teaching various categories of students. The feedback from students who have benefited from these sequences inspired the author to document them. The symptoms of any discomfort have been observed, studied and discussed with friends who are doctors and psychotherapists.

UNDERSTANDING METABOLISM

- Metabolism is affected by the body's composition, more specifically the amount of muscles versus the amount of fat.
- People who are active and fit have a higher metabolic rate. In medical terms, metabolism is the rate at which you burn calories. The symptoms of slow metabolism include fatigue, feeling cold, dry skin, constipation, low blood pressure.
- The endocrine system is responsible for balanced metabolic activity. The thyroid gland produces the hormones that normalise metabolism.

DEPLETED CHAKRAS

Manipura and Vishuddha

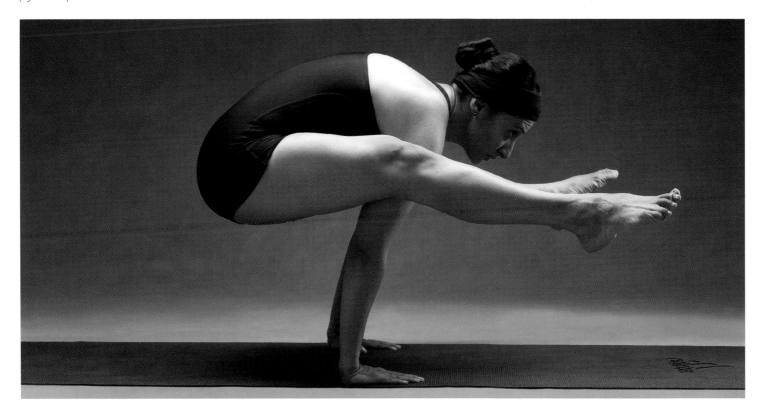

STANDING ASANA SEQUENCE

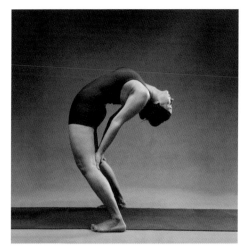

13. TRIANGA MUKHOTTASANA

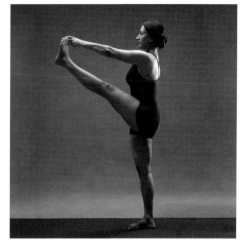

14. UTTHITA HASTA PADANGUSTASANA

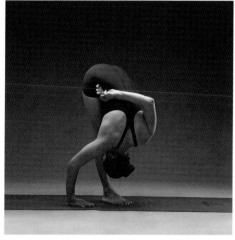

15. ARDHA BADDHA PADMOTTANASANA

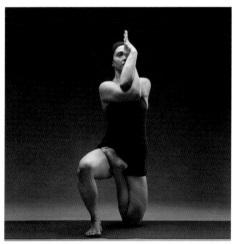

16. GARUDASANA / VATAYANASANA

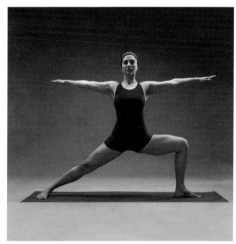

17. VEERABHADRASANA 3

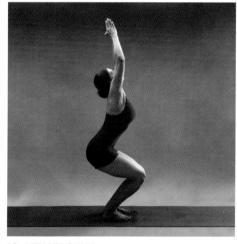

18. UTKATASANA

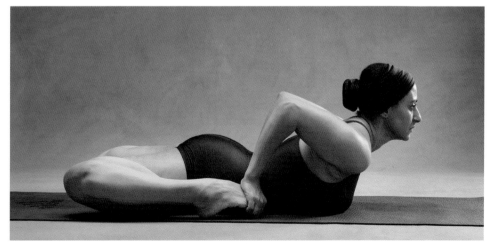

19. BAKASANA

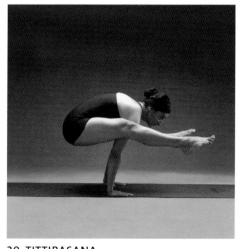

20. TITTIBASANA
Featured asana

FLOOR ASANA SEQUENCE

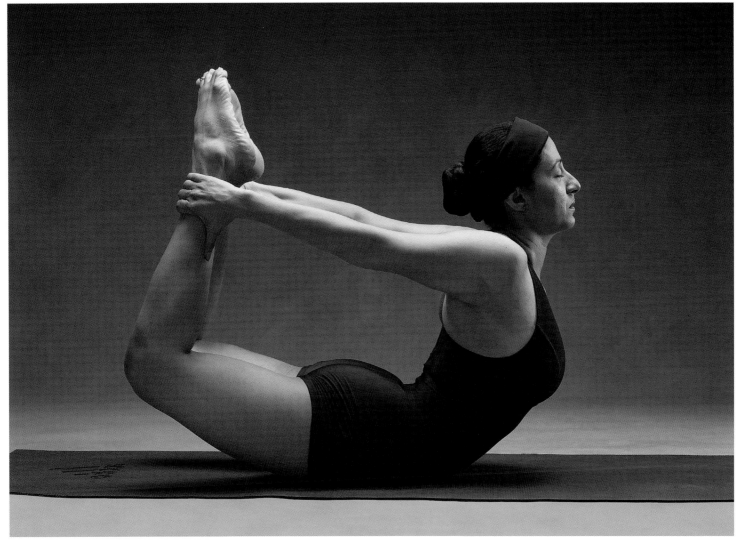

5. DHANURASANA
Follow with relaxing the back. Lie with chest down and move feet up and down with bent knees.

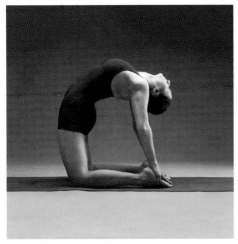

6. USHTRASANA

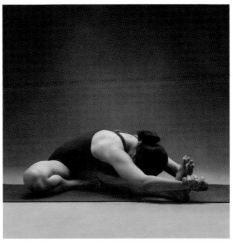

7. JANU SHIRSASANA

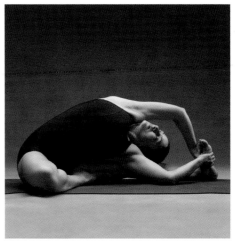

8. PARIVRTTA JANU SHIRSASANA

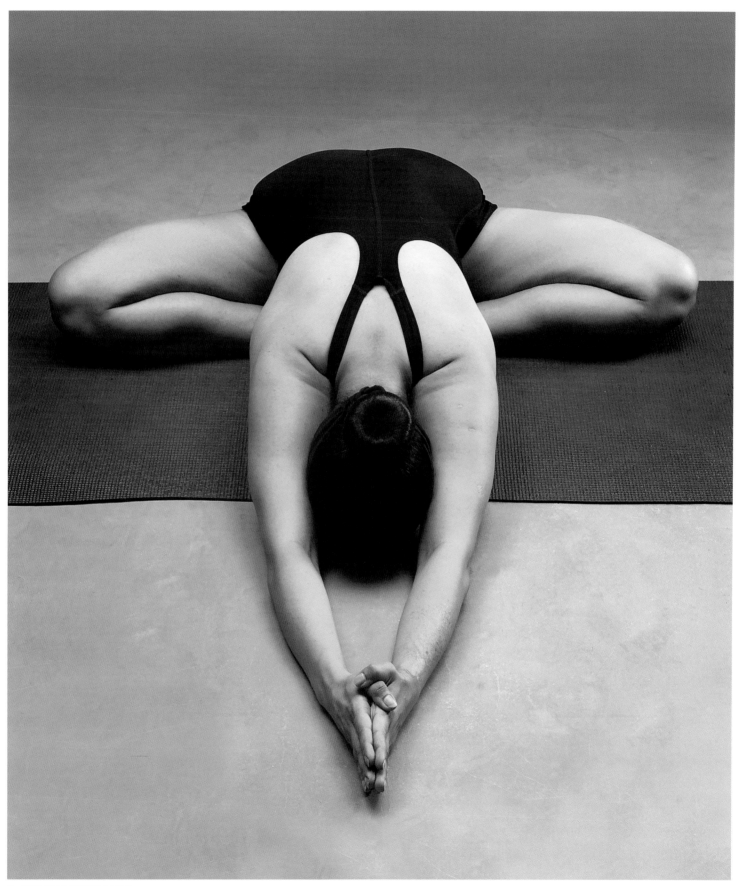

9. BADDHA KONASANA

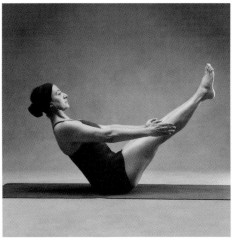

10. NAVASANA

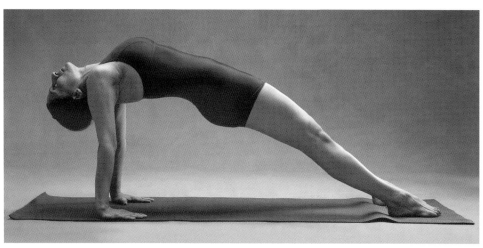

11. PURVOTTANASANANA

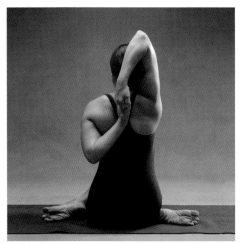

12. GOMUKHASANA

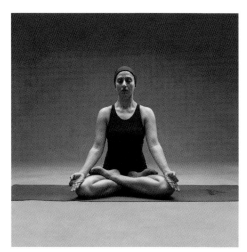

13. PADMASANA

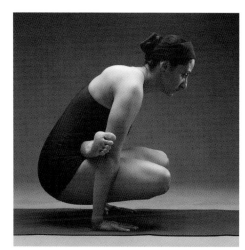

14. TOLASANA

COOLING DOWN

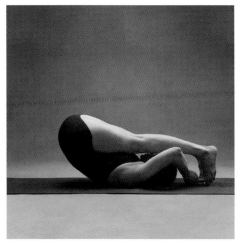

1. SUPTA PADANGUSTASANA 2

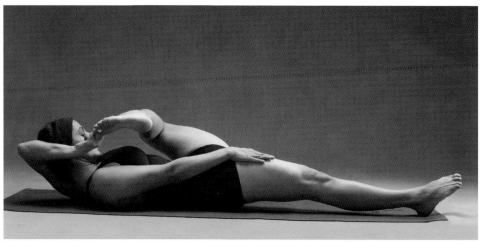

2. SUPTA PADANGUSTASANA 3

SEQUENCE TO KEEP THE BRAIN ACTIVE

WARM-UP ROUTINE

Perform soft rhythmic jumps 50 times.

Swing the arms forward and backward powerfully 10 times.

Circle the shoulders forward and backward 10 times.

Twist the waist with arms open and stretched 5 times each side.

Gently circle the knees, left & right sides, 5 times each.

Circle the ankles clockwise and anti-clockwise with the front sole pressed to the ground and heel raised 5 times each.

PRANAYAMA ROUTINE

Sit in a comfortable, relaxed position. Calm your mind and observe your thoughts.

Perform Ujjayee for 5 minutes.

Perform Ujjayee with Antara Kumbhaka (holding breath after inhaling) for 5 minutes.

Perform Anuloma Viloma for 10 minutes.

Perform Brahmari – 5 repetitions – with adequate rest in between.

Perform Kapalabhati – 300 blows – with adequate rest in between.

STANDING-ASANAS ROUTINE

1. Tadasana
2. Urdhva Tadasana
3. Vrikshasana
4. Santulanasana
5. Padangustasana
6. Surya Namaskara: Alternate between A & B – 5 times each.
7. Trikonasana
8. Parivrtta Trikonasana
9. Parsvakonasana
10. Parivrtta Parsvakonasana
11. Parsvottanasana
12. Prasarita Padottanasana
13. Utthita Hasta Padangustasana
14. Ardha Baddha Padmottanasana
15. Vatayanasana
16. Veerabhadrasana 1
17. Veerabhadrasana 2
18. Veerabhadrasana 3
19. Veerabhadrasana 4
20. Veerabhadrasana
21. Utkatasana

FLOOR-ASANAS ROUTINE

1. Chaduranga Dandasana
2. Urdhva Mukha Svanasana
3. Adho Mukha Svanasana
4. Adho Mukha Shavasana
5. Dhanurasana: Follow with relaxing the back. Lie with chest down and move feet up and down with bent knees.
6. Ushtrasana
7. Vajrasana
8. Shirsasana
9. Marichyasana 1
10. Marichyasana 2
11. Gomukhasana
12. Navasana – Featured Asana
13. Purvottanasana

COOLING-DOWN ROUTINE

1. Sarvangasana
2. Halasana
3. Setu Bandhasana
4. Urdhva Dhanurasana
5. Matsyasana
6. Shavasana – 5 min

Sit in Padmasana for a count of 5 breaths before leaving the mat.

IMPORTANT

Please make sure that all the asanas and Pranayama techniques have been taught to you by your yoga guru. A doctor's permission could be essential in some cases. Before starting on this sequence, it is imperative that the practitioner follows the Warm-up Exercises, Surya Namaskara (A&B) (Section B, Chapter 5) and Asanas (Section B, Chapters 3 & 4; Section C, Chapter 9).

Add Brahmari and Kapalabhati to the Pranayama Routine.

UNDERSTANDING THE HUMAN BRAIN

The human brain's most important and vital functions are considered to be intelligence and memory, thus making it active. During the course of a lifetime, the brain registers a multitude of information and experiences. If these experiences are not managed well, they remain cluttered in the mind, leading to issues like lack of concentration, absent-mindedness, lack of awareness and judgement, etc.

It is important that before beginning the asana practice sequence, the mind is calmed first. For example:

- Memorise a mantra and repeat it 21 times, practising focus and concentration.
- Relax the mind with thoughts of nature, like a beautiful landscape, a calm blue sky, a gentle sea, snow-capped mountains, etc.
- Sleep well and eat at the right time.

There are many techniques which can be adopted, depending on your personal liking.

DEPLETED CHAKRAS

Sahasrara and Ajna

The sequence prescribed is based on self-study and years of experience teaching various categories of students. The feedback from students who have benefited from these sequences inspired the author to document them. The symptoms of any discomfort have been observed, studied and discussed with friends who are doctors and psychotherapists.

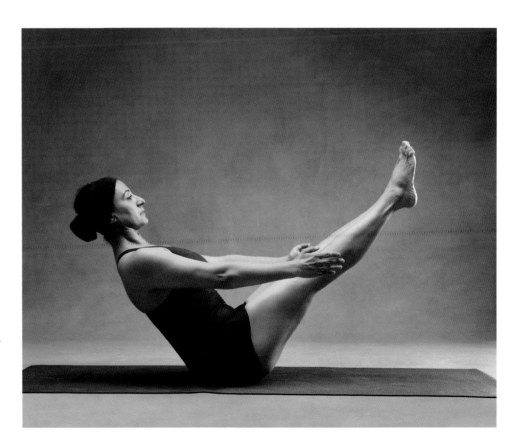

STANDING ASANA SEQUENCE

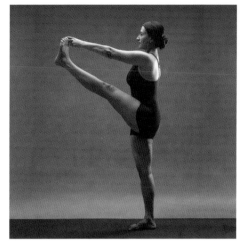

13. UTTHITA HASTA PADANGUSTASANA

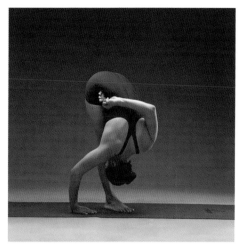

14. ARDHA BADDHA PADMOTTANASANA

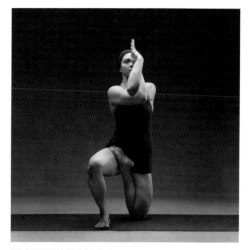

15. VATAYANASANA

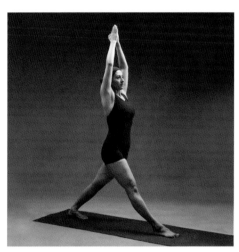

16. VEERABHADRASANA 1

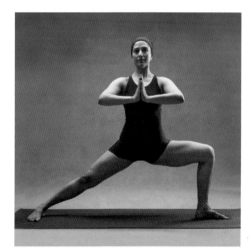

17. VEERABHADRASANA 2

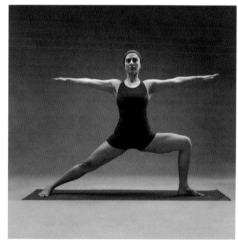

18. VEERABHADRASANA 3

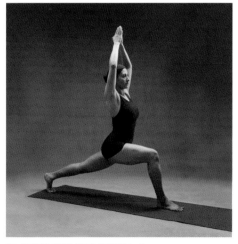

19. VEERABHADRASANA 4

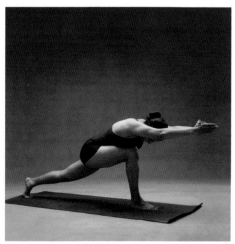

20. VEERABHADRASANA

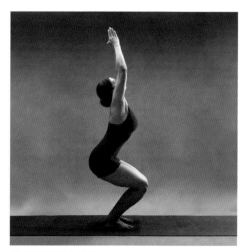

21. UTKATASANA

FLOOR ASANA SEQUENCE

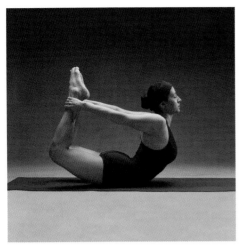

5. DHANURASANA
Follow with relaxing the back. Lie with chest down and move feet up and down with bent knees.

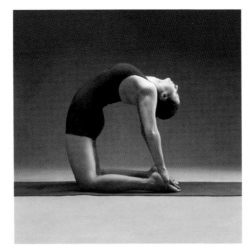

6. USHTRASANA

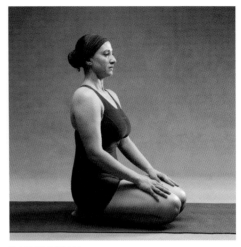

7. VAJRASANA

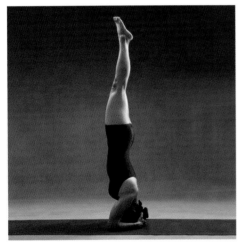

8. SHIRSASANA

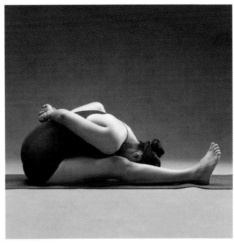

9. MARICHYASANA 1

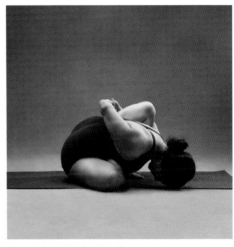

10. MARICHYASANA 2

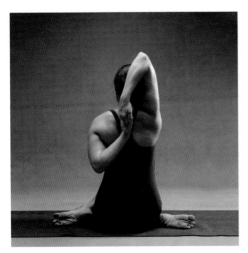

11. GOMUKHASANA

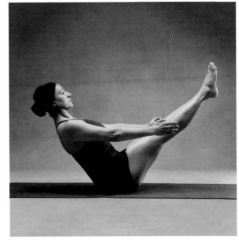

12. NAVASANA
Featured asana

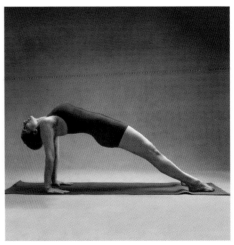

13. PURVOTTANASANA

SEQUENCE FOR INCREASING STAMINA

WARM-UP ROUTINE

Perform soft rhythmic jumps 50 times.
Swing the arms forward and backward powerfully 10 times.
Circle the shoulders forward and backward 10 times.
Twist the waist with arms open and stretched 5 times each side.
Gently circle the knees, left & right sides, 5 times each.
Circle the ankles clockwise and anti-clockwise with the front sole pressed to the ground and heel raised 5 times each.

PRANAYAMA ROUTINE

Sit in a comfortable, relaxed position. Calm your mind and observe your thoughts.
Perform Ujjayee for 5 minutes.
Perform Ujjayee with Antara Kumbhaka (holding breath after inhaling) for 5 minutes.
Perform Anuloma Viloma for 10 minutes.
Perform Brahmari 5 times. with adequate rest in between
Perform Kapalabhati – 300 blows – with adequate rest in between.

STANDING-ASANAS ROUTINE

1.	Tadasana
2.	Urdhva Tadasana
3.	Vrikshasana
4.	Santulanasana
5.	Padangustasana
6.	Surya Namaskara: Alternate between A & B – 5 times each.
7.	Trikonasana
8.	Parivrtta Trikonasana
9.	Parsvakonasana
10.	Parivrtta Parsvakonasana
11.	Parsvottanasana
12.	Prasarita Padottanasana
13.	Utthita Hasta Padangustasana
14.	Ardha Baddha Padmottanasana
15.	Vatayanasana
16.	Veerabhadrasana 3
17.	Utkatasana
18.	Natarajasana
19.	Vashistasana
20.	Kala Bhairavasana

FLOOR-ASANAS ROUTINE

1.	Chaduranga Dandasana
2.	Urdhva Mukha Svanasana
3.	Adho Mukha Svanasana
4.	Adho Mukha Shavasana
5.	Shalabhasana
6.	Dhanurasana: Follow with relaxing the back. Lie with chest down and move feet up and down with bent knees.
7.	Ushtrasana
8.	Vajrasana
9.	Paryankasana
10.	Baddha Konasana
11.	Kurmasana
12.	Navasana

COOLING-DOWN ROUTINE

1.	Sarvangasana
2.	Halasana
3.	Setu Bandhasana
4.	Urdhva Dhanurasana
5.	Chakrasana 2
6.	Matsyasana
7.	Viparita Dandasana – Featured Asana
8.	Matsyasana 2
9.	Shavasana – 5 min
Sit in Padmasana for a count of 5 breaths before leaving the mat.	

IMPORTANT

Please make sure that all the asanas and Pranayama techniques have been taught to you by your yoga guru. A doctor's permission could be essential in some cases. Before starting on this sequence, it is imperative that the practitioner follows the Warm-up Exercises, Surya Namaskara (A&B) (Section B, Chapter 5) and Asanas (Section B, Chapters 3 & 4; Section C, Chapter 9).

Add Brahmari and Kapalabhati to the Pranayama Routine.

The sequence prescribed is based on self-study and years of experience teaching various categories of students. The feedback from students who have benefited from these sequences inspired the author to document them. The symptoms of any discomfort have been observed, studied and discussed with friends who are doctors and psychotherapists.

IMPROVING STAMINA

Lack of energy or stamina is linked either to lifestyle factors, physical conditions or even psychological conditions.

- Lifestyle factors could be poor eating habits, use of caffeine and alcohol, sleep deprivation, and a sedentary lifestyle.
- Physical factors are allergies, persistent muscular pains, diabetes, overactive or underactive thyroid, obesity, nutritional deficiencies, etc.
- Psychological conditions can make the body become weak and tired when dealing with depression or grief; boredom with the current state of affairs could add to the lack of energy.

DEPLETED CHAKRAS

Anahata and Svadhisthana

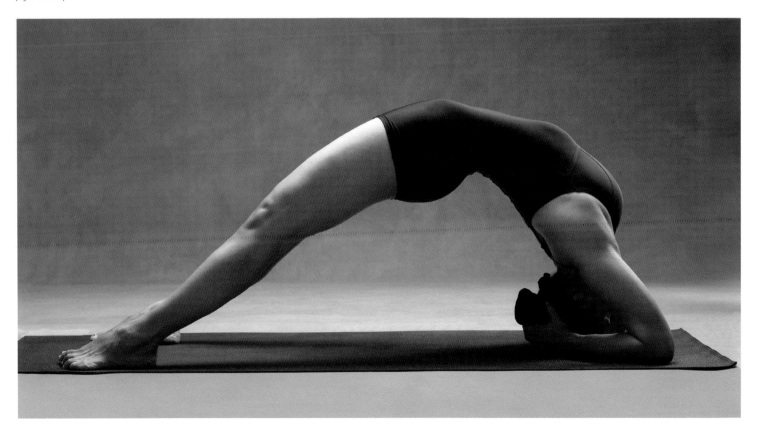

STANDING ASANA SEQUENCE

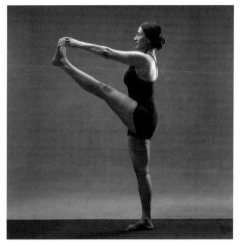

13. UTTHITA HASTA PADANGUSTASANA

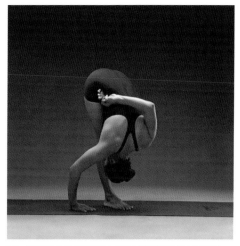

14. ARDHA BADDHA PADMOTTANASANA

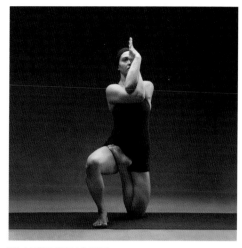

15. VATAYANASANA

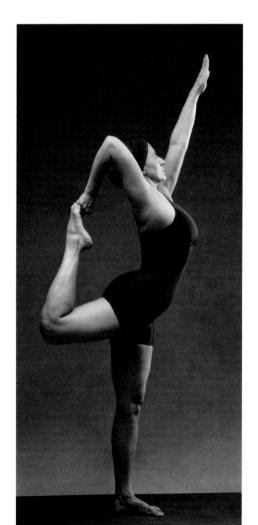

18. NATARAJASANA

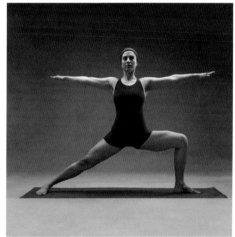

16. VEERABHADRASANA 3

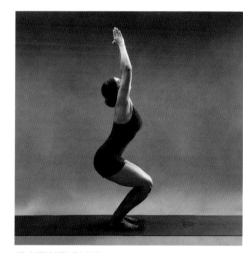

17. UTKATASANA

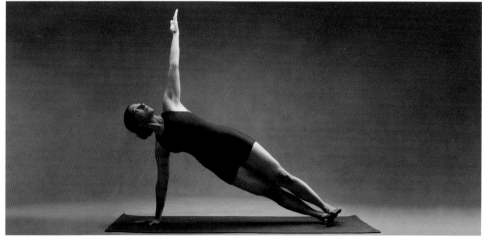

19. VASHISTASANA

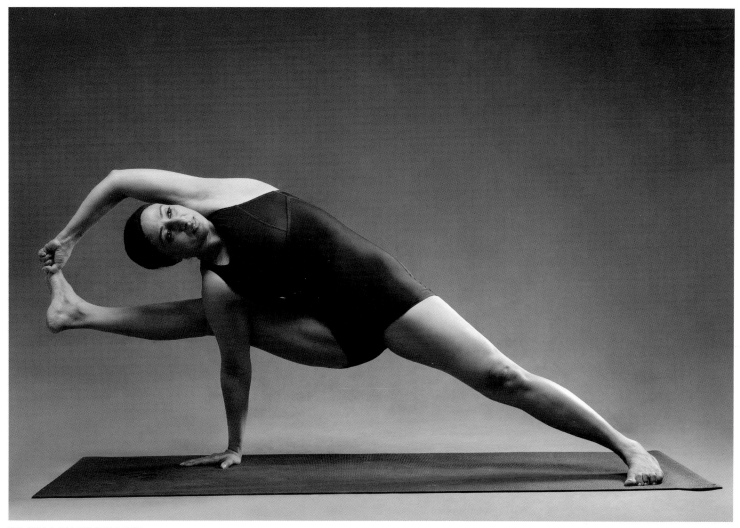

20. KALA BHAIRAVASANA

FLOOR ASANA SEQUENCE

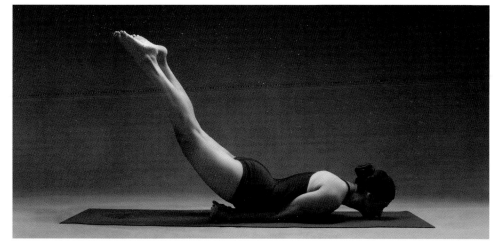

5. SHALABHASANA

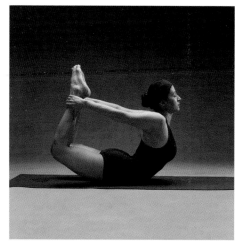

6. DHANURASANA
Follow with relaxing the back. Lie with chest down and move feet up and down with bent knees.

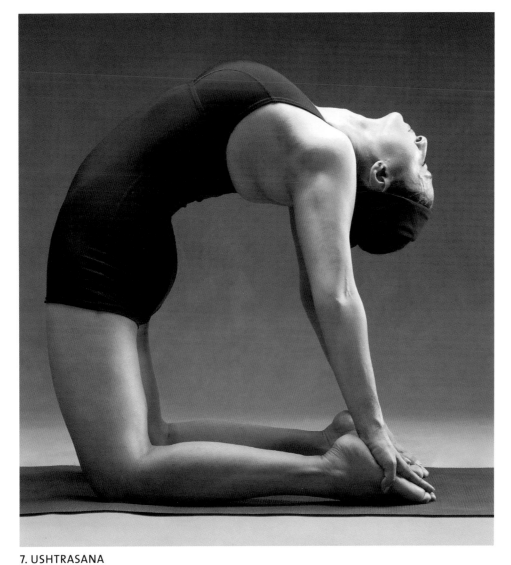

7. USHTRASANA

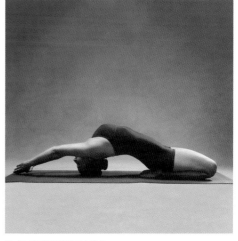

8. VAJRASANA

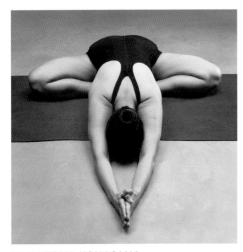

9. PARYANKASANA

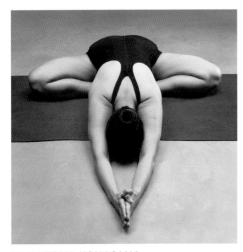

10. BADDHA KONASANA

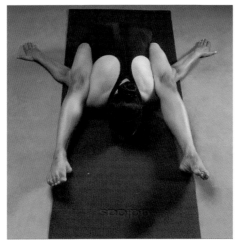

11. KURMASANA

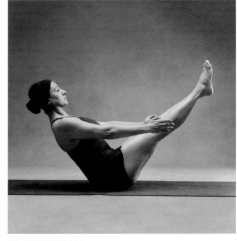

12. NAVASANA

COOLING DOWN

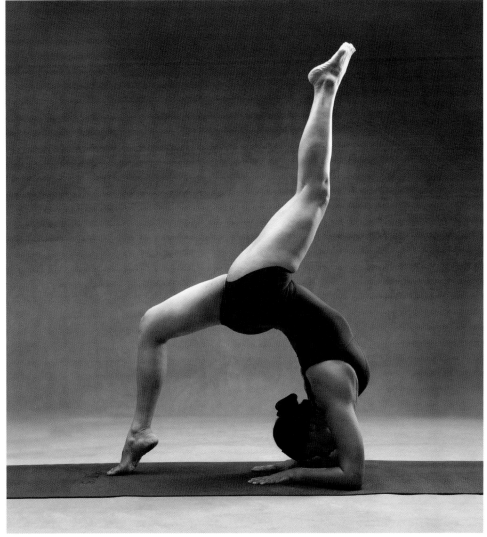

5. CHAKRASANA 2
Also called Eka Pada Viparita Dandasana

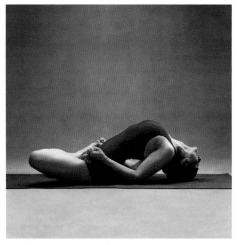

6. MATSYASANA

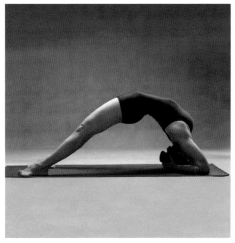

7. VIPARITA DANDASANA
Featured asana

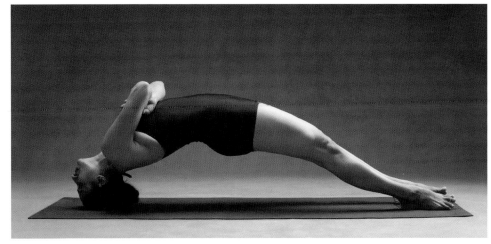

8. MATSYASANA 2

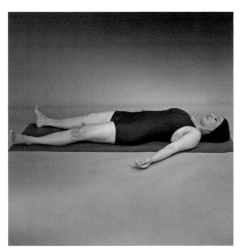

9. SHAVASANA
5 min

DAILY PRACTICE SEQUENCE – MONDAY

WARM-UP ROUTINE

Perform soft rhythmic jumps 50 times.

Swing the arms forward and backward powerfully 10 times.

Circle the shoulders forward and backward 10 times.

Twist the waist with arms open and stretched 5 times each side.

Gently circle the knees, left & right sides, 5 times each.

Circle the ankles clockwise and anti-clockwise with the front sole pressed to the ground and heel raised 5 times each.

PRANAYAMA ROUTINE

Sit in a comfortable, relaxed position. Calm your mind and observe your thoughts.

Perform Ujjayee for 5 minutes.

Perform Ujjayee with Antara Kumbhaka (holding breath after inhaling) for 5 minutes.

Perform Anuloma Viloma for 5 minutes.

Perform Anuloma Viloma with Antara Kumbhaka (holding breath after inhaling) for 10 minutes.

STANDING-ASANAS ROUTINE

1. Tadasana
2. Urdhva Tadasana
3. Vrikshasana
4. Santulanasana
5. Padangustasana
6. Surya Namaskara: Alternate between A & B – 5 times each.
7. Trikonasana
8. Parivrtta Trikonasana
9. Parsvakonasana
10. Parivrtta Parsvakonasana
11. Parsvottanasana
12. Prasarita Padottanasana
13. Utthita Hasta Padangustasana
14. Ardha Baddha Padmottanasana
15. Vatayanasana
16. Veerabhadrasana 3
17. Utkatasana
18. Natarajasana
19. Chakrasana 1
20. Pada Hastasana 1 – Featured Asana

FLOOR-ASANAS ROUTINE

1. Chaduranga Dandasana
2. Urdhva Mukha Svanasana
3. Adho Mukha Svanasana
4. Adho Mukha Shavasana
5. Shalabhasana
6. Urdhva Shalabhasana
7. Dhanurasana 2
8. Dhanurasana 3: Follow with relaxing the back. Lie with chest down and move feet up and down with bent knees.
9. Ushtrasana
10. Vajrasana
11. Supta Veerasana
12. Baddha Konasana
13. Kurmasana
14. Navasana
15. Ubhaya Paschimottanasana
16. Gomukhasana
17. Garbha Pindasana

COOLING-DOWN ROUTINE

1. Suptha Padangustasana 1
2. Suptha Padangustasana 2
3. Supta Trivikramasana
4. Sarvangasana
5. Halasana
6. Setu Bandhasana
7. Urdhva Dhanurasana
8. Eka Pada Urdhva Dhanurasana
9. Matsyasana
10. Baddha Padmasana
11. Yoga Mudrasana
12. Shavasana – 5 min

Sit in Padmasana for a count of 5 breaths before leaving the mat.

IMPORTANT

Please make sure that all the asanas and Pranayama techniques have been taught to you by your yoga guru. A doctor's permission could be essential in some cases. Before starting on this sequence, it is imperative that the practitioner follows the Warm-up Exercises, Surya Namaskara (A&B) (Section B, Chapter 5) and Asanas (Section B, Chapters 3 & 4; Section C, Chapter 9).

Add Antara Kumbhaka to Anuloma Viloma in the Pranayam Routine.

The sequence prescribed is based on self-study and years of experience teaching various categories of students. The feedback from students who have benefited from these sequences inspired the author to document them. The symptoms of any discomfort have been observed, studied and discussed with friends who are doctors and psychotherapists.

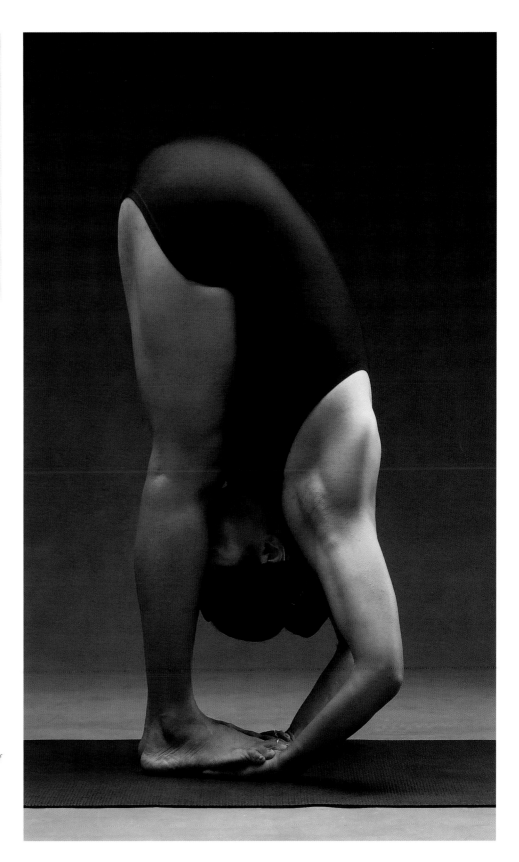

STANDING ASANA SEQUENCE

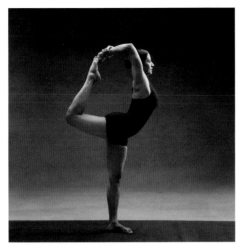

18. NATARAJASANA

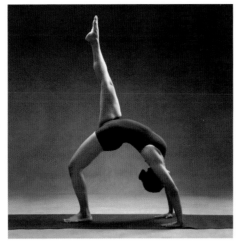

19. CHAKRASANA 1

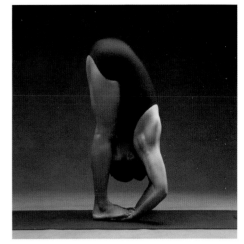

20. PADA HASTASANA 1
Featured aasana

FLOOR ASANA SEQUENCE

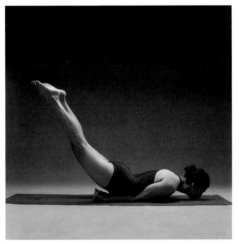

5. SHALABHASANA

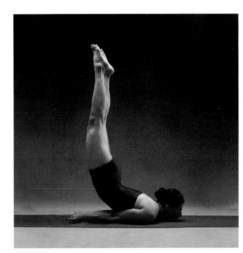

6. URDHVA SHALABHASANA

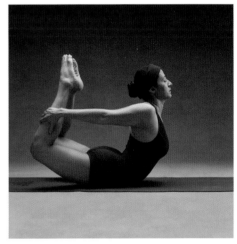

7. DHANURASANA 2

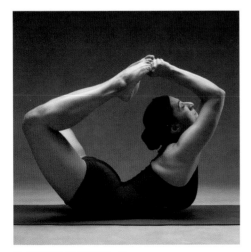

8. DHANURASANA 3
*Follow with relaxing the back. Lie with chest down
and move feet up and down with bent knees.*

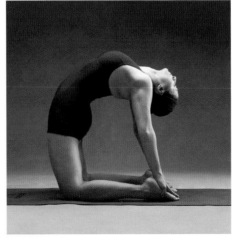

9. USHTRASANA

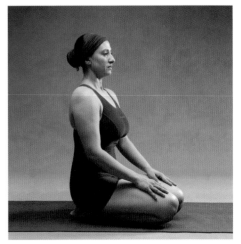

10. VAJRASANA

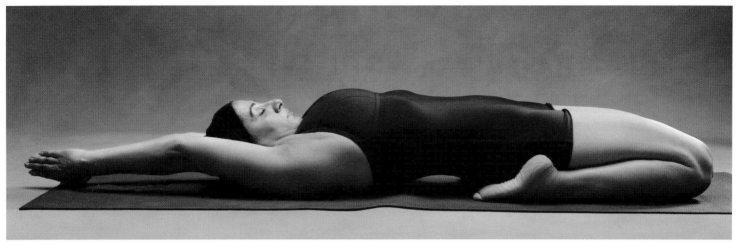

11. SUPTA VEERASANA

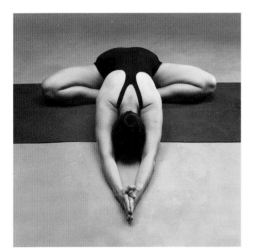

12. BADDHA KONASANA

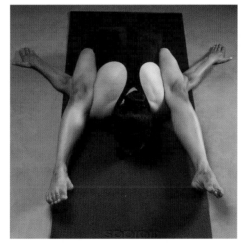

13. KURMASANA

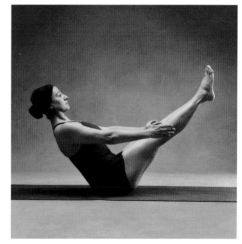

14. NAVASANA

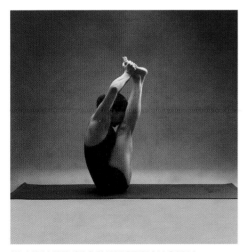

15. UBHAYA PASCHIMOTTANASANA

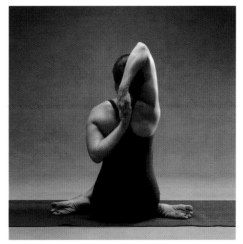

16. GOMUKHASANA

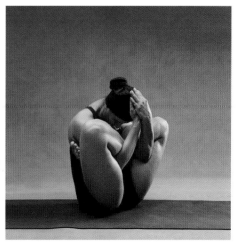

17. GARBHA PINDASANA

DAILY PRACTICE SEQUENCE – TUESDAY

WARM-UP ROUTINE

Perform soft rhythmic jumps 50 times.
Swing the arms forward and backward powerfully 10 times.
Circle the shoulders forward and backward 10 times.
Twist the waist with arms open and stretched 5 times each side.
Gently circle the knees, left & right sides, 5 times each.
Circle the ankles clockwise and anti-clockwise with the front sole pressed to the ground and heel raised 5 times each.

PRANAYAMA ROUTINE

Sit in a comfortable, relaxed position. Calm your mind and observe your thoughts.
Perform Ujjayee for 5 minutes.
Perform Ujjayee with Antara Kumbhaka (holding breath after inhaling) for 5 minutes.
Perform Anuloma Viloma for 10 minutes.
Perform Brahmari 5 times. with adequate rest in between

STANDING-ASANAS ROUTINE

1.	Tadasana
2.	Urdhva Tadasana
3.	Vrikshasana
4.	Santulanasana
5.	Padangustasana
6.	Surya Namaskara: Alternate between A & B – 5 times each.
7.	Trikonasana
8.	Parivrtta Trikonasana
9.	Parsvakonasana
10.	Ardha Chandrasana
11.	Parivrtta Ardha Chandrasana
12.	Parsvottanasana
13.	Prasarita Padottanasana
14.	Utthita Hasta Padangustasana
15.	Ardha Baddha Padmottanasana
16.	Vatayanasana
17.	Veerabhadrasana 3
18.	Utkatasana
19.	Upadasana
20.	Bakasana
21.	Tittibasana
22.	Eka Pada Kapotasana – Featured Asana
23.	Hanumanasana
24.	Parivrtta Hanumanasana
25.	Vishwamitrasana

FLOOR-ASANAS ROUTINE

1.	Chaduranga Dandasana
2.	Urdhva Mukha Svanasana
3.	Adho Mukha Svanasana
4.	Adho Mukha Shavasana
5.	Paschimottanasana
6.	Purvottanasana
7.	Baddha Konasana
8.	Upavishtakonasana
9.	Gomukhasana
10.	Bhardwajasana
11.	Navasana
12.	Ubhaya Upavishtakonasana
13.	Roll backward to Urdhva Mukha Upavishtakonasana

COOLING-DOWN ROUTINE

1.	Sarvangasana
2.	Halasana
3.	Setu Bandhasana
4.	Urdhva Dhanurasana
5.	Matsyasana
6.	Baddha Padmasana
7.	Yoga Mudrasana
8.	Shavasana – 5 min
Sit in Padmasana for a count of 5 breaths before leaving the mat.	

IMPORTANT

Please make sure that all the asanas and Pranayama techniques have been taught to you by your yoga guru. A doctor's permission could be essential in some cases. Before starting on this sequence, it is imperative that the practitioner follows the Warm-up Exercises, Surya Namaskara (A&B) (Section B, Chapter 5) and Asanas (Section B, Chapters 3 & 4; Section C, Chapter 9).

Add Brahmari to the Pranayama Routine.

The sequence prescribed is based on self-study and years of experience teaching various categories of students. The feedback from students who have benefited from these sequences inspired the author to document them. The symptoms of any discomfort have been observed, studied and discussed with friends who are doctors and psychotherapists.

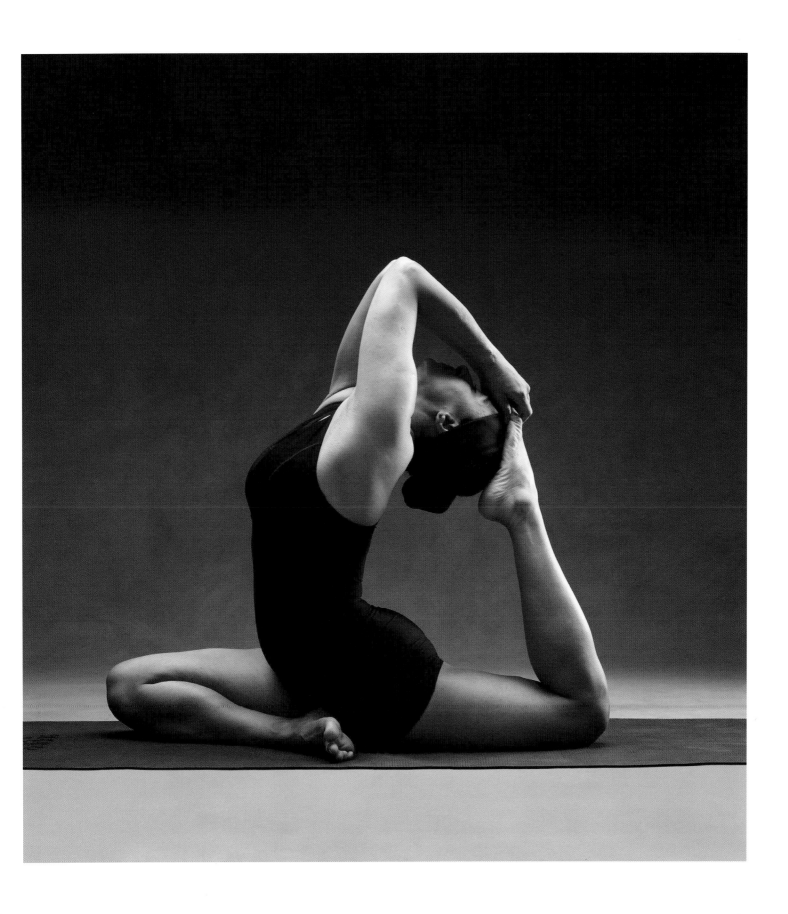

STANDING ASANA SEQUENCE

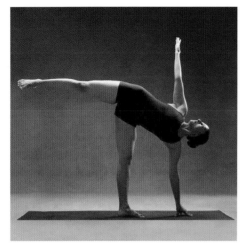

10. ARDHA CHANDRASANA

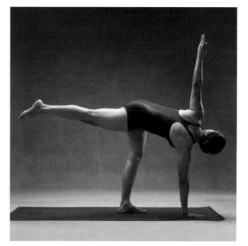

11. PARIVRTTA ARDHA CHANDRASANA

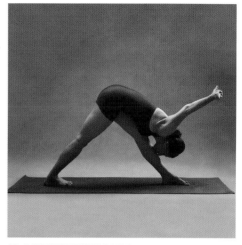

12. PARSVOTTANASANA

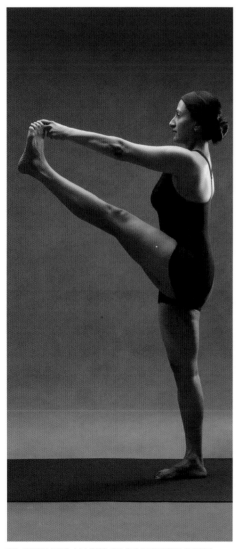

14. UTTHITA HASTA PADANGUSTASANA

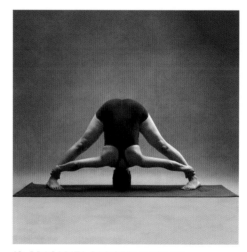

13. PRASARITA PADOTTANASANA

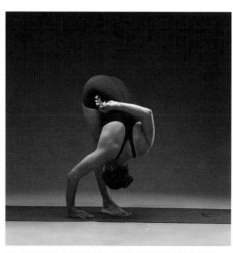

15. ARDHA BADDHA PADMOTTANASANA

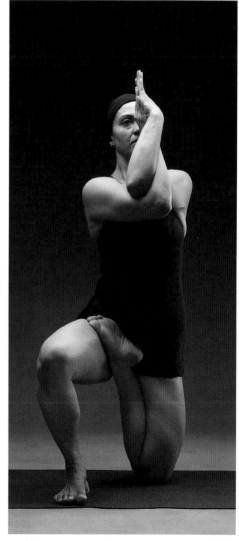

16. VATAYANASANA

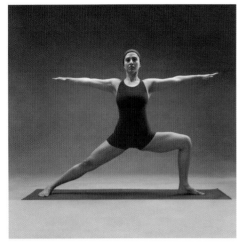

17. VEERABHADRASANA 3

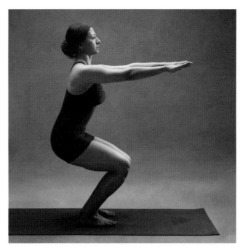

18. UTKATASANA

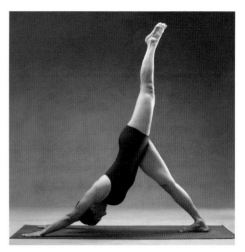

19. UPADASANA

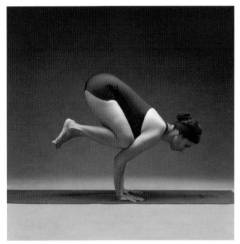

20. BAKASANA

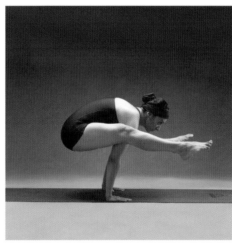

21. TITTIBASANA

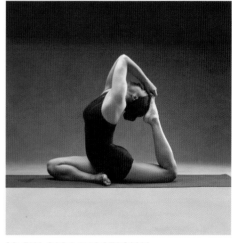

22. EKA PADA KAPOTASANA
Featured asana

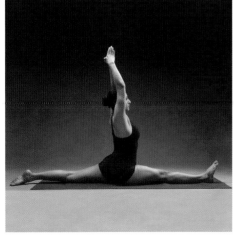

23. HANUMANASANA

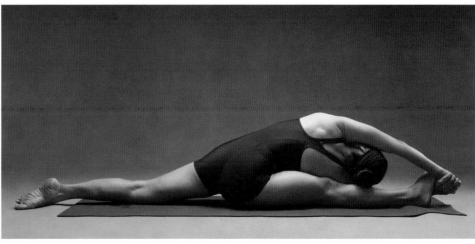

24. PARIVRTTA HANUMANASANA

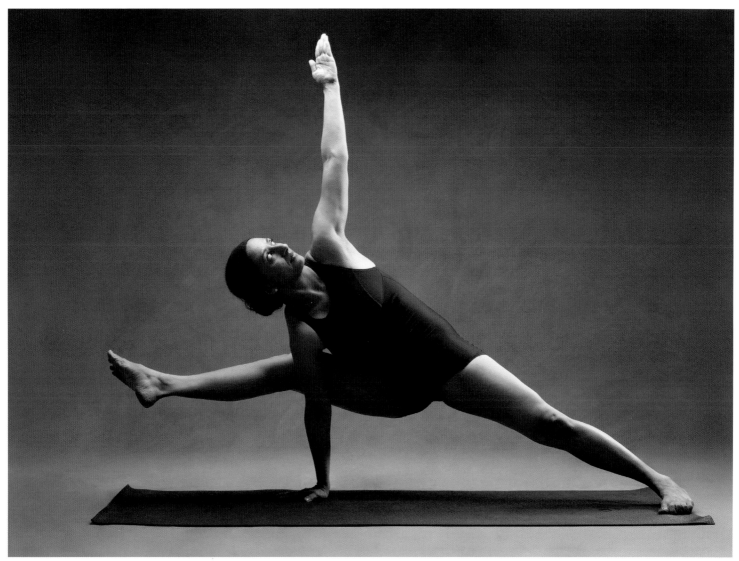

25. VISHWAMITRASANA

FLOOR ASANA SEQUENCE

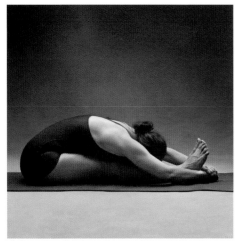

5. PASCHIMOTTANASANA

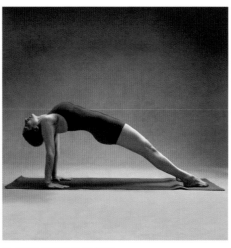

6. PURVOTTANASANA

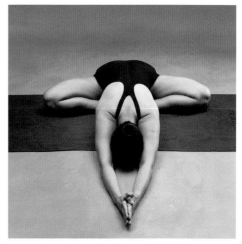

7. BADDHA KONASANA

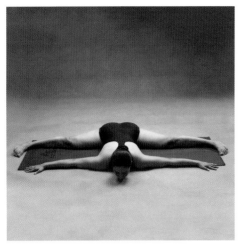

8. UPAVISHTAKONASANA

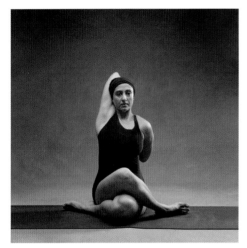

9. GOMUKHASANA

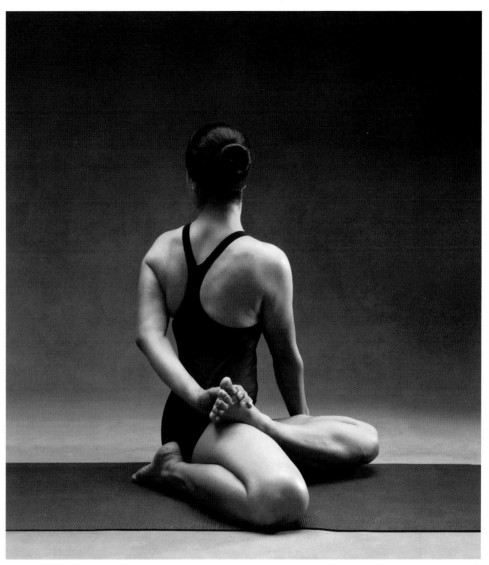

10. BHARADWAJASANA

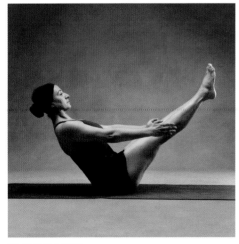

11. NAVASANA

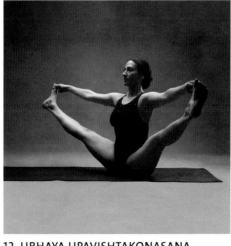

12. UBHAYA UPAVISHTAKONASANA

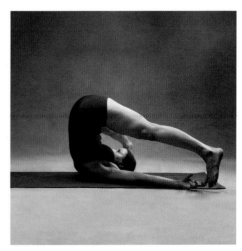

13. URDHVA MUKHA
UPAVISHTAKONASANA
Roll backward to this asana.

DAILY PRACTICE SEQUENCE – WEDNESDAY

WARM-UP ROUTINE

Perform soft rhythmic jumps 50 times.
Swing the arms forward and backward powerfully 10 times.
Circle the shoulders forward and backward 10 times.
Twist the waist with arms open and stretched 5 times each side.
Gently circle the knees, left & right sides, 5 times each.
Circle ankles clockwise and anti-clockwise with front sole pressed to the ground and heel raised – 5 times each

PRANAYAMA ROUTINE

Sit in a comfortable relaxed position. Calm your mind and observe your thoughts.
Perform Ujjayee for 5 minutes.
Perform Ujjayee with Antara Kumbhaka (holding breath after inhaling) for 5 minutes.
Perform Anuloma Viloma for 10 minutes.
Perform Kapalabhati – 300 blows – with adequate rest in between.

STANDING-ASANAS ROUTINE

1.	Tadasana
2.	Urdhva Tadasana
3.	Vrikshasana
4.	Santulanasana
5.	Padangustasana
6.	Upadasana
7.	Surya Namaskara: Alternate between A & B – 5 times each.
8.	Trikonasana
9.	Parivrtta Trikonasana
10.	Parsvakonasana
11.	Parivrtta Parsvakonasana
12.	Parsvottanasana
13.	Prasarita Padottanasana
14.	Utthita Hasta Padangustasana
15.	Ardha Baddha Padmottanasana
16.	Vatayanasana
17.	Trianga Mukhottasana
18.	Utkatasana
19.	Parivrtta Utkatasana
20.	Vashistasana 1
21.	Vashistasana 2
22.	Vishwamitrasana
23.	Kala Bhairavasana – Featured Asana

FLOOR-ASANAS ROUTINE

1.	Chaduranga Dandasana
2.	Urdhva Mukha Svanasana
3.	Adho Mukha Svanasana
4.	Adho Mukha Shavasana
5.	Shalabhasana
6.	Urdhva Shalabhasana
7.	Shayanasana
8.	Ananta Shayanasana
9.	Veerasana
10.	Supta Veerasana
11.	Ushtrasana
12.	Vajrasana
13.	Shirsasana
14.	Marichyasana 1
15.	Marichyasana 3
16.	Baddha Konasana
17.	Upavishtakonasana
18.	Navasana
19.	Ubhaya Upavishtakonasana
20.	Roll backward to Urdhva Mukha Upavishtakonasana.

COOLING-DOWN ROUTINE

1.	Sarvangasana
2.	Halasana
3.	Setu Bandhasana
4.	Urdhva Dhanurasana
5.	Matsyasana
6.	Baddha Padmasana
7.	Yoga Mudrasana
8.	Shavasana – 5 min
Sit in Padmasana for a count of 5 breaths before leaving the mat.	

IMPORTANT

Please make sure that all the asanas and Pranayama techniques have been taught to you by your yoga guru. A doctor's permission could be essential in some cases. Before starting on this sequence, it is imperative that the practitioner follows the Warm-up Exercises, Surya Namaskara (A&B) (Section B, Chapter 5) and Asanas (Section B, Chapters 3 & 4; Section C, Chapter 9).

Add Kapalabhati to the Pranayama Routine.

The sequence prescribed is based on self-study and years of experience teaching various categories of students. The feedback from students who have benefited from these sequences inspired the author to document them. The symptoms of any discomfort have been observed, studied and discussed with friends who are doctors and psychotherapists.

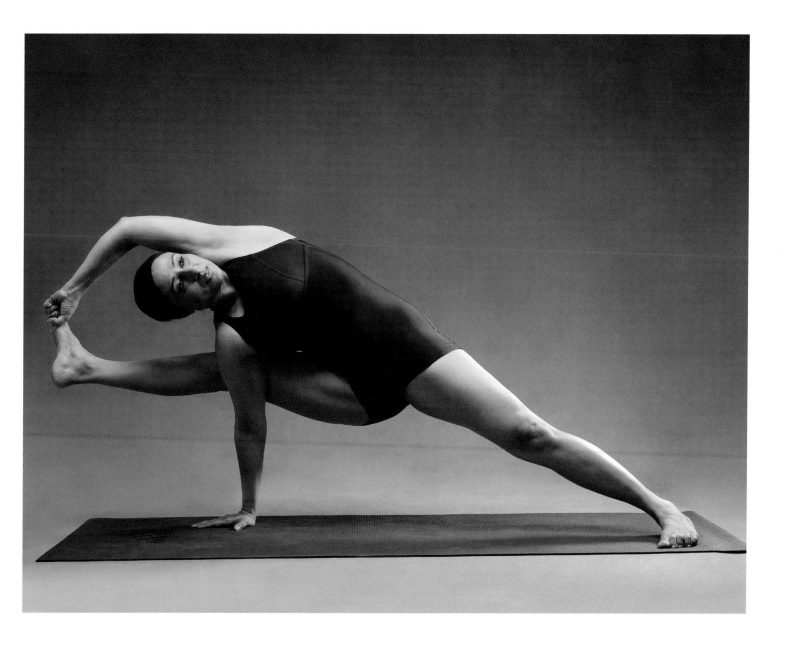

STANDING ASANA SEQUENCE

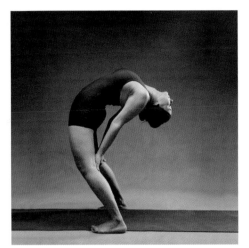

17. TRIANGA MUKHOTTASANA

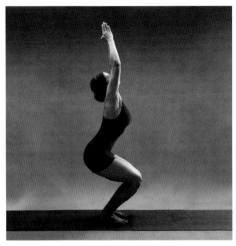

18. UTKATASANA

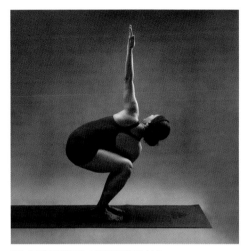

19. PARIVRTTA UTKATASANA

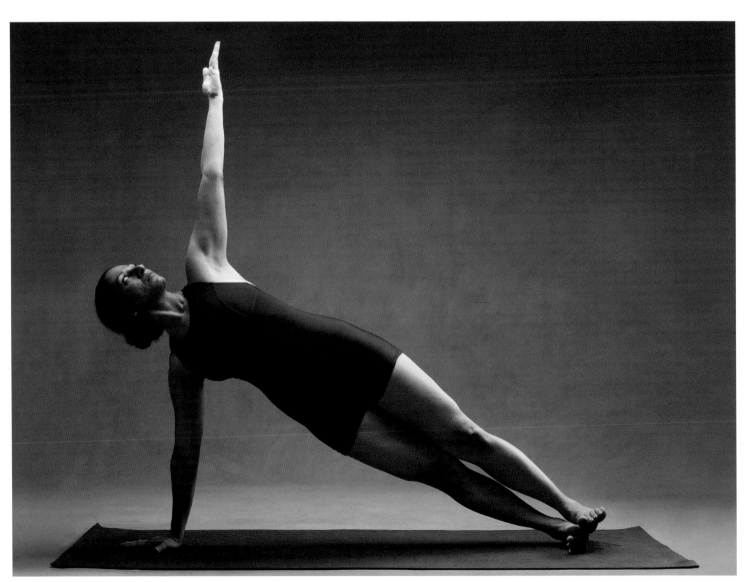

20. VASHISTASANA 1

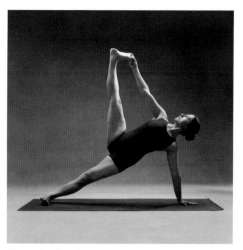

21. VASHISTASANA 2

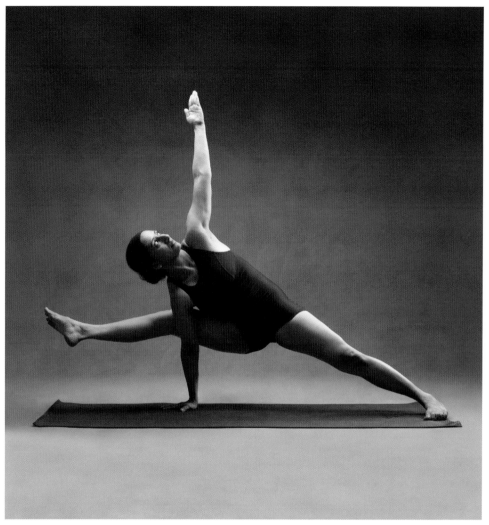

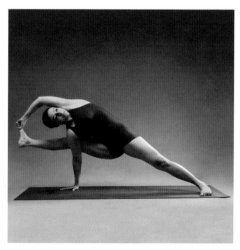

22. VISHWAMITRASANA

23. KALA BHAIRAVASANA
Featured asana

FLOOR ASANA SEQUENCE

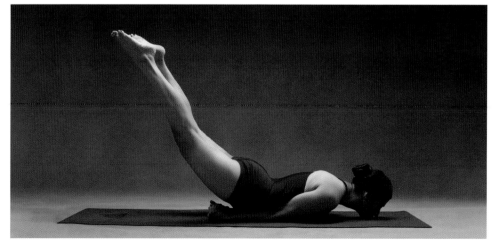

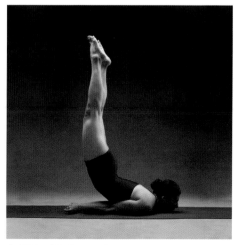

5. SHALABHASANA

6. URDHVA SHALABHASANA

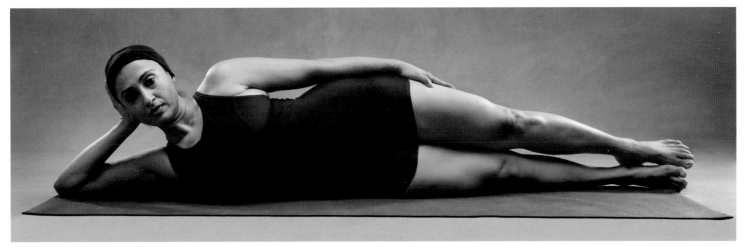

7. SHAYANASANA

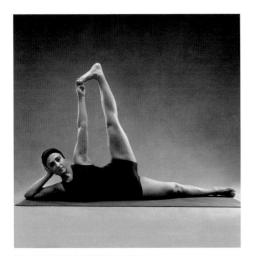

8. ANANTA SHAYANASANA

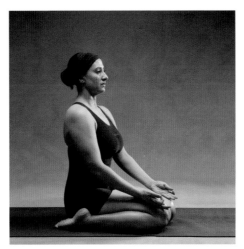

9. VEERASANA

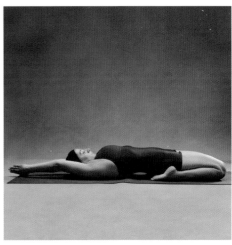

10. SUPTA VEERASANA

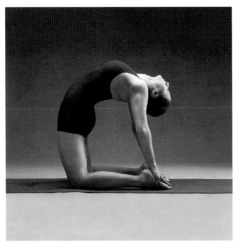

11. USHTRASANA

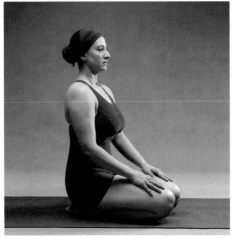

12. VAJRASANA

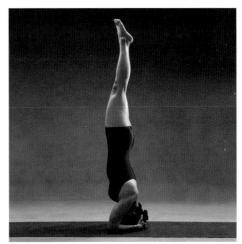

13. SHIRSASANA

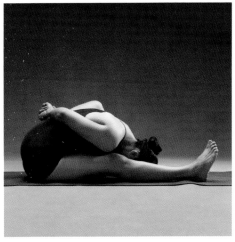

14. MARICHYASANA 1

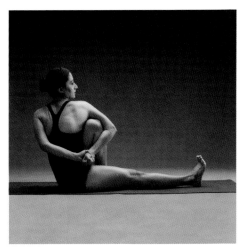

15. MARICHYASANA 3

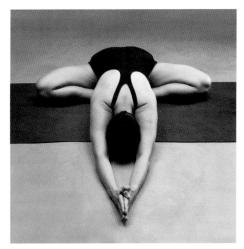

16. BADDHA KONASANA

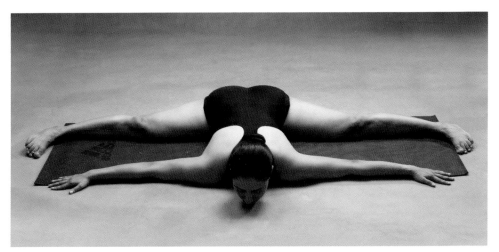

17. UPAVISHTAKONASANA

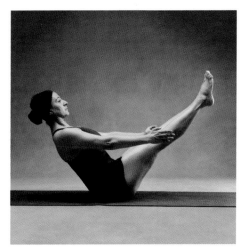

18. NAVASANA

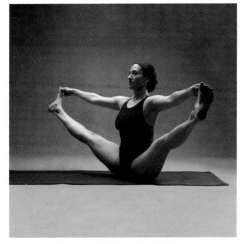

19. UBHAYA UPAVISHTAKONASANA

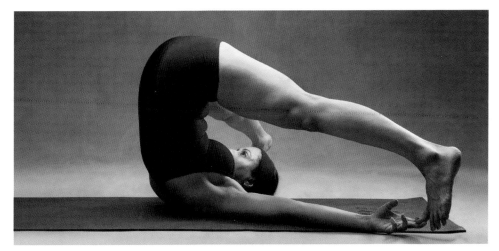

20. URDHVA MUKHA UPAVISHTAKONASANA
Roll backward to this asana.

DAILY PRACTICE SEQUENCE – THURSDAY

WARM-UP ROUTINE

Perform soft rhythmic jumps 50 times.

Swing the arms forward and backward powerfully 10 times.

Circle the shoulders forward and backward 10 times.

Twist the waist with arms open and stretched 5 times each side.

Gently circle the knees, left & right sides, 5 times each.

Circle the ankles clockwise and anti-clockwise with the front sole pressed to the ground and heel raised 5 times each.

PRANAYAMA ROUTINE

Sit in a comfortable relaxed position. Calm your mind and observe your thoughts.

Perform Ujjayee for 5 minutes.

Perform Ujjayee with Antara Kumbhaka (holding breath after inhaling) for 5 minutes.

Perform Anuloma Viloma for 10 minutes.

Perform Bhastrika – 50 blows – with adequate rest in between.

STANDING-ASANAS ROUTINE

1. Tadasana
2. Urdhva Tadasana
3. Vrikshasana
4. Santulanasana
5. Padangustasana
6. Surya Namaskara: Alternate between A & B – 5 times each.
7. Trikonasana
8. Parivrtta Trikonasana
9. Parsvakonasana
10. Parivrtta Parsvakonasana
11. Parsvottanasana
12. Prasarita Padottanasana
13. Utthita Hasta Padangustasana
14. Ardha Baddha Padmottanasana
15. Vatayanasana
16. Veerabhadrasana 5
17. Veerabhadrasana 6
18. Utkatasana
19. Chakrasana 1
20. Chakrasana 2
21. Pada Hastasana 2
22. Eka Pada Uttanasana

FLOOR-ASANAS ROUTINE

1. Chaduranga Dandasana
2. Urdhva Mukha Svanasana
3. Adho Mukha Svanasana
4. Adho Mukha Shavasana
5. Pashasana
6. Paschimottanasana
7. Purvottanasana – Featured Asana
8. Baddha Konasana
9. Gomukhasana
10. Vajrasana
11. Paryankasana
12. Ardha Matsyendrasana
13. Navasana
14. Ubhaya Paschimottanasana
15. Purvottanasana

COOLING-DOWN ROUTINE

1. Supta Padangustasana 1
2. Supta Padangustasana 2
3. Supta Padangustasana 3
4. Kapilasana
5. Sarvangasana
6. Halasana
7. Setu Bandhasana
8. Urdhva Dhanurasana
9. Matsyasana
10. Baddha Padmasana
11. Yoga Mudrasana
12. Shavasana – 5 min

Sit in Padmasana for a count of 5 breaths before leaving the mat.

IMPORTANT

Please make sure that all the asanas and Pranayama techniques have been taught to you by your yoga guru. A doctor's permission could be essential in some cases. Before starting on this sequence, it is imperative that the practitioner follows the Warm-up Exercises, Surya Namaskara (A&B) (Section B, Chapter 5) and Asanas (Section B, Chapters 3 & 4; Section C, Chapter 9).

Add Bhastrika to the Pranayama Routine.

The sequence prescribed is based on self-study and years of experience teaching various categories of students. The feedback from students who have benefited from these sequences inspired the author to document them. The symptoms of any discomfort have been observed, studied and discussed with friends who are doctors and psychotherapists.

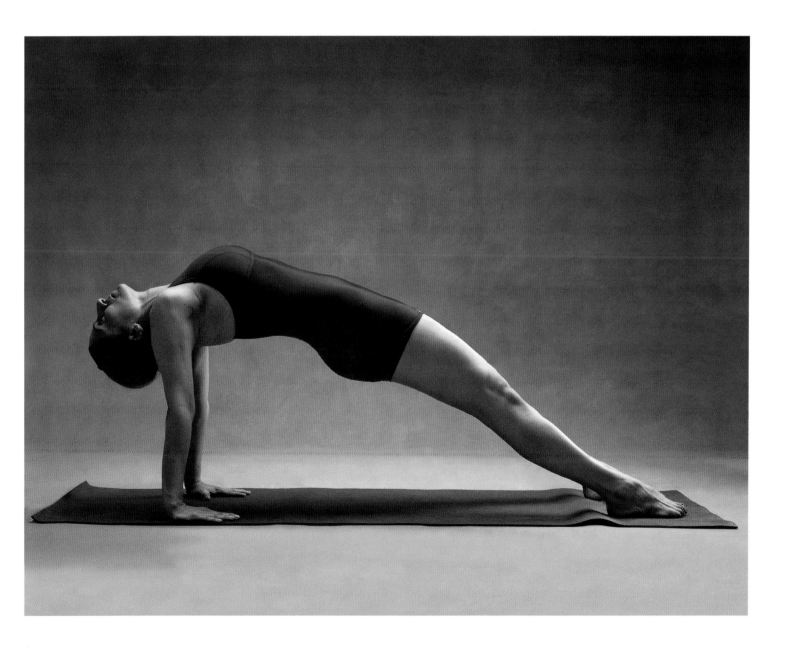

STANDING ASANA SEQUENCE

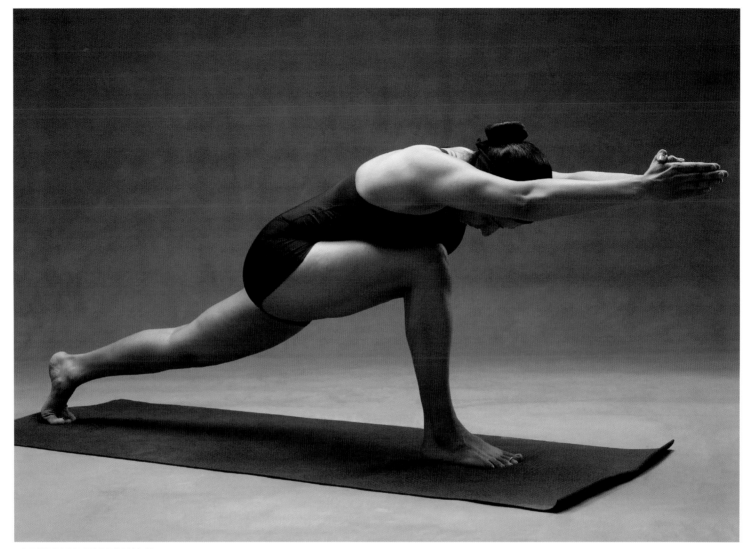

16. VEERABHADRASANA 5

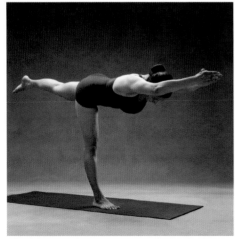

17. VEERABHADRASANA 6

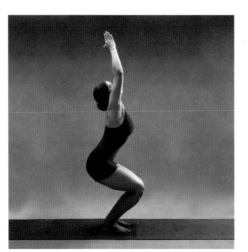

18. UTKATASANA

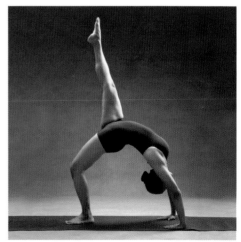

19. CHAKRASANA 1

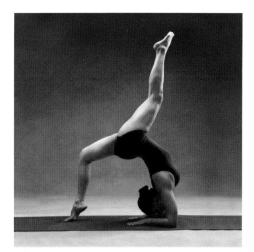

20. CHAKRASANA 2

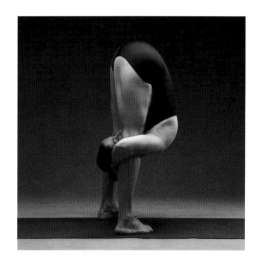

21. PADA HASTASANA 2

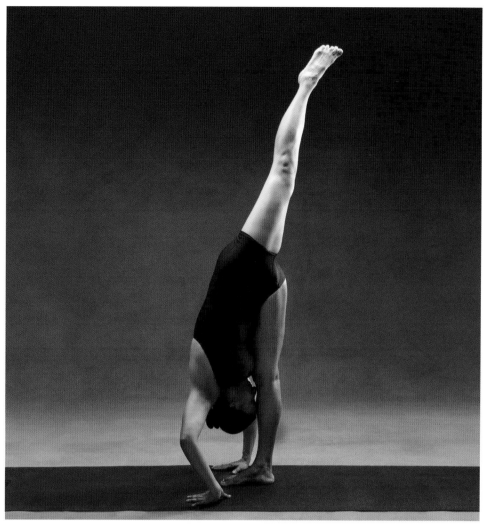

22. EKA PADA UTTANASANA

FLOOR ASANA SEQUENCE

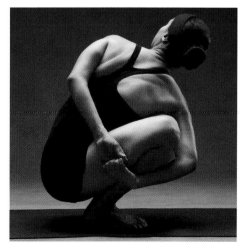

5. PASHASANA

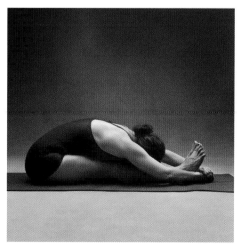

6. PASCHIMOTTANASANA

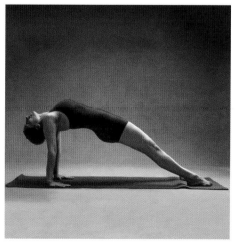

7. PURVOTTANASANA
Featured asana

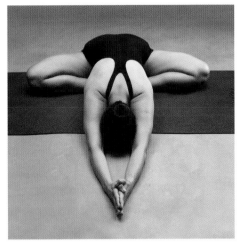

8. BADDHA KONASANA

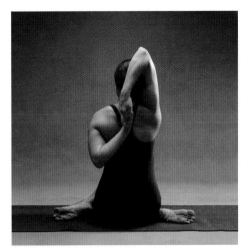

9. GOMUKHASANA

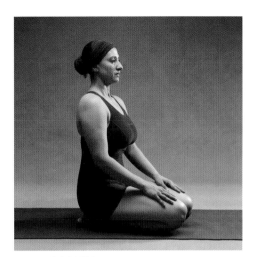

10. VAJRASANA

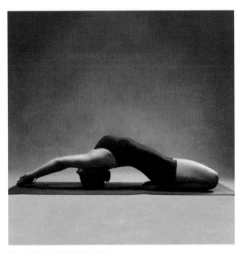

11. PARYANKASANA

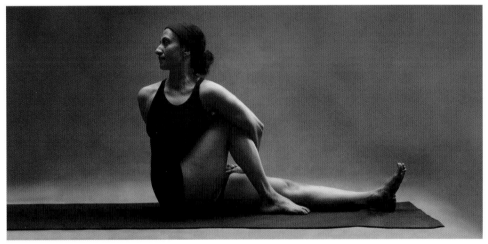

12. ARDHA MATSYENDRASANA

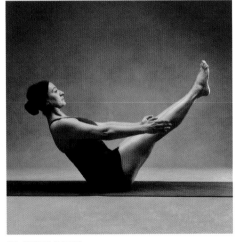

13. NAVASANA

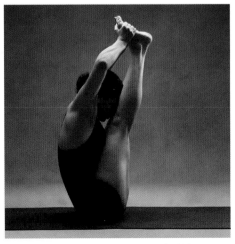

14. UBHAYA PASCHIMOTTANASANA

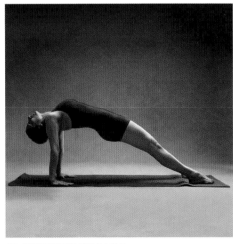

15. PURVOTTANASANA

COOLING DOWN

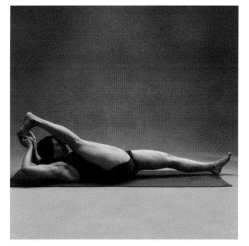

1. SUPTA PADANGUSTASANA 1

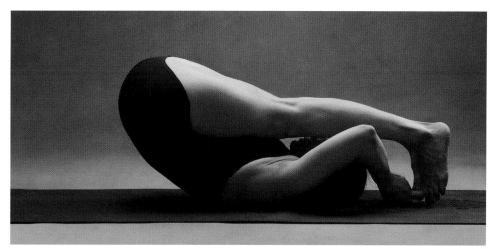

2. SUPTA PADANGUSTASANA 2

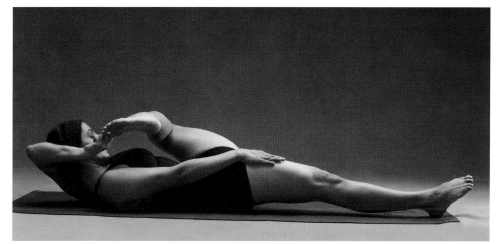

3. SUPTA PADANGUSTASANA 3

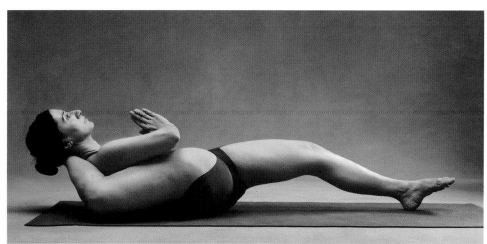

4. KAPILASANA

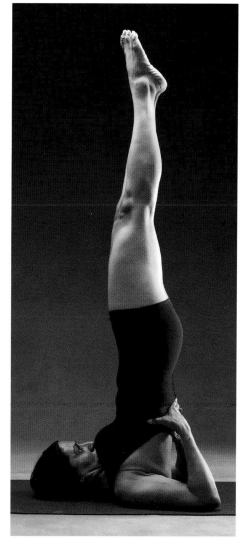

5. SARVANGASANA

DAILY PRACTICE SEQUENCE – FRIDAY

WARM-UP ROUTINE

Perform soft rhythmic jumps 50 times.

Swing the arms forward and backward powerfully 10 times.

Circle the shoulders forward and backward 10 times.

Twist the waist with arms open and stretched 5 times each side.

Gently circle the knees, left & right sides, 5 times each.

Circle the ankles clockwise and anti-clockwise with the front sole pressed to the ground and heel raised 5 times each.

PRANAYAMA ROUTINE

Sit in a comfortable, relaxed position. Calm your mind and observe your thoughts.

Perform Ujjayee for 5 minutes.

Perform Ujjayee with Antara Kumbhaka (holding breath after inhaling) for 5 minutes.

Perform Anuloma Viloma for 10 minutes.

Perform Omkara breathing 5-21 times.

STANDING-ASANAS ROUTINE

1. Tadasana
2. Urdhva Tadasana
3. Vrikshasana
4. Santulanasana
5. Padangustasana
6. Surya Namaskara: Alternate between A & B – 5 times each.
7. Trikonasana
8. Parivrtta Trikonasana
9. Parsvakonasana
10. Parivrtta Parsvakonasana
11. Ardha Chandrasana
12. Parsvottanasana
13. Prasarita Padottanasana
14. Utthita Hasta Padangustasana
15. Ardha Baddha Padmottanasana
16. Vatayanasana
17. Veerabhadrasana 3
18. Utkatasana
19. Bakasana
20. Eka Pada Bakasana
21. Dwi Pada Koundinyasana
22. Adho Mukha Tadasana
23. Pincha Mayurasana

FLOOR-ASANAS ROUTINE

1. Chaduranga Dandasana
2. Urdhva Mukha Svanasana
3. Adho Mukha Svanasana
4. Adho Mukha Shavasana
5. Shalabhasana
6. Dhanurasana: Follow with relaxing the back. Lie with chest down and move feet up and down with bent knees.
7. Ushtrasana
8. Kapotasana 1
9. Kapotasana 2
10. Vajrasana
11. Baddha Konasana
12. Ubhaya Paschimottanasana
13. Purvottanasana
14. Veerasana
15. Krounchasana
16. Akarna Dhanurasana – Featured Asana
17. Eka Pada Shirsasana
18. Chakorasana

COOLING-DOWN ROUTINE

1. Supta Padangustasana 1
2. Supta Padangustasana 2
3. Supta Trivikramasana
4. Yoga Nidrasana
5. Urdhva Mukha Paschimottanasana
6. Sarvangasana
7. Halasana
8. Setu Bandhasana
9. Urdhva Dhanurasana
10. Matsyasana
11. Baddha Padmasana
12. Yoga Mudrasana
13. Shavasana – 5 min

Sit in Padmasana for a count of 5 breaths before leaving the mat.

IMPORTANT

Please make sure that all the asanas and Pranayama techniques have been taught to you by your yoga guru. A doctor's permission could be essential in some cases. Before starting on this sequence, it is imperative that the practitioner follows the Warm-up Exercises, Surya Namaskara (A&B) (Section B, Chapter 5) and Asanas (Section B, Chapters 3 & 4; Section C, Chapter 9).

Add Omkara (Om chanting at every exhale, 5-21 times) to the Pranayama Routine.

The sequence prescribed is based on self-study and years of experience teaching various categories of students. The feedback from students who have benefited from these sequences inspired the author to document them. The symptoms of any discomfort have been observed, studied and discussed with friends who are doctors and psychotherapists.

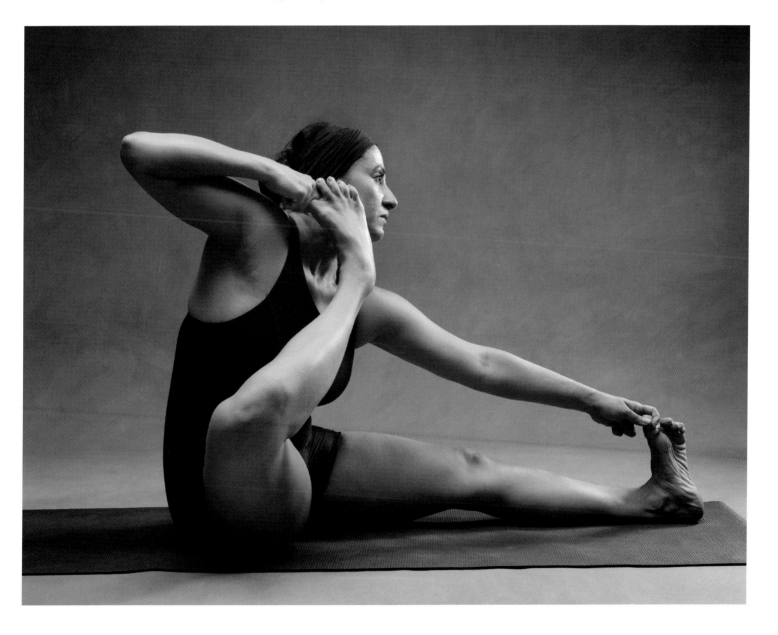

STANDING ASANA SEQUENCE

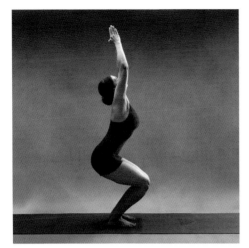

18. UTKATASANA

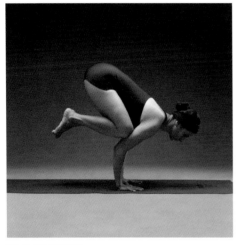

19. BAKASANA

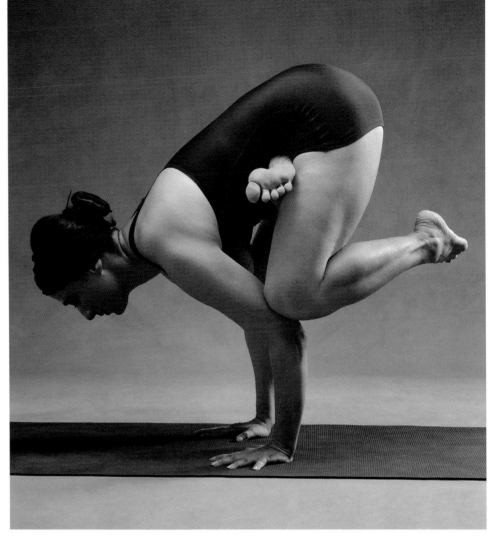

20. EKA PADA BAKASANA

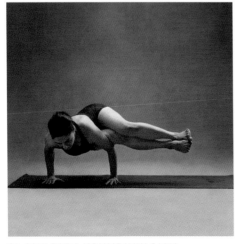

21. DWI PADA KOUNDINYASANA

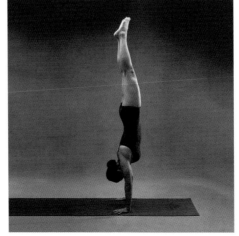

22. ADHO MUKHA TADASANA

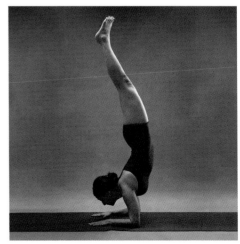

23. PINCHA MAYURASANA

FLOOR ASANA SEQUENCE

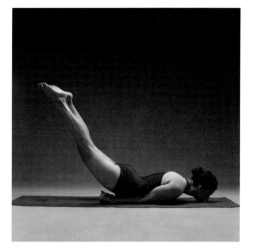

5. SHALABHASANA

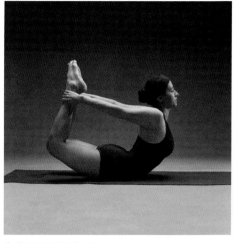

6. DHANURASANA
Follow with relaxing the back. Lie with chest down and move feet up and down with bent knees.

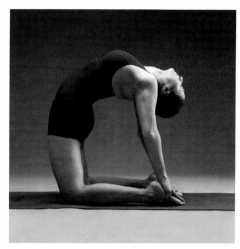

7. USHTRASANA

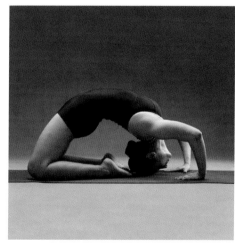

8. KAPOTASANA 1

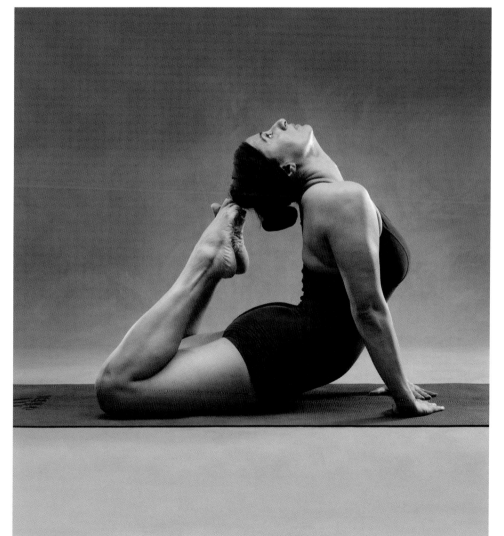

9. KAPOTASANA 2

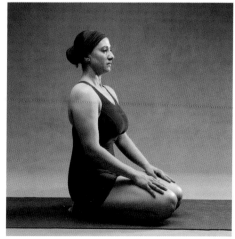

10. VAJRASANA

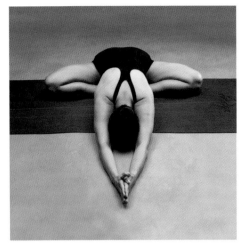

11. BADDHA KONASANA

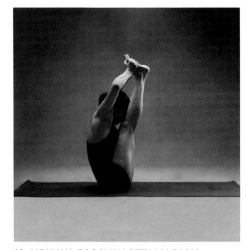

12. UBHAYA PASCHIMOTTANASANA

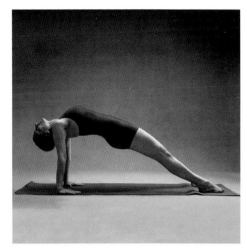

13. PURVOTTANASANA

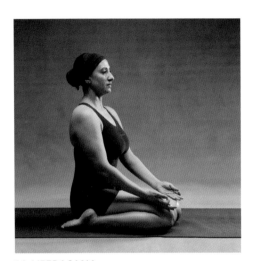

14. VEERASANA

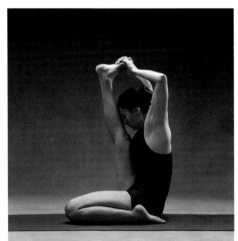

15. KROUNCHASANA

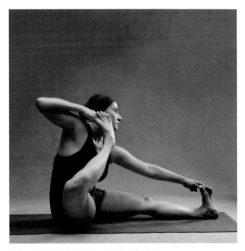

16. AKARNA DHANURASANA
Featured asana

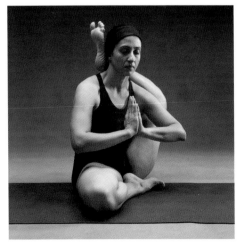

17. EKA PADA SHIRSASANA

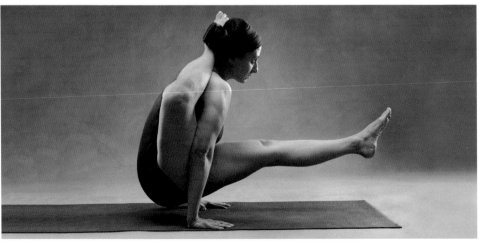

18. CHAKORASANA

COOLING DOWN

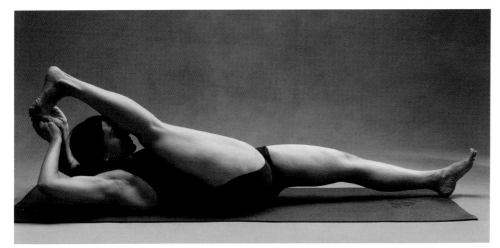

1. SUPTA PADANGUSTASANA 1

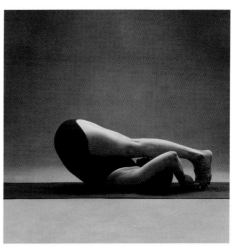

2. SUPTA PADANGUSTASANA 2

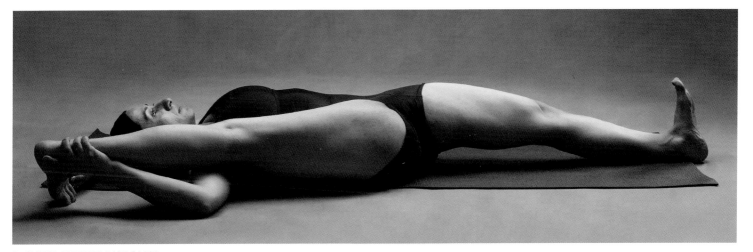

3. SUPTA TRIVIKRAMASANA

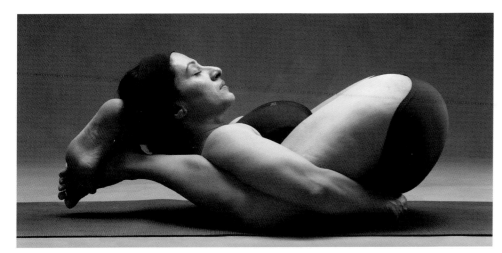

4. YOGA NIDRASANA

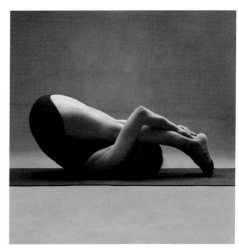

5. URDHVA MUKHA
PASCHIMOTTANASANA

DAILY PRACTICE SEQUENCE – SATURDAY

WARM-UP ROUTINE
Perform soft rhythmic jumps 50 times.
Swing the arms forward and backward powerfully 10 times.
Circle the shoulders forward and backward 10 times.
Twist the waist with arms open and stretched 5 times each side.
Gently circle the knees, left & right sides, 5 times each.
Circle the ankles clockwise and anti-clockwise with the front sole pressed to the ground and heel raised 5 times each.

PRANAYAMA ROUTINE
Sit in a comfortable, relaxed position. Calm your mind and observe your thoughts.
Perform Ujjayee for 5 minutes.
Perform Ujjayee with Anthar Khumbaka (holding breath after inhaling) for 5 minutes.
Perform Anuloma Viloma for 10 minutes.
Perform Shitali 5 times.

STANDING-ASANAS ROUTINE
1. Tadasana
2. Urdhva Tadasana
3. Vrikshasana
4. Santulanasana
5. Padangustasana
6. Surya Namaskara: Alternate between A & B – 5 times each.
7. Trikonasana
8. Parivrtta Trikonasana
9. Parsvakonasana
10. Parivrtta Parsvakonasana
11. Parsvottanasana
12. Prasarita Padottanasana
13. Utthita Hasta Padangustasana
14. Ardha Baddha Padmottanasana
15. Vatayanasana
16. Veerabhadrasana 1
17. Veerabhadrasana 2
18. Veerabhadrasana 3
19. Veerabhadrasana 4
20. Veerabhadrasana 5
21. Veerabhadrasana 6
22. Trivikramasana
23. Natarajasana
24. Ardha Chandra Natarajasana
25. Utkatasana

FLOOR-ASANAS ROUTINE
1. Chaduranga Dandasana
2. Urdhva Mukha Svanasana
3. Adho Mukha Svanasana 1
4. Adho Mukha Shavasana
5. Shalabhasana
6. Dhanurasana: Follow with relaxing the back. Lie with chest down and move feet up and down with bent knees.
7. Vajrasana
8. Supta Veerasana
9. Trianga Mukhapeeda Paschimottanasana
10. Ardha Baddha Paschimottanasana
11. Janu Shirsasana 1
12. Janu Shirsasana 2
13. Parivrtta Janu Shirsasana
14. Marichyasana 2
15. Marichyasana 4
16. Matsyendrasana – Featured Asana
17. Gomukhasana

COOLING-DOWN ROUTINE
1. Supta Padangusthasana 1
2. Supta Padangusthasana 2
3. Supta Trivikramasana
4. Sarvangasana
5. Halasana
6. Setu Bandhasana
7. Urdhva Dhanurasana
8. Matsyasana
9. Baddha Padmasana
10. Yoga Mudrasana
11. Shavasana – 5 min
Sit in Padmasana for a count of 5 breaths before leaving the mat.

IMPORTANT

Please make sure that all the asanas and Pranayama techniques have been taught to you by your yoga guru. A doctor's permission could be essential in some cases. Before starting on this sequence, it is imperative that the practitioner follows the Warm-up Exercises, Surya Namaskara (A&B) (Section B, Chapter 5) and Asanas (Section B, Chapters 3 & 4; Section C, Chapter 9).

Add Shitali to the Pranayama Routine.

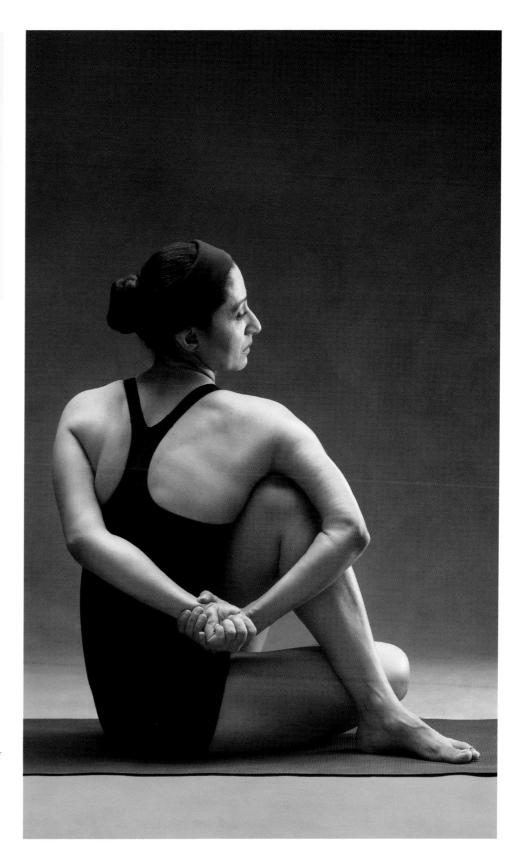

The sequence prescribed is based on self-study and years of experience teaching various categories of students. The feedback from students who have benefited from these sequences inspired the author to document them. The symptoms of any discomfort have been observed, studied and discussed with friends who are doctors and psychotherapists.

STANDING ASANA SEQUENCE

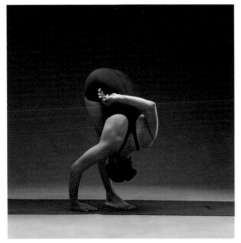

14. ARDHA BADDHA PADMOTTANASANA

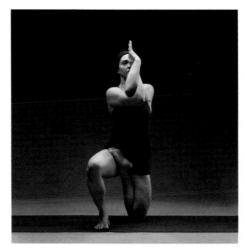

15. VATAYANASANA

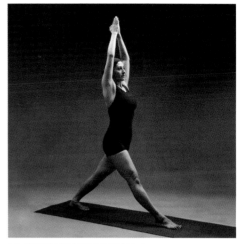

16. VEERABHADRASANA 1

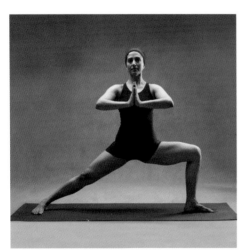

17. VEERABHADRASANA 2

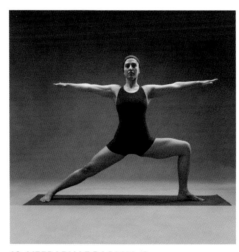

18. VEERABHADRASANA 3

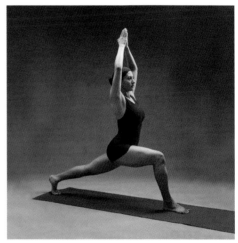

19. VEERABHADRASANA 4

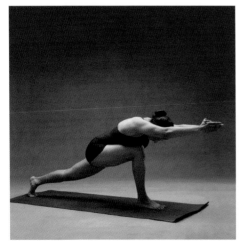

20. VEERABHADRASANA 5

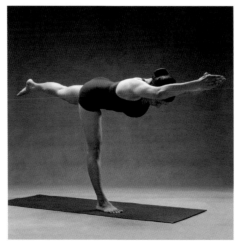

21. VEERABHADRASANA 6

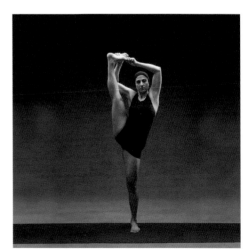

22. TRIVIKRAMASANA

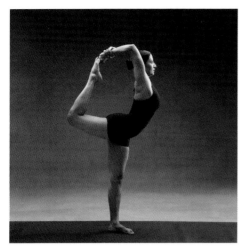

23. NATARAJASANA

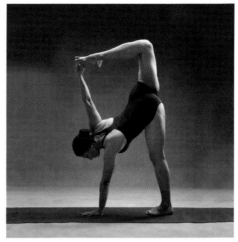

24. ARDHA CHANDRA NATARAJASANA

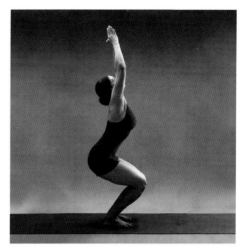

25. UTKATASANA

FLOOR ASANA SEQUENCE

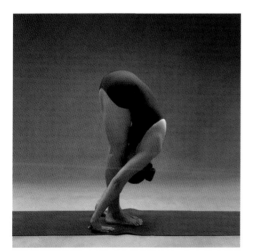

1. CHADURANGA DANDASANA

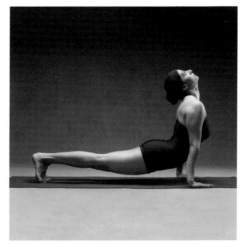

2. URDHVA MUKHA SVANASANA

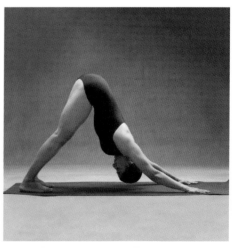

3. ADHO MUKHA SVANASANA 1

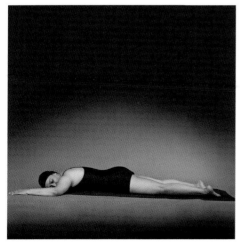

4. ADHO MUKHA SHAVASANA

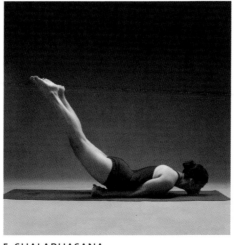

5. SHALABHASANA

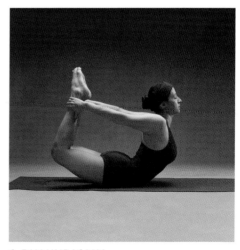

6. DHANURASANA
Follow with relaxing the back. Lie with chest down and move feet up and down with bent knees.

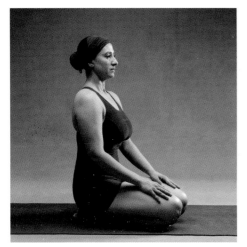

7. VAJRASANA

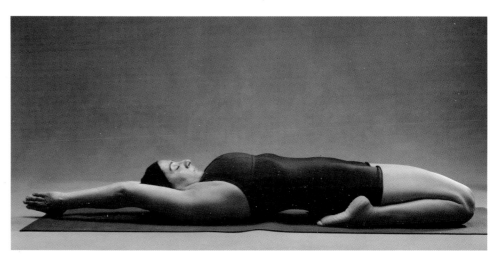

8. SUPTA VEERASANA

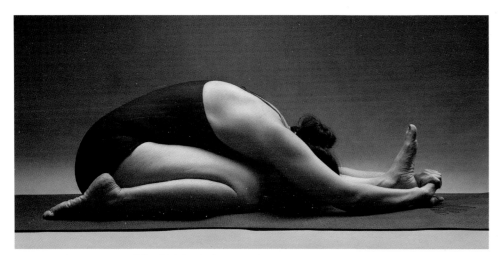

9. TRIANGA MUKHAPEEDA PASCHIMOTTANASANA

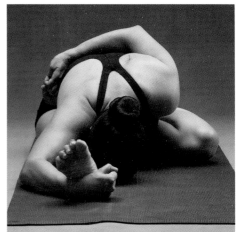

10. ARDHA PADMA PASCHIMOTTANASANA

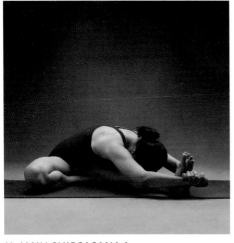

11. JANU SHIRSASANA 1

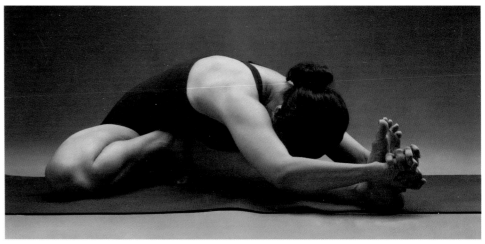

12. JANU SHIRSASANA 2

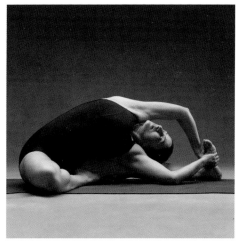

13. PARIVRTTA JANU SHIRSASANA

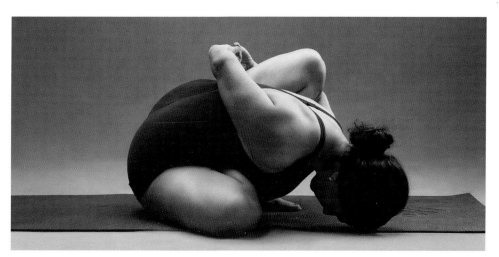

14. MARICHYASANA 2

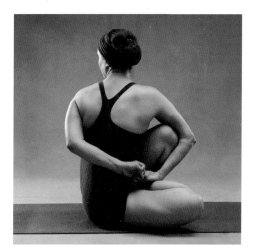

15. MARICHYASANA 4

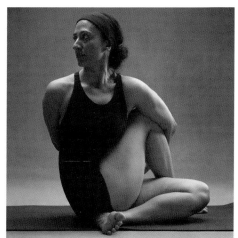

16. MATSYENDRASANA
Featured asana

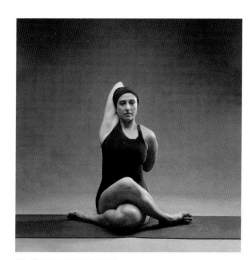

17. GOMUKHASANA

COOLING DOWN

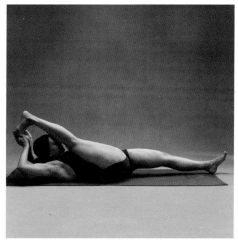

1. SUPTA PADANGUSTASANA 1

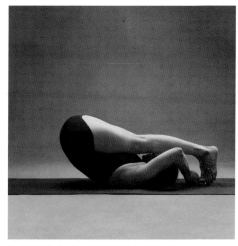

2. SUPTA PADANGUSTASANA 2

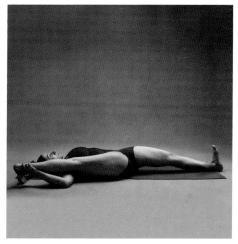

3. SUPTA TRIVIKRAMASANA

CHAPTER 7
SHAVASANA (SYSTEMIC RELAXATION)

- Lie down on the floor with the chest towards the ceiling. Release the tension from all the muscles of the body by blowing out strongly through the mouth. (like blowing out birthday candles).
- Take a few moments to settle down and allow the body to soften into the ground.
- Watch the breath and observe your heart rate settling down to a steady and rhythmic pace.
- Draw awareness to the crown, head, forehead, temples, eyebrows, eyelids, eyes, cheeks, jaws, mouth and chin.
- Rest attention on the nose and breathe normally (but at the same steady pace) 5 times.
- Now focus on the hollow of the throat, the back of the neck, shoulders, back of the shoulders, upper arm, centre of the shoulders, lower arms, wrists, hands and fingers. Make sure the wrists and the finger tips are facing the ceiling.
- Breathe 5 deep breaths (Ujjayee) and trace the flow of air from the nose to your fingertips.
- Continuing Ujjayee breathing, draw awareness to the chest, rib cage, abdomen, hips, buttocks, pelvic floor, upper legs, lower legs, feet and toes.
- Inhale visualising the breath flow down to the heart centre and exhale through the nostrils.
- Reverse the sequence by drawing awareness up the body, from the toes to the head. Be aware of breathing and relax into Shavasana.

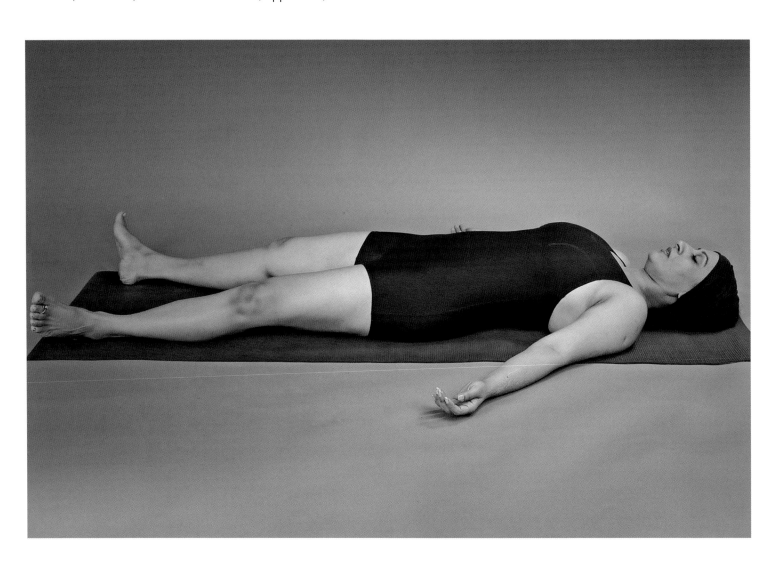

CAUTION

- Be careful when the mind wanders and you feel that you are falling asleep. Dring awareness back to the moment and flow into the sequence where you had stopped before your mind wandered.
- Remind yourself that you are determined to stay awake.
- Sometimes awareness is all it takes to reestablish the focus.

SIMPLE RELAXATION TIPS

Relaxation helps the body to deal with a chronic pain. Plonking on a sofa or watching television does not constitute relaxation. Systematic relaxation is a technique that should be done mindfully and sincerely.

- Lie on your back and settle the spine to a comfortable position. Place the hand and feet at a comfortable distance.
- Close your eyes with your mouth slightly open, focusing on relaxing the face.
- Pay complete attention to the breathing. Watch the movement of the diaphragm as it fills in and expels air. Studies note that this activates the parasympathetic nervous system which relaxes the body.
- Pay attention to the wandering mind and focus on drawing it back to observing the breathing.
- In a few minutes of settling down, the body will start to completely relax. Observe the body getting heavy and almost sinking to the ground.
- Maintain this state of rest for at least 5 minutes.
- Chanting 5 times the sound 'HAM' (activating mantra of Vishuddha or Throat Chakra) in this state will deepen the relaxation and calm the mind.

At the beginning of the practice of systematic relaxation, it is common to feel that the body is not relaxing. The reasons for this are circumstantial – overactive schedule, stale food, sedentary lifestyle, etc. A little planning and rescheduling the routine would give sufficient time to focus on the all-important relaxation.

EASY TECHNIQUES TO STABILISE THE MIND

- Focus on a single object of your liking. Select the object that calms your mind. It could be a lamp, a flower, a spiritual symbol, etc.
- Learn mantras from your guru and try chanting them.
- Visualise beautiful scenes from nature with eyes closed.
- Focus on deep breathing.
- Keep the mind alert during the above practice so as to deal with distractions without getting agitated or reactive.
- Work on handling distracting thoughts, images and emotions by drawing back focus to your breath or an object.
- Monitor the pattern of thoughts that are mostly disturbing.
- Listen to pleasant music and sounds, or a mantra that calms the mind.

CHAPTER 9
INDIVIDUAL ASANAS – BENEFITS AND PRACTICE TIPS

While step-by-step instructions for getting into an asana is beyond the scope of this book, the present chapter focuses on the finer aspects of each asana, provides tips on achieving proper alignment, indicates its benefits and also lists the precautions one has to take to avoid injuries. To understand how to do an asana, it is advisable to seek guidance from a qualified yoga guru.

1. ADHO MUKHA SVANASANA
DRISHTI – Nabigrai

TIPS
* Push the hip and the buttock bones up, high and backward. Press the heels down into the ground to establish this stretch.
* Release the shoulders wide by opening up the shoulder blades and pressing them inwards towards the back, while gently pressing the chest inwards towards the thighs.
* Keep the abdominal muscles drawn towards the spine and strengthen the hold with the Uddiyana Bandha.
* Keep your chin pointed towards the neck.

CAUTION
* If there is a problem of high blood pressure or frequent headaches, try to avoid this asana.
* If there is shoulder pain, do not rotate the shoulder into the body. Keep the arms straight and release tension in the area.
* This asana should not be practised during advanced stages of pregnancy.

BENEFITS
* Rushes blood circulation towards the head and rejuvenates the brain cells and invigorates the brain by relieving fatigue.
* Removes tiredness from the body and mind by stimulating the nerves.
* The chest region gets a rich supply of blood without any strain on the heart.
* Reduces stiffness in the shoulders and arms.
* Lengthens, strengthens and tones the legs and ankles.
* Relieves pain in the ankles.
* Prevents menstrual cramps and also hot flushes during menopause.

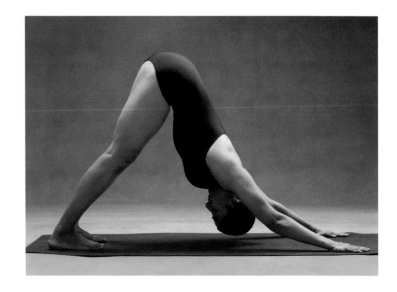

ENERGY FLOW
* The upward flow of the breath benefits all the chakras and conserves energy.

INDIVIDUAL ASANAS – BENEFITS AND PRACTICE TIPS 161

2. ADHO MUKHA SHAVASANA
DRISHTI – Nasagrai

TIPS

- Lie down on the floor with chest downwards facing the ground. Release the tension from all the muscles of the body by blowing out strongly through the mouth.
- Give a few moments to settle down and allow the body to feel like it is sinking into the ground.
- Watch the breath and observe your heart rate settling down to a steady and rhythmic pace.
- Work on a regular and steady Ujjayee breathing. At the same time, draw awareness to the chest, rib cage, abdomen, hips, buttocks, pelvic floor, upper legs, lower legs, feet and toes.
- Draw awareness to the crown, head, forehead, temples, eyebrows, eyelids, eyes, cheeks, jaws, mouth and chin.
- Rest attention on the nose and breathe normally (but with the same steady pace) 5 times.
- Now focus on the hollow of the throat, back of the neck, shoulders, back of the shoulders, upper arms, centre of the shoulders, lower arms, wrists, hands and fingers. Make sure the wrists and the finger tips fall softly on the floor.
- Take 5 deep breaths (Ujjayee).
- Inhale visualising the breath flowing deep into your chest and expanding against the floor and exhale through the nostrils.
- Watch the body settle down into the coolness of the floor while the back muscles gently rest into the rhythm of the breathing.

BENEFITS

- Relaxes the back completely.
- Settles the breathing rhythm to a very comfortable pace.
- The heart beating against the floor pumps in a good blood supply.
- Oxygenates and relaxes the chest.

CAUTION

- As the diaphragm is pressed against the floor in this asana, it could shorten breath.
- Do no attempt this asana if you are suffering from asthama or other respiratory disorders.
- Do not attempt this asana during pregnancy.
- Do not attempt this asana if you have chest congestion.

ENERGY FLOW

- All the chakras benefit from this asana. Energy flows downwards towards the ground, relaxing any stressed chakra.

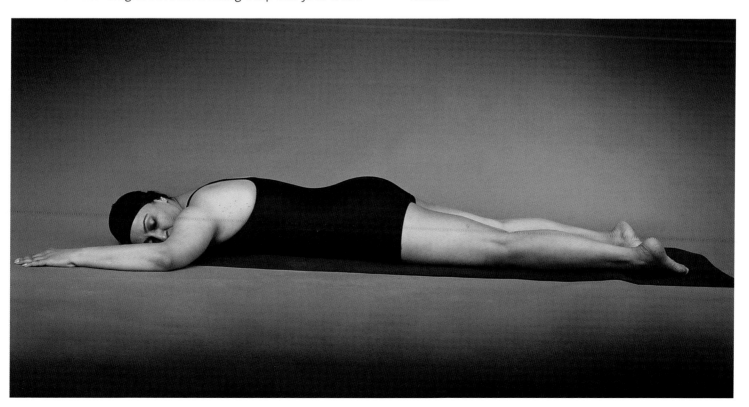

3. ADHO MUKHA TADASANA
DRISHTI – Bhoomigrai

TIPS
- When attempting this asana for the first time, place the palm a foot away from the wall so that when swinging the leg up, it would be against the wall.
- Do not keep the hands far away from the wall as during the swing, the back might curve, which will make you unstable.

BENEFITS
- All inverted asanas have similar benefits.
- In addition, this asana develops strength in the shoulders and back, as this asana demands core support.
- It improves focus and concentration.

CAUTION
- Attempt this asana after sufficient practice of inverted asanas such as Shirsasana.
- Take support of the wall in the initial stages of the practice.

ENERGY FLOW
- Same as in most inverted asanas.

NOTE
This challenging asana has lots of benefits but requires proper preparation. After adequate practice of all the basic asanas, the body gets tuned and ready for the Vishesha or extreme asanas. Master the Preceding and Succeeding asanas mentioned below before attempting this asana.

Preceding asanas
Surya Namaskara, Chaduranga Dandasana, Utkatasana, Bakasana.

Succeeding asanas
Paschimottanasana, Purvottansasana, Bharadwajasana, Sarvangasana, Halasana, Matsyasana.

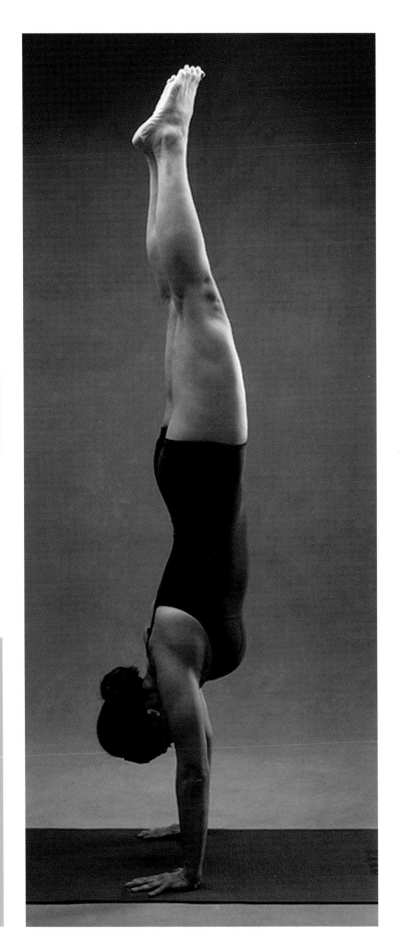

4. AKARNA DHANURASANA
DRISHTI – Sama

TIPS
- Reach forward and hold the toes with both hands.
- Exhale completely, deflating the stomach and hold your breath while pulling one toe towards the ear.
- Keep the shoulders strong and rotated backward.
- Open up the inner thighs and lift the chest up, with the head looking straight.

BENEFITS
- Helps align hip joints and rectifies minor deformities.
- Relaxes the lower back.
- The position contracts the abdominal muscles which further improves bowel movements.

CAUTION
- Keep the stretched leg pressed to the ground and do not let the hip tilt.
- Do the asana with complete awareness of the lower back and knees.

ENERGY FLOW
- Manipura Chakra and Svadhisthana Chakra are activated in this asana.

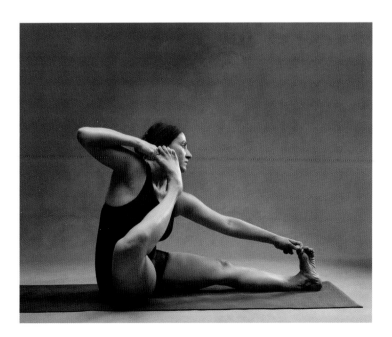

5. ANANTA SHAYANASANA
DRISHTI – Sama

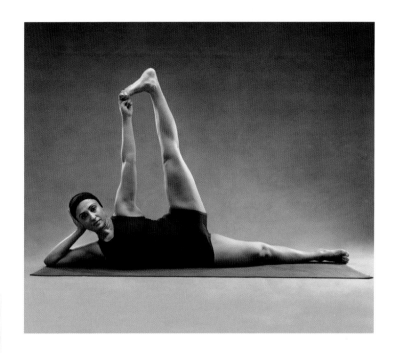

TIPS
- Lie face down on the floor. Stretch the entire length of the body with a forward movement before turning to the side.
- Carefully bend the knee and grab the toes. Extend the leg towards the ceiling until the leg is completely stretched upward.
- Constantly stabilise the hips by tucking the pelvis in and keeping the navel tucked in.

BENEFITS
- The stretch in the pelvic region relaxes the muscles of the area.
- The organs around the area get good blood supply, and thus benefit the reproductive and digestive organs.
- Relieves menstrual cramps and leg cramps.

CAUTION
- Do not attempt lifting the legs until the hip is well aligned and in balance.
- Once the legs are lifted, make sure the hip does not tilt.

ENERGY FLOW
- The Muladhara Chakra freely releases energy to other chakras, especially Svadhistana Chakra.

6. ARDHA PADMA PADANGUSTASANA
DRISHTI – Nasagrai

TIPS
- Exhale deep when bending forward.
- Pull the thigh muscles of your standing leg firmly upward.
- The sole of the standing foot should be spread strongly to the ground to create a firm foundation.

BENEFITS
- Cures stiffness of the knees.
- Pressing of the lower heel to the lower abdomen increases the peristaltic activity which helps to eliminate toxins and increases digestive powers.
- The binding of the arm increases the opening of the shoulders and further expands the chest, encouraging deep breathing.

CAUTION
- Do not attempt this asana if there is a spinal disc disorder, or if you feel dizzy or suffer from acidity.
- Keep the back concave throughout the asana and do not force the stretch, but wait for the stretch to progress.

ENERGY FLOW
- The heel pressing the lower abdomen, the seat of Muladhara Chakra, makes the energy flow to the other chakras powerful.

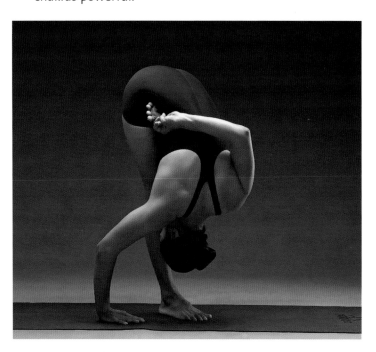

7. ARDHA PADMA PASCHIMOTTANASANA
DRISHTI – Bhoomigrai

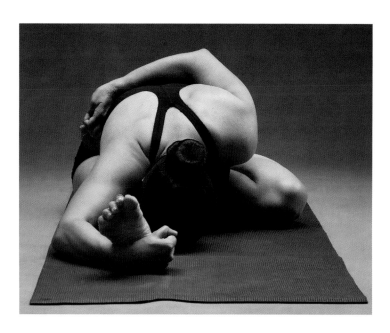

TIPS
- Keep the leg fully stretched throughout the asana.
- Exhale and widen elbows while leaning forward towards the length of the thigh.
- Keep the neck elongated and free. Do not allow the stretched foot to tilt.
- Focus on both sides of the torso being in line so that the back gets an even stretch.

BENEFITS
- Tones the liver, spleen, kidneys and aids digestion.
- Benefit people with an enlarged prostate.
- Relieves stiffness in the legs, knees, hip, pelvis and develops suppleness around these area.
- Eases the effects of stress on the heart and mind.

CAUTION
- Avoid rounding of the shoulders and back and keep the spine straight and erect.
- Do not allow the knees to tilt and keep them evenly stretched on both sides to avoid injury along the hamstrings.

ENERGY FLOW
- The Muladhara Chakra and Svadhisthana Chakra are energised in this asana.

8. ARDHA CHANDRA NATARAJASANA
DRISHTI – Padayoragrai

TIPS
* Same as Natarajasana.
* You can progress in the asana from the Ardha Chandrasana stretch.
* While bending forward, keep the knee of the standing leg slightly bent until the hand reaches the floor and then straighten the knee.

BENEFITS
* Same as Natarajasana.
* The vertebral joints get a rich supply of blood during downward the stretch.
* Forward bending of the asana intensifies the stretch even further into the hamstring and the back, increasing circulation and flexibility in the area.
* There is a huge supply of blood to the brain.
* Reduces physical exhaustion.
* Slows down the heartbeat.

CAUTION
* Keep the stretched leg pressed to the ground and do not let the hip tilt.
* Do the asana with complete awareness of the lower back and knees.

NOTE
This challenging asana has lots of benefits but requires proper preparation. After adequate practice of all the basic asanas, the body gets tuned and ready for the Vishesha or extreme asanas. Master the Preceding asanas and Succeeding asanas mentioned below before attempting this asana.

Preceding asanas
Uttitha Hasta Padangustasana Series, Ardha Chandrasana, Natarajasana, Ardha Chandra Natarajasana

Succeeding asanas
Ardha Badha Padangustasana, Utkatasana, Garudasana

ENERGY FLOW
* The forward tilt of the asana benefits all the chakras with a strong flow of prana.

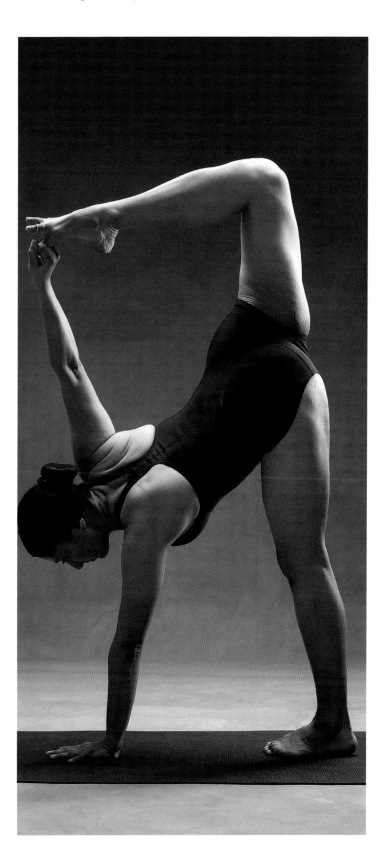

9. ARDHA CHANDRASANA
DRISHTI – Hastagrai

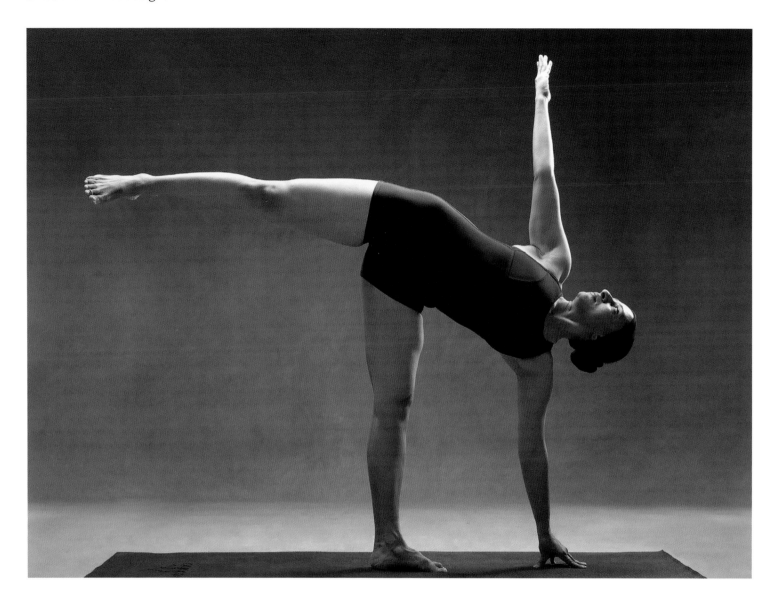

TIPS

- Ideally, start this asana as you would Parsvakonasana. However, if you find difficulty in straightening the knees, then tilt sideward from the standing position (Trikonasa).
- Place the hand opposite to the tilting side on the hip until you achieve balance.
- Keep the chest open and not tilted towards the floor.
- The weight of the body is borne by the grounded foot and hip. The other hand is only a support to control the balance.

BENEFITS

- Helps strengthen the legs.
- Tones lower regions of the spine and the nerves connected to it.
- Cures gastric troubles.

CAUTION

Do not attempt this asana if the knees are weak.

ENERGY FLOW

- The flow of energy of this asana is from the Muladhara Chakra into the two ends of the body, both towards the head, and the foot rooted to the floor.

10. BADDHA PADMASANA
DRISHTI – Nasagrai

TIPS
- Press the knees in towards each other and ensure the feet are sufficiently crossed on the thighs.
- Inhale deeply and expand the chest, feeling the shoulder blades drop into the body, while opening the entire area of the collarbones.
- Secure the hands in a tight grip.
- Lengthen the spine, adjusting the hip position by tucking the tail bone more towards the thigh and not towards the back.

BENEFITS
- Does not allow the spine to slop, which benefits the smooth flow of energy though the spine.
- Aids concentration and keep the mind alert and attentive.

CAUTION
- People who are not used to sitting on the floor might find this asana a little challenging on the knees.
- Try to practise Padmasana, sitting on a pillow for the first few times.
- Practise half Padmasana by placing one foot first, e.g. the right one on the root of the left foot and flap to loosen the knee and ankle. Repeat the same on the left. This exercise would help release the tightness in the knees.

- Keeps the length of the abdomen and the spine toned and healthy.
- Releases stiffness in the knees and the ankles.
- Benefits the entire lumbar regions.

ENERGY FLOW
- Activates all the chakras of the body.

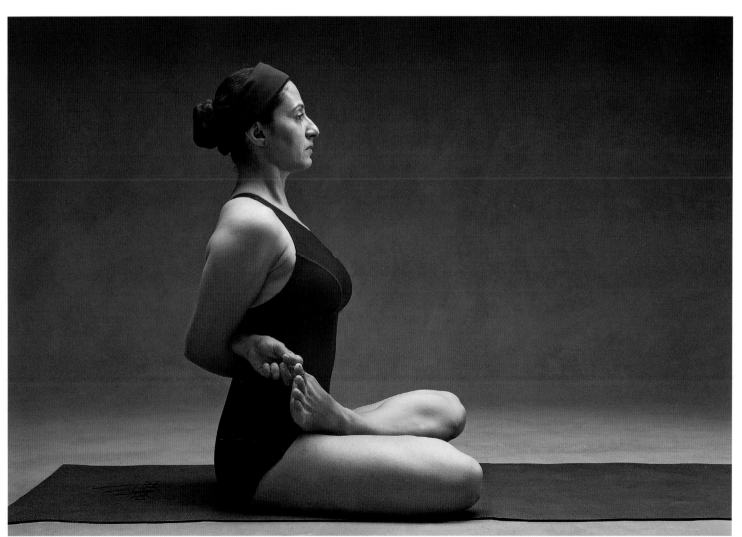

11. BADDHA KONASANA
DRISHTI – Nasagrai

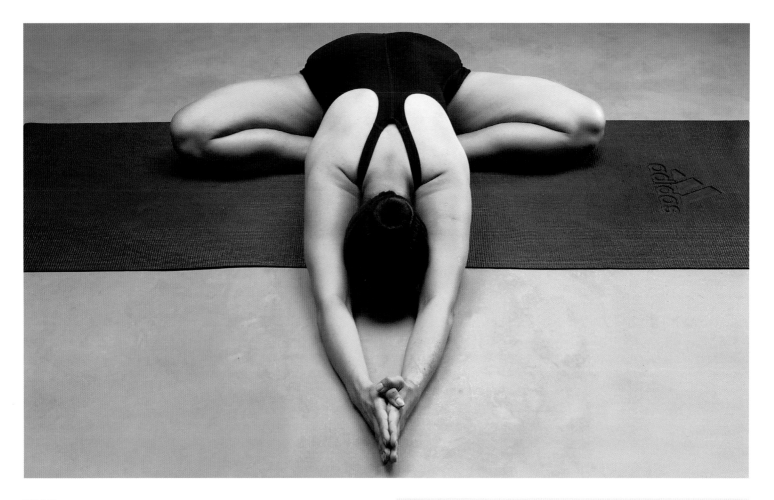

TIPS

- Make sure your sitting posture is correct with the back erect, chest up and the seat bones anchored firmly to the ground.
- Engage Uddiyana Bandha in this position.
- As you inhale, lengthen your spine.
- Try not to get into the asana in one go. Pause at every point of resistance and lengthen the back with every breath.
- Open up the inner length of the legs and keep the knees in line with each other. Try tucking the elbows into the inner thighs to gently put pressure on the legs to deepen the stretch.
- Reach forward by folding at your hip and adjust it, using small and gentle tilts to the left and right, to reach as far as possible.

BENEFITS

- Benefits the pelvic region and the length of the legs by improving blood circulation.

CAUTION

- Do not collapse the back at any point of time.
- Hold the shoulders wide and open.
- Breathe deep into the asana.
- Avoid bending forward during pregnancy.

- Rejuvenates the kidneys and keeps the prostate and the urinary bladder healthy.
- Regularizes menstrual flow and also stimulates the ovaries.
- Pregnant women can safely practise this asana as it helps pelvic flexibility and reduces chances of varicose veins.
- Relaxes a strained back.

ENERGY FLOW

- This position frees up energy from the Muladhara Chakra and rejuvenates the Svadhisthana Chakra.

12. BAKASANA
DRISHTI – Bhoomigrai

TIPS
- If it is uncomfortable to place the knees on the triceps, keep them placed by the sides of the upper arm, close to the arm pit.
- Do not lift the hip too high while trying to position the body.
- Keep the abdominal muscles contracted and maintain the length of the front of the body.
- Try to release the hunch in the back as you start lifting the toes above the ground.

BENEFITS
- Strengthens the arms and shoulders.
- Tones the abdominal muscles.
- Makes the intestines stronger and function better.

CAUTION
- Do not collapse the back at any point of time.
- Hold the shoulders wide and open.
- Breathe deep into the asana.

ENERGY FLOW
- This position frees up energy from the Muladhara Chakra and rejuvenates the Svadhisthana Chakra.

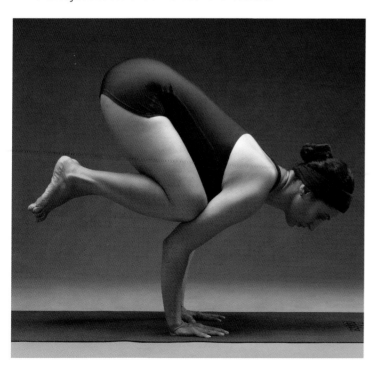

13. BEKASANA
DRISHTI – Sama

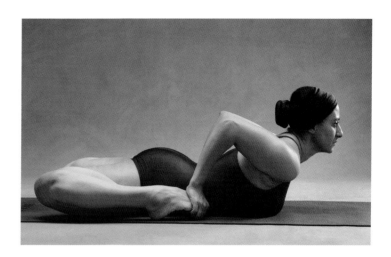

TIPS
- While lying face down, fold the knees and move the legs back and forth gently around 20 times to warm up the knees and to loosen them.
- Exhale and lift the trunk up from the floor and look up.
- Turn the hands so that it is easier to get hold of the upper part of the feet and pull the feet forward.
- Adjust or rotate the palms gently so that both toes and fingers point towards the head.
- The final pull of the feet towards the ground has to be done very progressively and not with a jerk.

BENEFITS
- The challenge imposed on the trunk and chest builds up strength in the respiratory region.
- Abdominal organs will benefit from the challenge.
- Knees and ankles will gain flexibility and strength.
- Relieves any rheumatic pain.
- Very beneficial to those who have flat feet.

CAUTION
- This asana has to be performed very carefully as it is a very intense stretch for the knees.
- Any indication of pain in the knees while preparing for the asana should not be ignored.

ENERGY FLOW
- This asana benefits the Svadhisthana Chakra and Muladhara Chakra.

14. BHARADWAJASANA
DRISHTI – Sama

TIPS
* Make sure your spine is erect. Ensure that your body does not lean back.
* Seat bones should be firmly on the ground.
* Keep the hip and the opposite shoulder in line while the torso should be kept erect.
* Keep both knees pressed to the ground. That helps to lengthen the spine.

BENEFITS
* Relieves pain in the back, shoulders and neck.

CAUTION
Do not attempt this asana if you have:
* Stress-related headache, migraine, eye-strain or high blood pressure.
* An upset stomach or are recovering from dysentery.

* Works on the dorsal and lumbar regions of the spine.
* Increases the flexibility of the shoulders and the hip.
* Expands the chest completely.

ENERGY FLOW
* The Manipura Chakra is highly energised along with Vishuddha Chakra and Ajna Chakra.

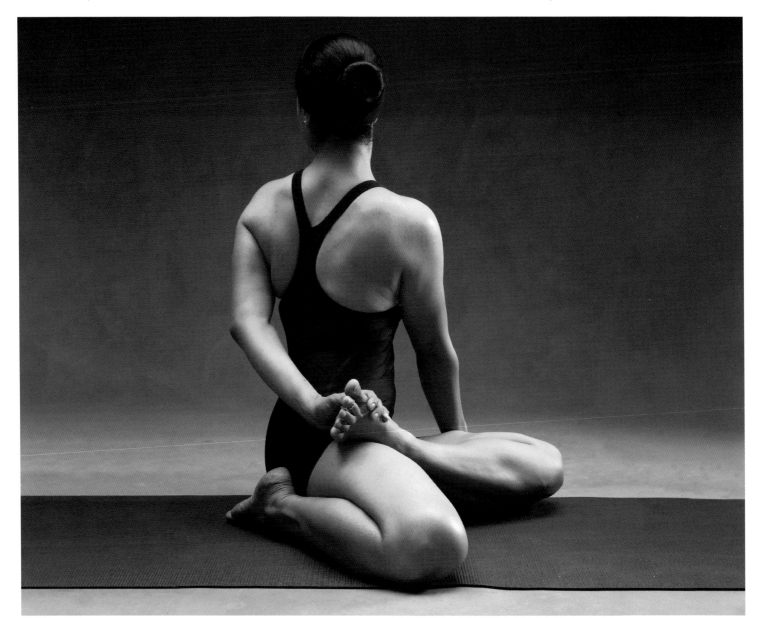

15. BHUJANGASANA
DRISHTI – Nasagrai

TIPS
- Lie down with chest facing the floor (Adho Mukha Shavasana).
- Exhale completely and gently lift up from the midriff, expanding the shoulders and chest.
- Lift the head up and look at the tip of your nose.
- Expand the collarbone and fold the hands backwards.
- Pin the hip bones to the ground and press the upper part of the feet to the floor.
- Stay in position and release tension before breathing.

BENEFITS
- Strengthens the lower back region along with the abdominal area.
- The complete expansion of the midriff builds strength around the chest.

CAUTION
- Do not use the neck instead of the midriff in the first stage of the asana, which is the lifting up of the chest.
- Do not keep the legs suspended while doing this asana.
- Breathing is challenging in this position, therefore, do not hold your breath at any point of the stretch and keep up a steady pace in the breathing (5 deep breaths would be ideal).

- Opened shoulders relax the neck, pectorals and the shoulders.
- Breathing in this asana strengthens the diaphragm.

ENERGY FLOW
- The chest and the abdominal region are activated in this asana which benefits the Muladhara Chakra , Svadhisthana Chakra and Anahata Chakra.

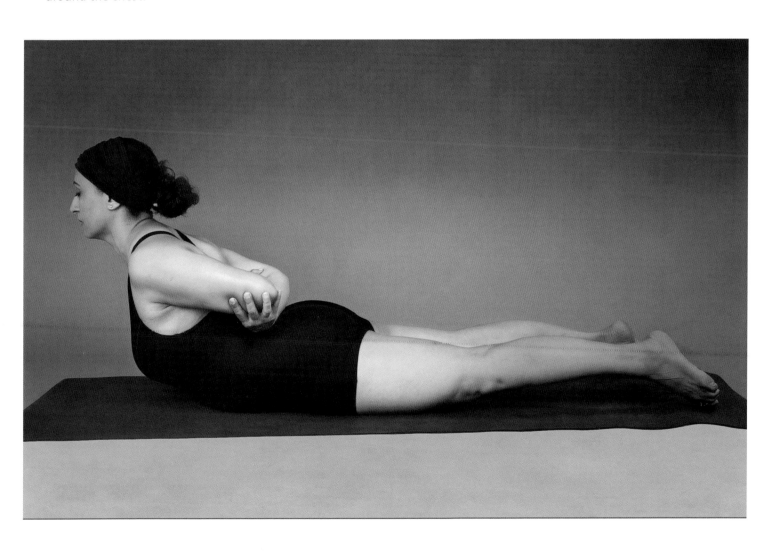

16. CHADURANGA DANDASANA
DRISHTI – Bhoomigrai

TIPS
- Hop backward into the asana to achieve a complete length of the body. If hopping is uncomfortable, stretch legs into its full length.
- Place the hands shoulder width apart to establish good shoulder support, open the fingers and press the palm to the floor.
- As the body is lowered to do the Chaduranga Dandasana, keep the elbows close to the ribs as if to support them to avoid collapsing.
- Keep the lower abdomen lifted off the floor as if to support the spine.
- Keep the thighs strong to avoid the hips collapsing.

BENEFITS
- Builds overall strength of the body.
- Helps strengthen arms, wrists and elbows.
- Aligns the spin and contracts the abdominal muscles.

ENERGY FLOW
- It energises the chakra power from the base of the spine to the head.

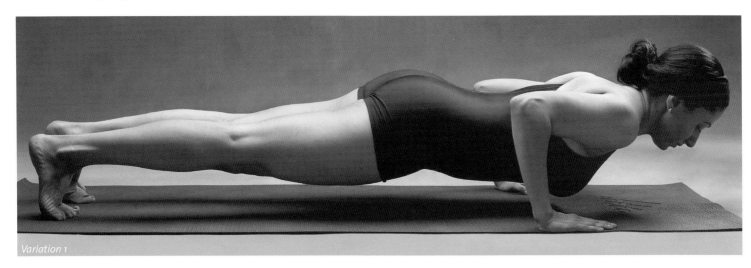

Variation 1

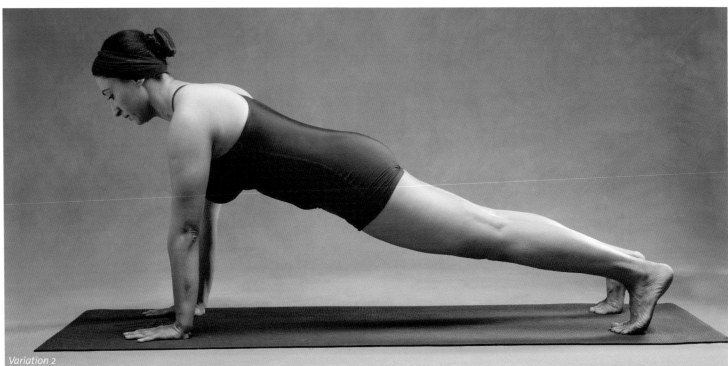

Variation 2

17. CHAKORASANA
DRISHTI – Sama

TIPS
- It would be easier to achieve this asana from the lying down position of Kapilasana and then pushing the body forward to a sitting posture.

NOTE
This challenging asana has lots of benefits but requires proper preparation. After adequate practice of all the basic asanas, the body gets tuned and ready for the Vishesha or extreme asanas. Master the Preceding asanas and Succeeding asanas mentioned below before attempting this asana.

Preceding asanas
Chaduranga Dandasana, Bakasana, Tittibasana, Navasana, Purvottanasana, Krounchasana, Eka Pada Shirsasana

Succeeding asanas
Pachimottanasana, Purvottanasana, Sarvangasana, Halasana, Matsyasana

- Raise the hip above the floor by keeping the palms for support by the sides.
- Keep the fingers open for greater grip of the floor, which would further strengthen the shoulders bearing the weight of the asana.

BENEFITS
- Tones the muscular, nervous and circulatory functions of the entire body.

CAUTION
- Breathing in this asana is challenging. Especially focus on the breathing out which makes the body supple and light to be comfortable in the lift.
- Progress into the asana and do not rush into it in the first attempt.
- A regular and consistent practice is the only way to master this asana.

ENERGY FLOW
- All the chakras benefit from this asana.

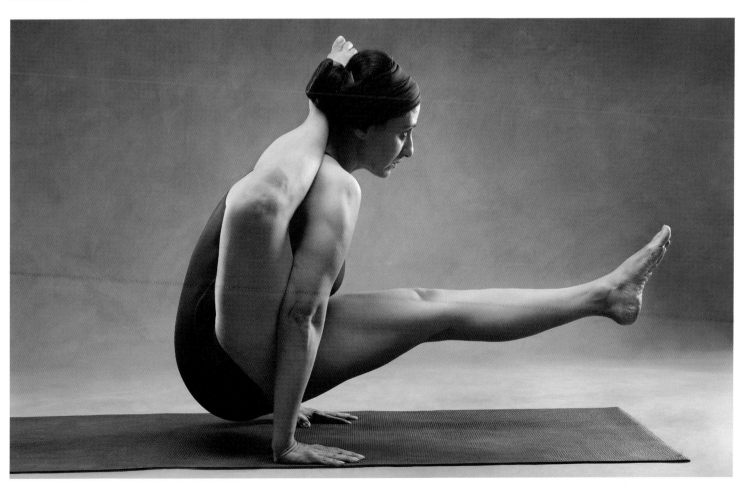

18. CHAKRASANA / URDHVA DHANURASANA

DRISHTI – Purva

TIPS

- Inhale to get your initial curve of the back and exhale as you intensify the curve, especially while reaching close to the ground.
- Straighten the elbows before your palms reach the ground. Lift and stretch the thighs towards the pelvis.
- Release the chest gently towards the head in the curve.
- While achieving the curve, ensure that the weight of the body shifts to the thighs and feet.
- Once the curve is achieved, make sure that the body weight is evenly distributed on the palms and feet.
- Keep the feet parallel to each other.
- Keep the inner edges of the feet pressed to the ground.

BENEFITS

- A well-toned and flexible spine.

CAUTION

Do not attempt this asana if you:
- Are tired or stressed.
- Have high blood pressure or low blood pressure.
- Have a headache / migraine.
- Have an upset stomach, constipation or diarrhoea.

- Expands the chest completely which is very beneficial to the heart.
- Strengthens the abdominal and pelvic organs.
- Improves blood circulation along the entire length of the body.
- Stimulates the thyroid glands.
- Keeps the uterus healthy and strong and prevents its prolapse.

ENERGY FLOW

- Energy moves from the Muladhara Chakra to all the parts of the body.

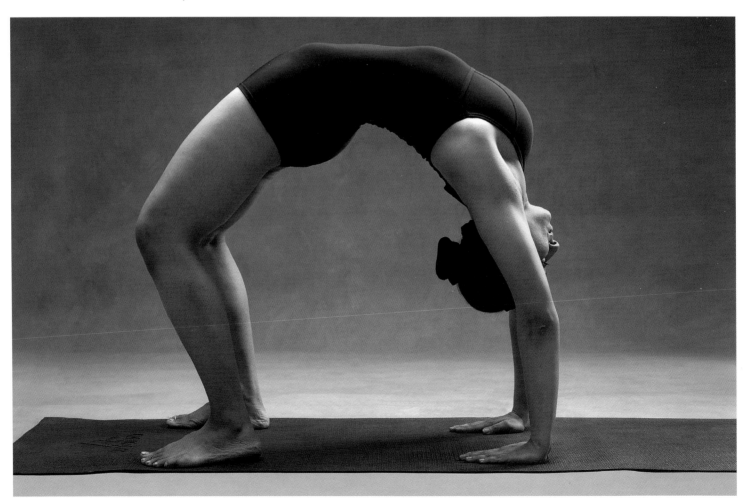

19. DHANURASANA
DRISHTI – Sama or Nasagrai

TIPS
- Maintain a firm grip of the ankles.
- Keep the knees apart till you achieve the full stretch.
- Keep the legs and the thighs stretched from the groin.
- Balance on the abdomen and not on the pelvic bones or the ribs.
- Keep breathing throughout the asana.
- Deepen the breathing and enjoy a gentle rocking of the body when the diaphragm stretches.
- Do not move the neck up and down to initiate the rock. It has to be achieved by breathing.

BENEFITS
- Helps correct posture.
- Brings elasticity to the spine.
- Increases blood circulation to all areas of the body.
- Tones the muscles of the back and spine.
- Safe for people suffering from slipped discs.
- The whole weight of the body falls on the centre of the abdomen, rushing large amount of blood around the abdominal organs.
- The shoulder blades are completely stretched which releases shoulder stiffness.
- Keeps the body trim and young.

CAUTION
- Prepare for the asana by getting comfortable with asanas like Bhujangasana and Shalabhasana.
- Do not practise this asana if you have an upset stomach, acidity, constipation or diarrhoea.
- Women suffering from problems of the uterus should not attempt this asana.

ENERGY FLOW
- All the chakras benefit from this asana. The Manipura Chakra and Anahata Chakra are especially energised.

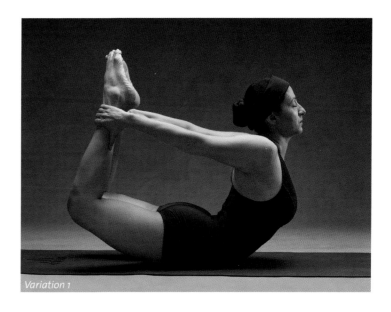
Variation 1

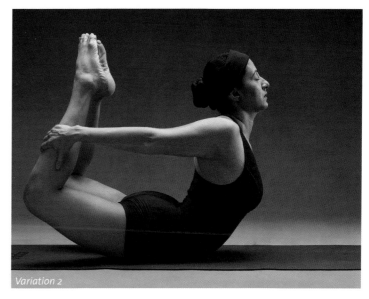
Variation 2

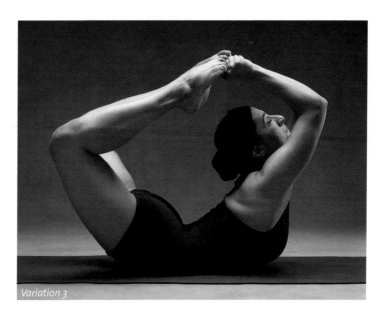
Variation 3

20. DWI PADA KOUNDINYASANA
DRISHTI – Bhoomigrai

TIPS
- Keep the palms firm, with all the fingers open on the floor.
- The shoulders should be wide open and strong.
- Establish strength at the core by keeping the navel tucked in.

NOTE
This challenging asana has lots of benefits but requires proper preparation. After adequate practice of all the basic asanas, the body gets tuned and ready for the Vishesha or extreme asanas. Master the Preceding asanas and Succeeding asanas before attempting this asana.

Preceding asanas
Chaduranga Dandasana, Bakasana, Tittibasana, Navasana, Purvottanasana, Krounchasana, Eka Pada Shirsasana

Succeeding asanas
Paschimottanasana, Purvottanasana, Sarvangasana, Halasana, Matsyasana

- Keep the lower back straight so that it accommodates strength in the hip.
- The entire lift of the leg has to be initiated by the hip, with a slight tilt to pull the feet off the floor.

BENEFITS
- Strengthens the arms, shoulders and chest.
- Strngthens the muscles of the abdomen.
- Benefits the abdominal organs.
- Makes the intestines stronger and function better.

CAUTION
- Make sure you are comfortable in Bakasana first.
- The arms and wrists have to be strong for this asana.
- This asana could strain your back if the hip is not placed properly.
- Do not practise this asana if recovering from diarrhoea or dysentery.
- Avoid this asana if you are trying to get pregnant.
- Do not attempt this asana if you have blood pressure or eye-strain.

ENERGY FLOW
- The Svadhisthana Chakra, Muladhara Chakra and Ajna Chakra benefit from this asana.

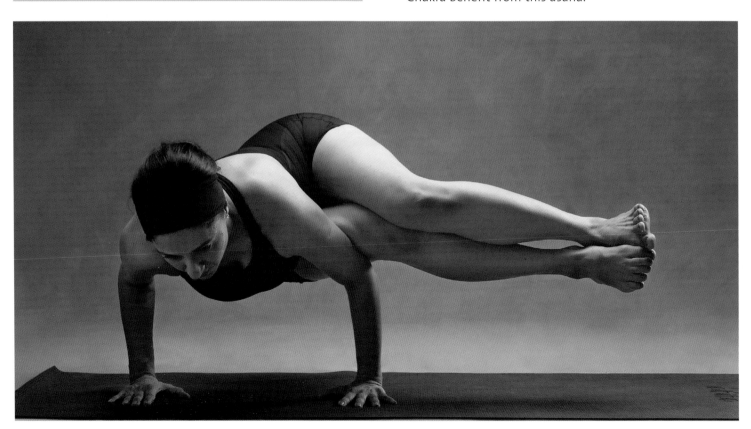

21. URDHVA SHALABHASANA
DRISHTI – Bhoomigrai

TIPS
* Same as in Shalabhasana.
* Press the shoulders to the ground and lift the legs up with more momentum.

BENEFITS
* Along with the benefits mentioned in Shalabhasana, also engages the shoulders which further challenges the diaphragm.

CAUTION
* Do not force the lift too much as it effects breathing.
* Do not practise this asana during pregnancy.

* Increases the blood flow into the heart benefiting its functions.

ENERGY FLOW
* The Anahata Chakra benefits from this asana but also engages all the chakras for power.

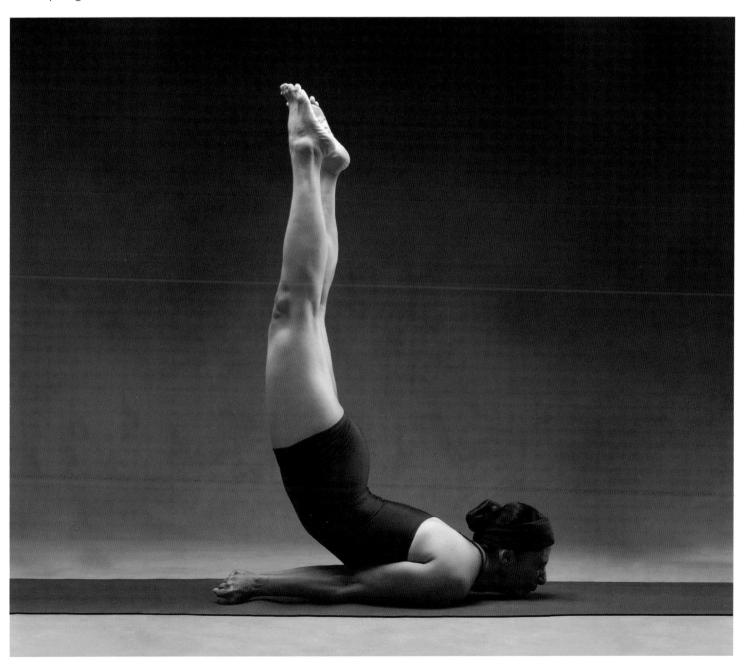

22. EKA PADA BAKASANA
DRISHTI – Bhoomigrai

TIPS

- Same as in Bakasana.
- Get into Eka Pada by folding one leg and placing it on the groin of the other, while in Tadasana.
- Bend down the body and also lower down the hips and place both the knees a little above the elbows.
- Pull in the lower abdomen.

BENEFITS AND ENERGY FLOW

- Same as in Bakasana.

CAUTION

- Do not collapse the back at any point of time.
- Hold the shoulders wide and open.
- Breathe deep into the asana.
- Avoid bending forward during pregnancy.

NOTE

This challenging asana has lots of benefits but requires proper preparation. After adequate practice of all the basic asanas, the body gets tuned and ready for the Vishesha or extreme asanas. Master the Preceding asanas and Succeeding asanas mentioned below before attempting this asana.

Preceding asanas

Adhomuka Swanasana, Parsvatanasana, Prasarita Padottanasana, Eka Pada Kapotasana, Upadasana, Bakasana, Eka Pada Bakasana

Succeeding asanas

Same as in Bakasana

- The difficulty with the folding of legs poses extra challenge to this asana, as this asana demands Mula energy.
- It trains the mind to impose balance.

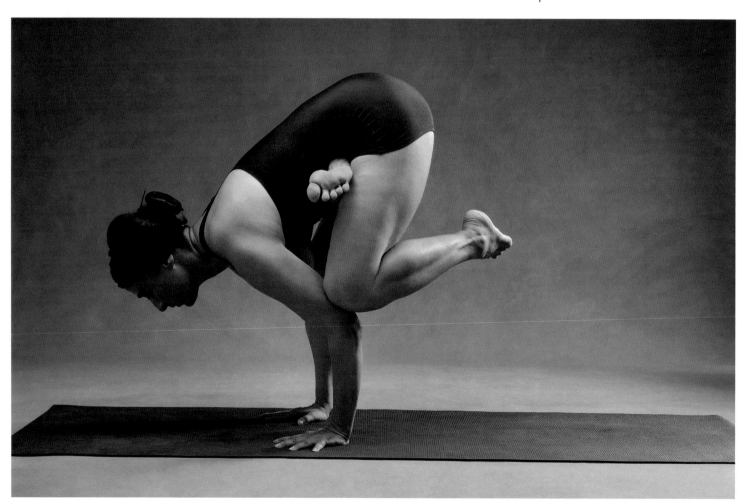

23. EKA PADA KAPOTASANA
DRISHTI – Urdhva

TIPS
- With the front leg in a folded position and the back leg stretched backward, keep the hip strongly pressed towards the floor to maintain balance.
- Keep the shoulder position in line with the hip and make sure there is no tilt to any side.
- Stretch the chest completely before stretching the neck and lifting the head up.
- While lifting the back leg up, keep its length perpendicular to the floor and reach the toe straight to the head.
- Inhale while stretching the chest and exhale while further stretching.

BENEFITS
- Rejuvenates the lower region of the spine.
- Increases circulation around the pelvic region and rejuvenates the pubic region, making them healthy.
- Benefits the neck and shoulder muscles.
- Provides a rich supply of blood to the thyroid and parathyroid glands, and adrenal glands thus increasing vitality.

CAUTION
- As the chest is intensely expanded, the breathing could feel restricted. Try to breathe normally.
- Prepare well for the asana before attempting it by mastering simple back-bend asanas like Dhanurasana.

ENERGY FLOW
- All the chakras benefit from this asana. The Svadhisthana Chakra, Muladara Chakra benefit from the downward flow of energy while the Manipura Chakra, Anahata Chakra and Vishuddha Chakra benefit from the upward flow of energy.

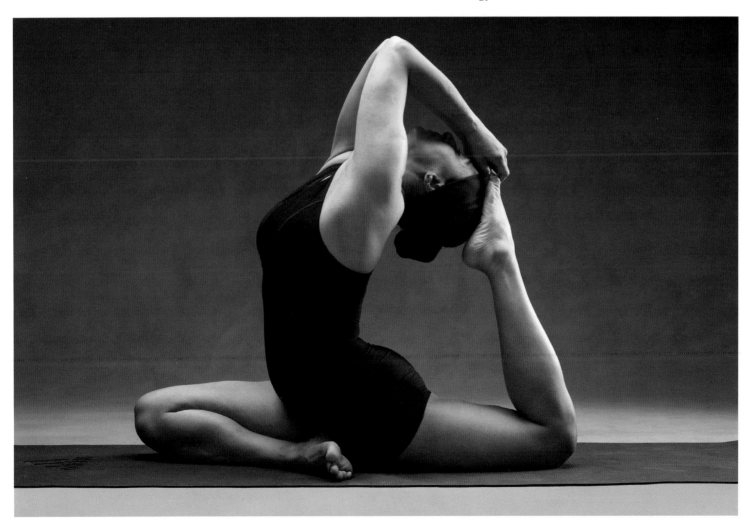

24. EKA PADA SHIRSASANA
DRISHTI – Sama

TIPS

* Try to get the shin on the shoulder so as to have the feet in front of the face by tucking the arms under the knees. Completely exhale in this position as it creates space and relaxes the stretch.
* Bend the trunk and the neck a little and place the ankle behind the neck.
* If leg is not placed properly, adjust the knees and point the toes upward. The leg should stay horizontally straight on the shoulder.
* Make sure you breathe deep.

BENEFITS

* Strengthens the neck as well as shoulders.
* Stretches the lower area of the thighs and also the hamstrings.

CAUTION

* Lack of flexibility in the knee and ankles would make this asana difficult to achieve.
* The asana needs a lot of practice and understanding about the pressure of the leg on the neck.

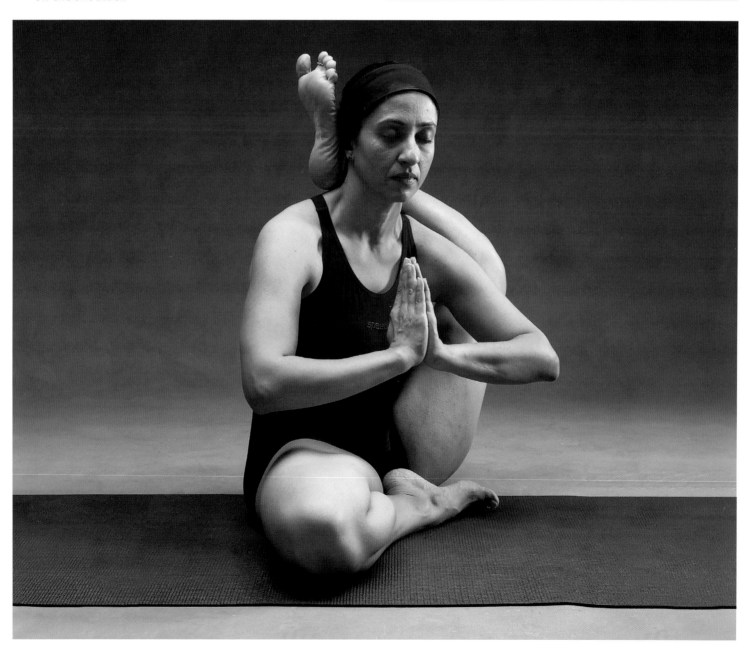

25. EKA PADA UTTANASANA
DRISHTI – Nasagrai

TIPS
- Same as in Uttanasana.
- Once Uttanasana is established, gently lift one leg up towards the ceiling.
- Try not to tilt the hip, but lengthen the spine instead towards the ground.
- Make sure the back is straight and does not curve at any point of this asana.

BENEFITS
- Same as in Uttanasana.
- Further increases the flexibility in the sacrum and hip rotators.
- More blood rushes into the head, benefiting the length of the spine.

CAUTION
- Same as in Uttanasana.

ENERGY FLOW
- Vital energy flow is from the Muladhara Chakra to Sahasrara Chakra.

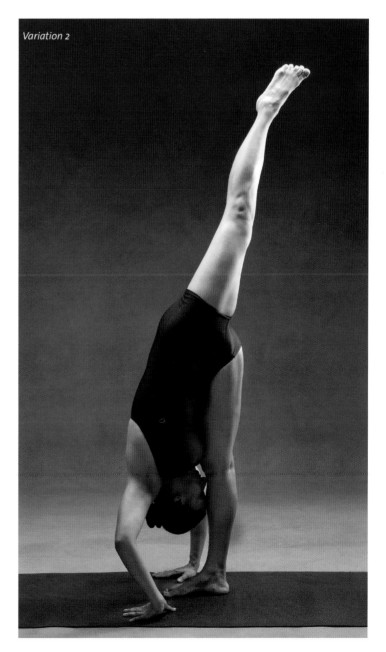

Variation 1

Variation 2

26. EKA PADA URDHVA DHANURASANA
DRISHTI – Purva

TIPS
- Inhale to get the initial curve of the back and exhale as you intensify the curve, especially while reaching the hands close to the ground.
- Straighten the elbows before your palms reach the ground. Lift and stretch the thighs towards the pelvis.
- Release the chest gently towards the head in the curve.
- While achieving the curve, ensure that the weight of the body shifts to the thighs and feet.
- Once the curve is achieved, make sure that the body weight is evenly distributed on the palms and feet.
- Keep the feet parallel to each other.
- Keep the inner edges of the feet pressed to the ground.
- Gently lift one leg up towards the ceiling without tilting the hip and shifting the weight to the other side.

BENEFITS
- Tones the spine well and makes it flexible.
- Expands the chest completely which is very beneficial to the heart.
- Strengthens the abdominal and pelvic organs.
- Improves blood circulation in the entire body.
- Stimulates the thyroid glands.
- Conditions the core muscles and strengthens the legs

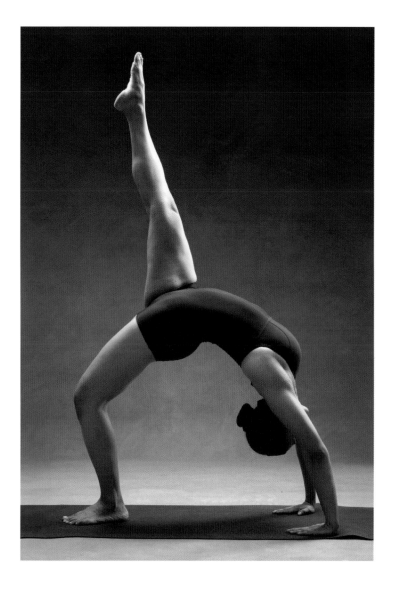

CAUTION
- Do not do attempt asana if you are tired or stressed.
- Do not attempt this asana if you have high blood pressure or low blood pressure.
- Do not attempt this asana if you have a headache / migraine.
- Do not attempt this asana if you have an upset stomach, constipation or diarrhoea.
- For the final lift of one leg, make sure weight of the body is equally distributed on both the palms and the leg which is touching ground. For this, control from the hip is necessary.
- Adjust the leg positioning in line with the hip bones.

ENERGY FLOW
- All the chakras are energised in this asana.

27. GARBHA PINDASANA
DRISHTI – Nasagrai

TIPS
- Relax in Padmasana by loosening the grip of the muscles between the thighs and calves.
- Exhale completely after inserting the arms between the thighs and calves, and inhale only after reaching them to the head.
- The Padmasana has to fold upward towards the head to achieve the final position.

BENEFITS
- Tones the abdominal area by increasing blood circulation.
- Contracts the abdominal organs, keeping the area trim and strong.
- Rocking a few times in a circle while holding the asana is a good massage for the spine and back muscles.

CAUTION
- Practise Lolasana before and after this asana.
- Breathing in this hold is challenging. However, Ujjayee has to be maintained in equal ratio breathing.

ENERGY FLOW
- All the chakras are rejuvenated in this position.

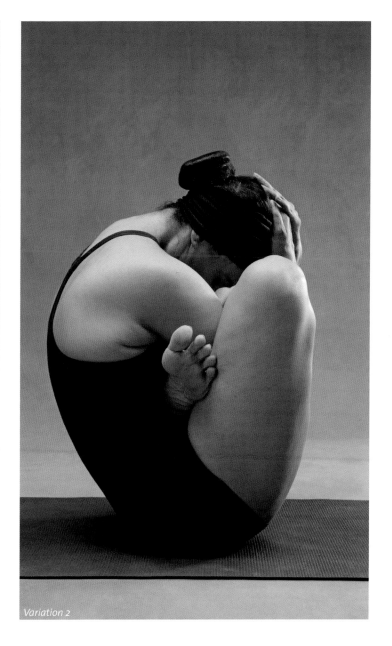

Variation 1

Variation 2

28. GOMUKHASANA
DRISHTI – Sama

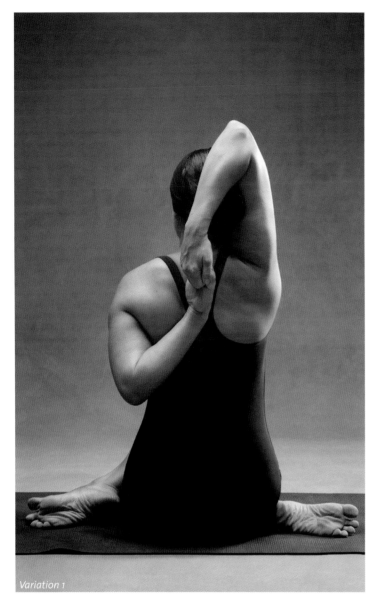

Variation 1

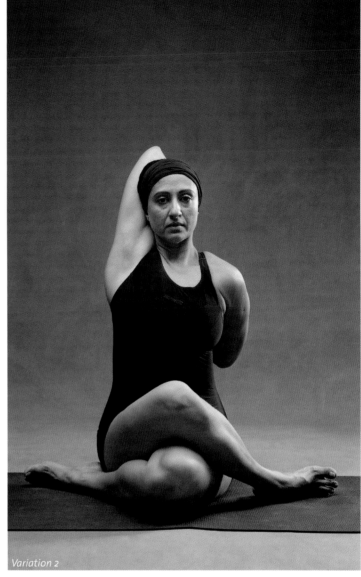

Variation 2

TIPS
- From Vajrasana, place one knee upon another and open up the feet to seat the hip on the floor firmly.
- Keep the spine straight by expanding the chest and stretching spine downwards.
- Keep the bicep close to the ear.

BENEFITS
- Benefits the legs and knees.
- Benefits the neck shoulders and the arms.
- The intense opening up stretch around the armpits activates the lymph nodes which in turn benefits the immune system.

- Releases fatigue or tamasic energy from the body.
- The lift in the midriff area deepens breathing.

CAUTION
- Once the asana is accomplished, release the tension in the muscles along the length of the shoulder and arms.
- Also, relax the tightness in the length of the legs and thighs.

ENERGY FLOW
- This asana aligns and rejuvenates all the depleted chakra energy.

29. HALASANA
DRISHTI – Nasagrai

TIPS
- Exhale and maintain a strong length in the abdomen while stretching the length of the legs to the floor behind the head.
- Keep exhaling to hollow the stomach, while lowering the legs to the floor.
- Keep the shoulders rolled down, away from the ears while in the stretch.
- Draw the collarbones wide and open your chest up and into your chin forming a Jalandhara Bandha.
- Look towards the chest through the tip of the nose.

BENEFITS
Along with the benefits of Sarvangasana it also:
- Rejuvenates the body, relieves fatigue and tension after a tiring day.
- Reaches blood to the head to maintain calmness and lightness in the brain.
- Rejuvenates the abdominal organs, thus helping in digestion and constipation.
- Improves the alignment of the shoulders and the length of the spine.
- Relieves backache as the spine receives a rich supply of blood.
- Provides relief to people suffering from stiff shoulders and elbows, lumbago and arthritis of the back find.
- Relieves stiffness in the fingers if the variation of interlocking of the fingers is practised.
- Relieves stomach pain due to gas.
- Is the best preparatory asana for Paschimottasana.
- Is good for people suffering from high blood pressure.

This asana should be held for three minutes before releasing it to Sarvangasana, so that the immediate blood rush into the brain is not felt.

CAUTION
- Do not practise this asana with severe headache, migraine, cervical spondylitis, upset stomach or diarrhoea.
- This asana will be uncomfortable during a cold or an attack of asthma.

ENERGY FLOW
- All the chakras benefit from this asana.

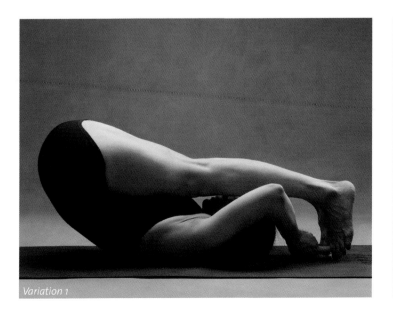
Variation 1

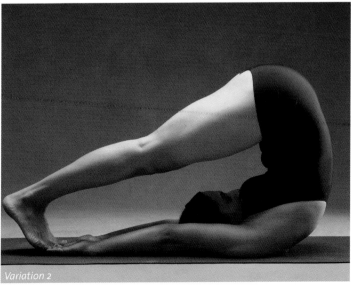
Variation 2

30. HANUMANASANA
DRISHTI – Sama or Urdhva

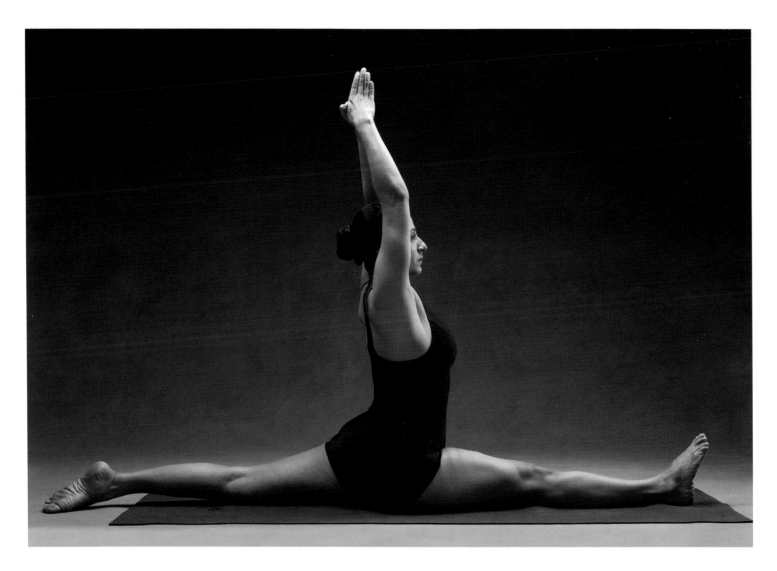

TIPS

- Achieve this asana very gradually over a period of time.
- Try the asana from Parsvatanasana. Bend forward and reach your hands to the floor.
- Slowly start stretching the back leg first and bend the front knee to achieve a lunge position.
- From here on, work on the stretching the front leg by straightening the knee to come to a split.
- To further the stretch, focus on gently stretching the back leg (rotating or sliding the leg from the hip) so that the hamstrings of the front leg are safe from tear.

BENEFITS

- Tones and relaxes the leg muscles.
- Lengthens the leg muscles and helps cure sciatica.

CAUTION
- Make sure that the hip and the leg area are well warmed up.
- To achieve this asana, flexibility of the groin is important.

ENERGY FLOW

- In this asana, the Mula Chakra is the central source of energy, which then flows into the lower limbs of the body and energises all the chakras above.

31. JANU SHIRSASANA
DRISHTI – Bhoomigrai

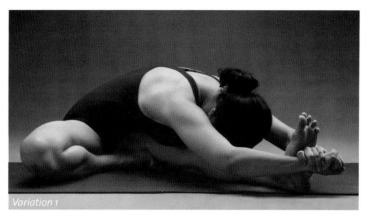

Variation 1

TIPS
- Exhale and widen the elbows while leaning forward along the length of the thigh.
- Keep the stretched leg straight with the calf touching the floor and do not allow the foot to tilt or the thigh to lift.
- Focus on both sides of the torso being in line, so that the back gets an even stretch, which would also expand the chest.

BENEFITS
- Balances and tones the liver, the spleen and the kidneys.
- Benefits people with enlarged prostate.
- Helps people suffering from prolonged fever.
- Relieves stiffness in the legs, knees, hip, pelvis and develops suppleness around these areas.
- Eases stiffness in the shoulders, hips, elbows and wrists.
- Eases the effects of stress on the heart and mind.

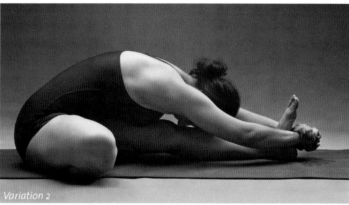

Variation 2

CAUTION
- If the asana is difficult to achieve, use a strap to prevent rounding of the shoulders and back. It will also aid to keep the spine straight.
- Do not allow the knees to tilt and keep them evenly stretched on both sides to avoid injury along the hamstrings.

ENERGY FLOW
- All the chakras benefit from this asana as forward-bending asanas binds the chakras and releases them.
- This helps increase the chakra energy due to the stress-and-release effect.

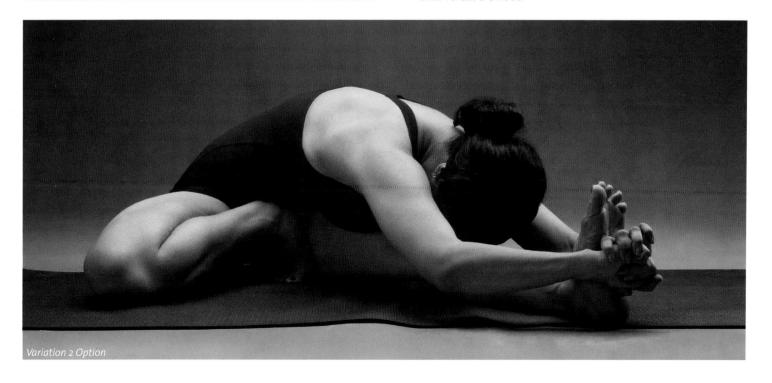

Variation 2 Option

32. KALA BHAIRAVASANA
DRISHTI – Urdhva

TIPS
Attempt this asana from Adho Mukha Svanasana into a Parsvakonasana stretch by:

- Pressing the palm to the floor and lifting the right leg off the floor and extending the left hand to grab the left toe.
- Stabilising in this position and then trying to extend the left leg as straight as possible.

BENEFITS
- Strengthens the arms, legs and abdominal muscles.

CAUTION
- This asana poses an extreme challenge to the hamstrings and, therefore, takes time and effort to achieve.
- Mastering Hanumanasana is mandatory before attempting this asana.

ENERGY FLOW
- This powerful asana energises all the chakras in the body.

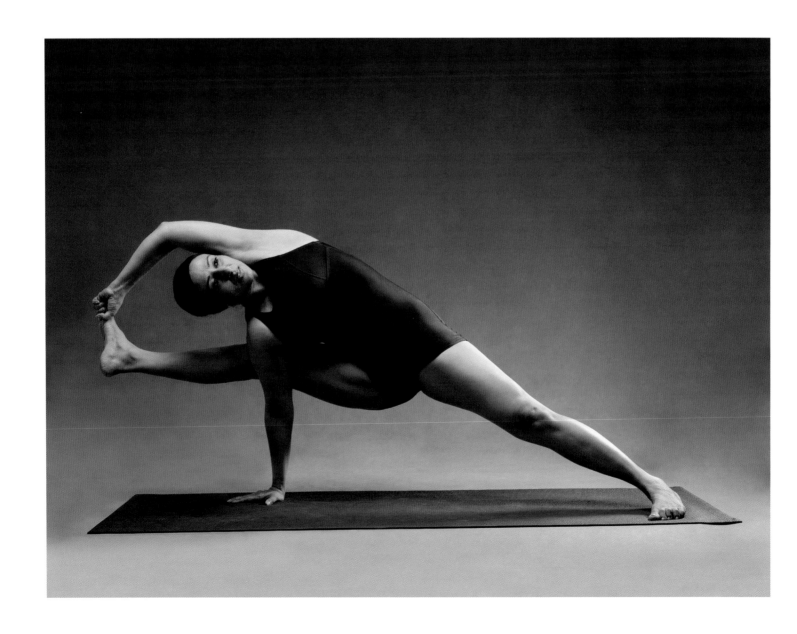

33. KAPILASANA
DRISHTI – Sama

TIPS
- From Eka Pada Shirsasana, recline backward towards the floor.
- Once the asana is achieved, relax the muscles as it makes the breathing easier to maintain in a rhythmic flow.

NOTE
This challenging asana has lots of benefits but requires proper preparation. After adequate practice of all the basic asanas, the body gets tuned and ready for the Vishesha or extreme asanas. Master the Preceding asanas and Succeeding asanas mentioned below before attempting this asana.

Preceding asanas
Parshvakonasana, Parivrtta Parsvakonasana, Parsvatanasana, Prasarita Padottanasana, Veerabhadrasana 3, Eka Pada Kapotasana

Succeeding asanas
Same as Chakorasana

BENEFITS
- Provides good flexibility to the spine.
- Provides a rich circulation of blood to the lower back.
- The compressed position of the chest poses a challenge for breathing which in turn helps the diaphragm muscles to get strong.

CAUTION
- Breathing in this asana is challenging. Especially focus on the breathing out, which makes the body supple and light to be comfortable in the lift.
- Progress into the asana and do not rush into it in the first attempt.
- A regular and consistent practice is the only way to master this asana.

ENERGY FLOW
- The Vishuddha Chakra, Anahata Chakra, Manipura Chakra, Svadhisthana Chakra and Muladhara Chakra are energised. As the nerve plexus are along the length of the spine, this asana benefits the health of the nadis.

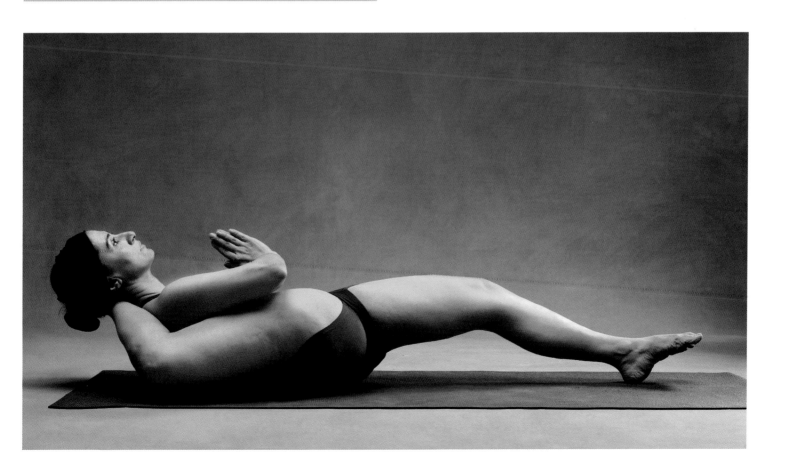

34. KAPOTASANA
DRISHTI – Urdhva

TIPS

- To achieve the right and deep curve, extend the length of the thighs backward and length of the abdomen forward and upward, which settles the groin into a position of hold on the floor.
- Maintain balance.
- Press the heel of the palms so that the wrists feel strong.
- Inhale while beginning the lift and expand the chest completely.

- Exhale completely once the lift is achieved and feel the spine relax.
- Breathing could become very fast and unsteady. Pay attention and try not to lose the rhythm of the breathing.
- Hold the pelvic region tight so that the spine does not collapse.

BENEFITS

- The nerves and the area around the spine receive good circulation of blood making it strong.
- The diaphragm feels completely lifted and the chest is fully expanded, strengthening the respiratory muscles and also increasing the flexibility of the ribs.
- The heart gets a massage when the chest is fully expanded, increasing supply of blood in the body.
- The pelvic region is also completely expanded.

CAUTION

- Practise Dhanurasana well before you attempt this stretch.
- Make sure the spine has acquired sufficient flexibility before attempting this challenging asana.
- The knees and the thighs have to be strong to hold this stretch.

ENERGY FLOW

- All the chakras benefit from this asana. The Svadhisthana Chakra, Muladhara Chakra benefit from the downward flow of energy while the Manipura Chakra, Anahata Chakra and Vishuddha Chakra benefit fom the upward flow of energy.

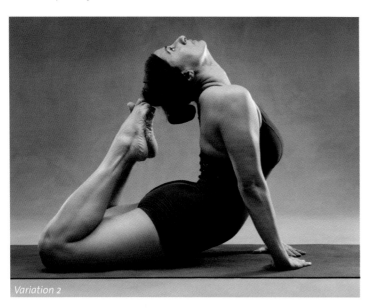
Variation 2

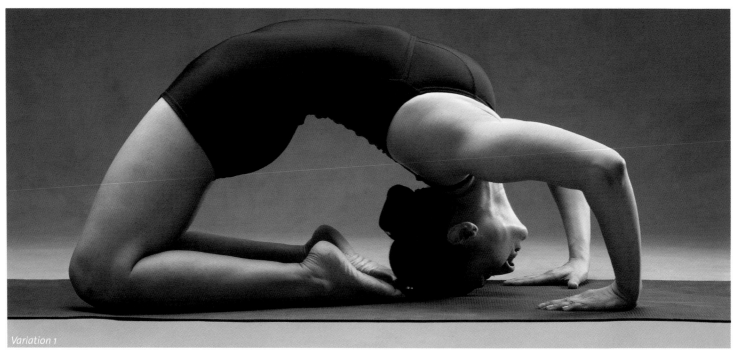
Variation 1

35. KARNA PEEDASANA
DRISHTI – Nasagrai

TIPS
- Initially dropping the knees to the floor would be a problem, so do not force it.
- Hug thighs from the back of the knees and hold that position.
- The spine will stretch more when knees are bent.
- Engage the bandhas one by one in this asana.

BENEFITS
- Same as in Halasana.
- However the spine is stretched more as the knees are bent and this helps more circulation of the blood around the area.

CAUTION
- Pay attention to the caution points mentioned in the Halasana.
- Do not force this asana in case of pain / injury in the neck.
- Do not try dropping the knees totally down towards the ground.
- While coming out of the asana, gently release the knees to the floor.

ENERGY FLOW
- All the chakras benefit from this asana. The Sahasrara Chakra feels relaxed and rejuvenated.

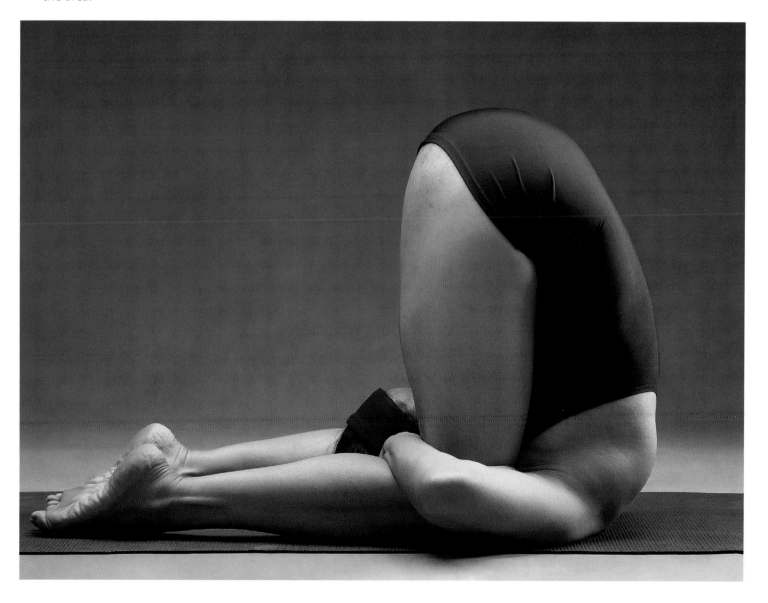

36. KROUNCHASANA
DRISHTI – Padayoragrai

TIPS
- Keep the stomach hollow so that you can extend the spine comfortably.
- Try to keep your back straight.
- Get your seat bones to be steady on the floor.

BENEFITS
- Stretches the muscles of the leg.
- Gently releases the hamstrings and the IT band.
- Benefits the lower back.
- Rejuvenates the abdominal organs.

CAUTION
- This is a safe asana. While it is a challenging asana, regular practice will help improve the forward-bending stretches like Paschimottanasana.

ENERGY FLOW
- The Muladhara Chakra receives maximum flow of energy.

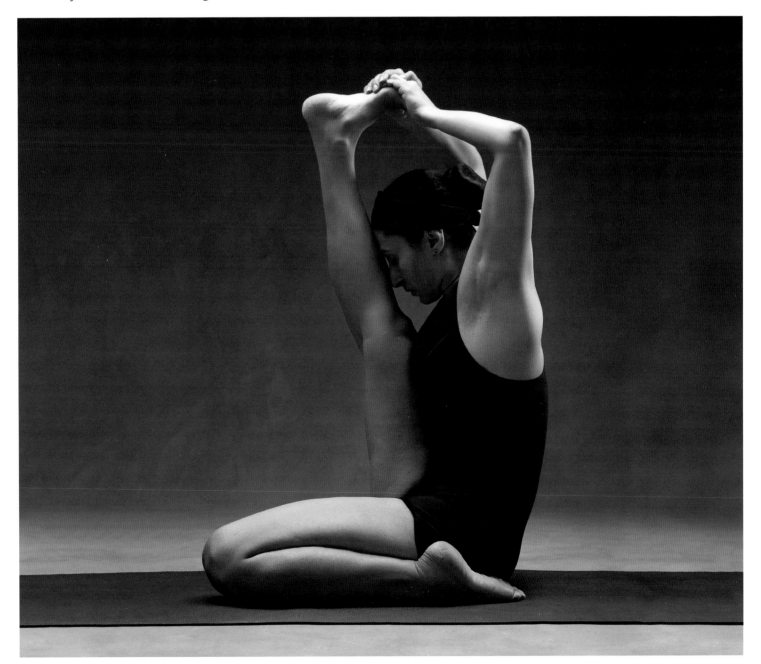

37. KURMASANA
DRISHTI – Bhrumadhya

TIPS
- Start this asana from Baddha Konasana.
- Insert the hands one by one under the thighs and place the knees over the shoulders.
- Instead of trying to bend forward, make the knees press the shoulders towards floor, which also opens up the chest.

BENEFITS
- Intensely lengthens the back muscles, opens up the shoulders and expands the chest.
- Releases tightness in the spine and sacrum.
- Improves the digestive system.
- Relaxes the mind and calms the senses.

CAUTION
- Be careful if you have a problem with your shoulders.
- Do not attempt this asana without a proper warm-up.
- Ease into the stretch and do not force the pressing of the leg until the muscles around your hip and legs feel supple.

ENERGY FLOW
- All the chakras are energised and energy flows back towards the spine, benefiting the backward / inward movement of the chakras, which are conical.

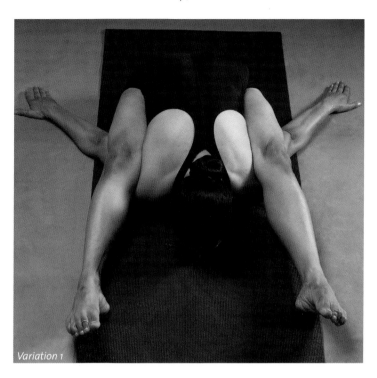

Variation 1

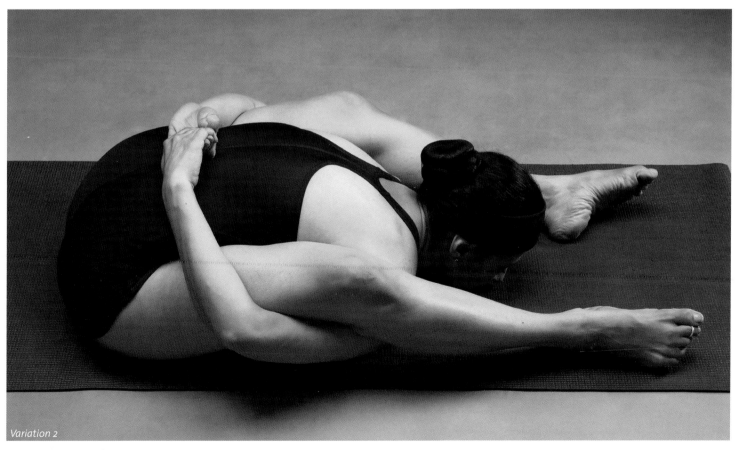

Variation 2

38. MALASANA
DRISHTI – Nasagrai

TIPS
- It is important to squat into this position gently.
- Root the soles of the feet to the ground.
- During practice, if it is difficult to place the feet on the ground, place a folded blanket or a rolled mat under the heels. This would train the calves and ankles to adjust into the stretch.
- Widen the knees and push the trunk forward, and exhale completely as you bend forward.

BENEFITS
- Stretches the spine and relaxes the back muscles.
- Relieves abdominal cramps and aids digestion.
- Tones the abdominal muscles.

CAUTION
- Do not bend forward in this asana if suffering from a headache.
- Do not attempt this asana if nauseous due to indigestion.

ENERGY FLOW
- Releases tension from the Muladhara Chakra which governs digestion.
- Benefits the Svadhisthana Chakra which governs the reproductive function of the body.

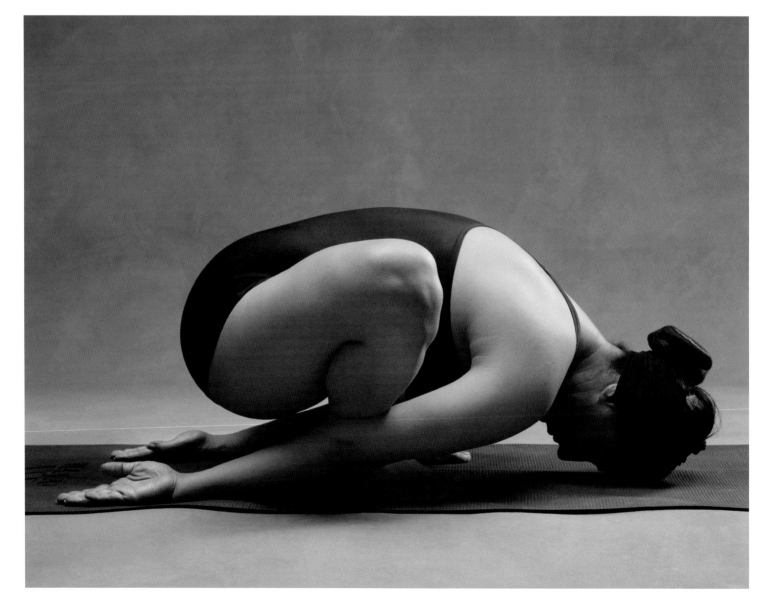

39. MANDUKASANA
DRISHTI – Nasagrai

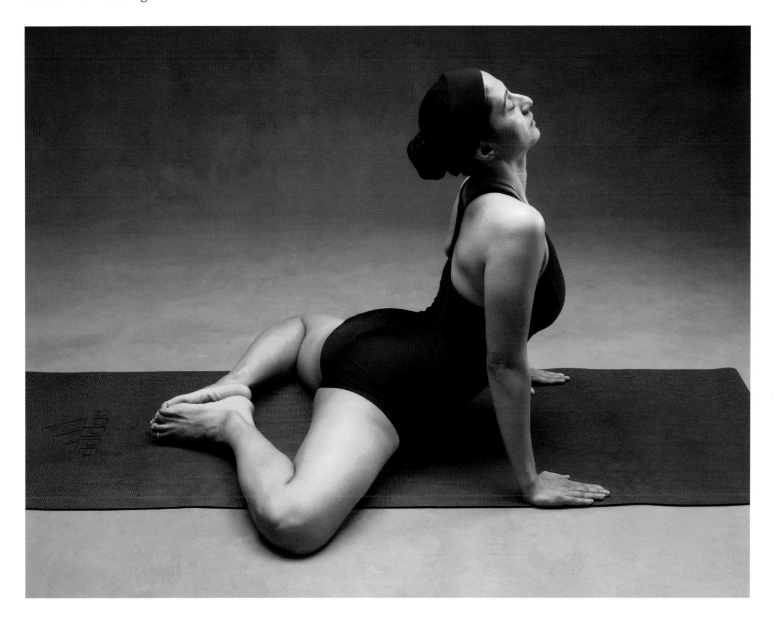

TIPS
- This asana is best achieved from Baddha Konasana.
- Lift the hips up and tilt the body forward, adjusting the feet to feel comfortable.
- Lower the hips forward with the hands supporting in the front.
- Press the hips towards the floor and relax the lower back, lifting the chest up.

BENEFITS
- A good hip opener.
- Benefits the area around the hips and reduces excess fat in this region.
- Activates the lymph nodes along the length of the groin, thus releasing toxins from the area.

CAUTION
- Do not attempt this asana if you have weak knees.
- Practise complete Baddha Konasana before attempting this asana.

ENERGY FLOW
- Benefits the Muladhara Chakra and Anahata Chakra, while the other chakras receive a rich supply of prana.

40. MARICHYASANA
DRISHTI – Nasagrai and Sama

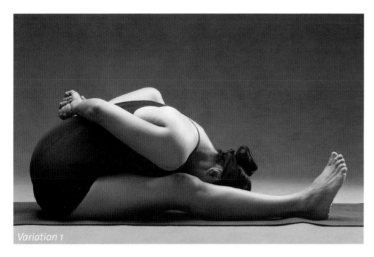

Variation 1

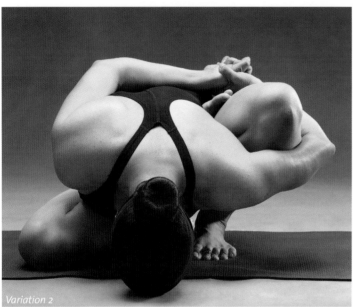

Variation 2

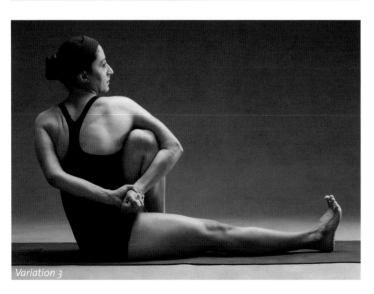

Variation 3

TIPS
- Adjust the foot position of the bent knee and make sure it is pointing straight.
- Place the foot in line with the hip bone.
- After binding the hands behind the back, make sure that the shoulders are square before leaning forward.
- While inhaling, lengthen the spine and while exhaling, stretch down deflating the stomach completely to accommodate a comfortable stretch.
- Uddiyana Bandha and Mula Bandha can be attempted in these asanas.

BENEFITS
- Helps relieve back problems.
- Helps reduce the waistline and makes it flexible.
- The forward bend moves the abdomen inwards, thus massaging and toning the abdominal organs and also reducing the size around this area.
- Benefits the liver and spleen.
- Tones the muscles of the back, shoulders and neck.
- Contracts the abdominal organs.

CAUTION
Do not practise this asana:
- After an upset stomach.
- If you have an acidity problem.
- If the body is tired.
- If you have conceived.

ENERGY FLOW
- The Muladhara Chakra, Svadhisthana Chakra, Manipura Chakra, Anahata Chakra and Vishuddha Chakra benefit from this asana.

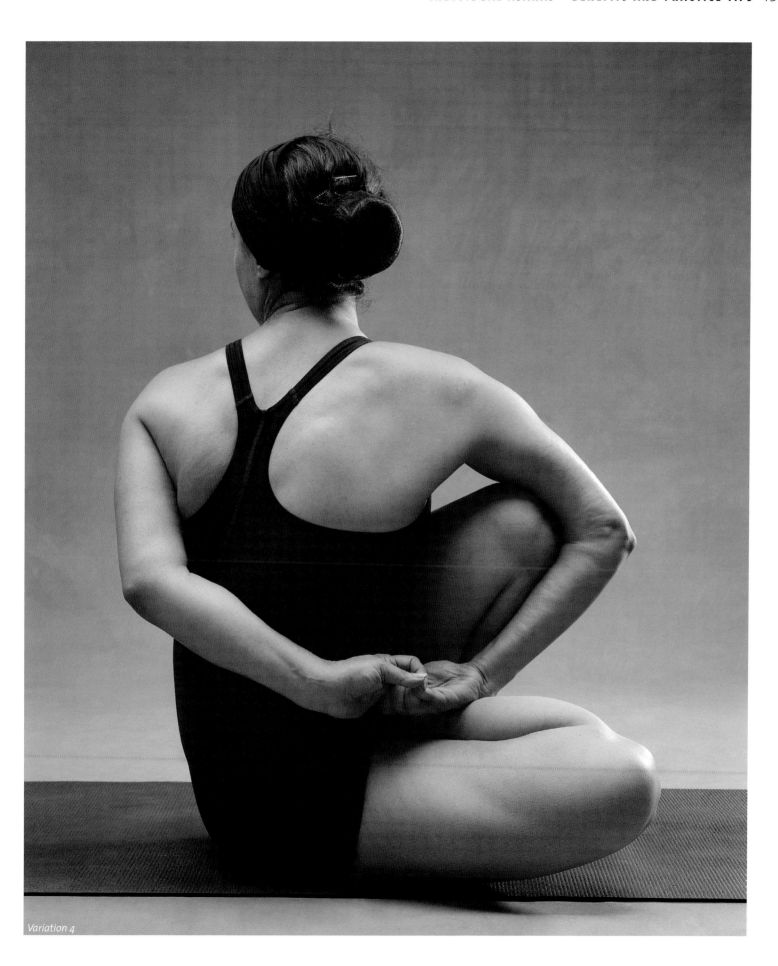

Variation 4

41. MATSYASANA
DRISHTI – Urdhva

TIPS
- Expand the chest fully and evenly on either side of the sternum.
- Keep the shoulder blades tucked in by keeping the elbows as close to each other as possible.

BENEFITS
- The thyroid benefits from the stretching of the neck.
- The chest is fully expanded and the entire dorsal region benefits from the stretch.
- The pelvic region becomes flexible and strong.
- Stretches the abdomen and works on the back.
- Reduces menstrual pains and helps treat disorders of the ovaries.

CAUTION
- Do not practise this asana if you have a cardiac condition, lower back problems or spinal disc disorders.
- If Padmasana feels strained, stretch the legs forward in a straight line, maintaining the lift of the chest, and the neck region.

ENERGY FLOW
- The Manipura Chakra, Anahata Chakra, Vishuddha Chakra, and the Ajna Chakra are energised in this asana.

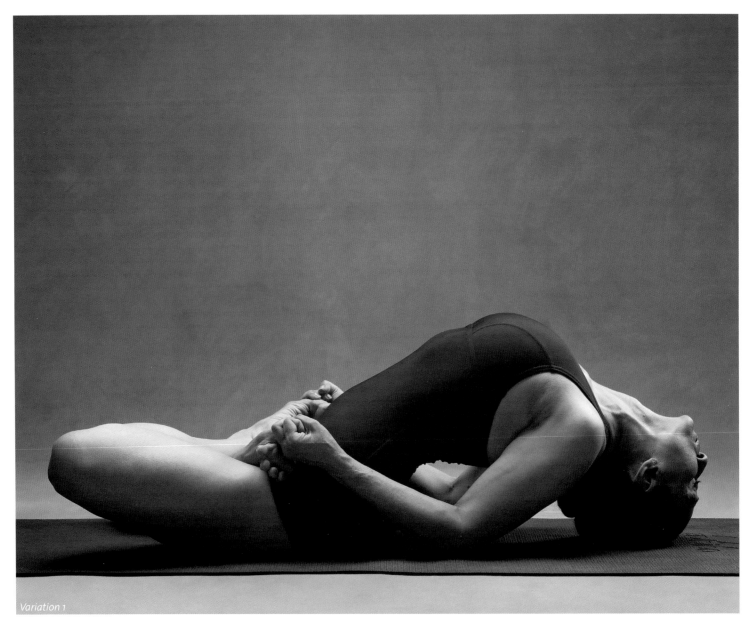

Variation 1

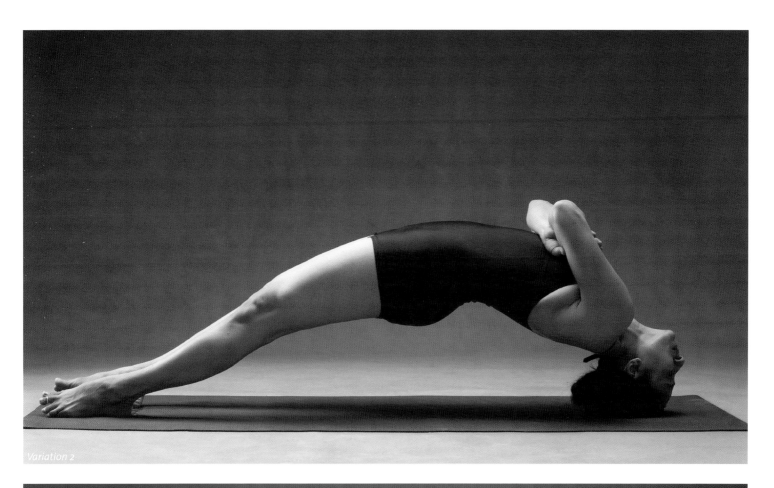

Variation 2

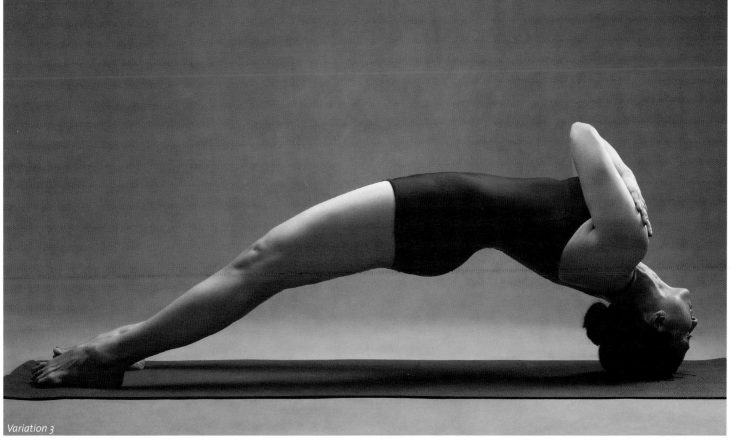

Variation 3

42. MATSYENDRASANA
DRISHTI – Sama

TIPS
- To twist the trunk completely, try to turn the shoulder 90° backward.
- Keep the neck in sync with the turn of the shoulders and make sure it is placed in line with the shoulders after the turn.
- Keep the trunk tall with the abdomen completely deflated.
- Keep the gaze steady and in a straight line.

BENEFITS
- Alleviates backache and relieves lumbago.
- Improves function of the liver, pancreas, intestines, kidney and lungs.
- Reduces fat around the waistline.
- Increases stamina.

CAUTION
- The spinal twist will compress the diaphragm and breathing could be restricted. However try to breathe normally.
- Do not practise this asana when you lack stamina or feel tired.
- If you have a cold, headache or migraine, or are suffering from dysentery or just recovering from an upset stomach, do not attempt this asana.
- The body should be well warmed up to do this stretch.

ENERGY FLOW
- The Anahata Chakra, Vishuddha Chakra, Ajna Chakra and Sahasrara Chakra benefit from this asana.

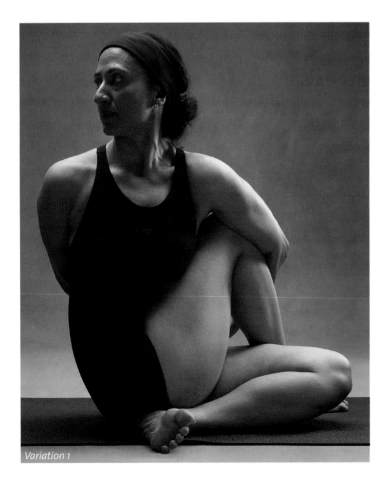
Variation 1

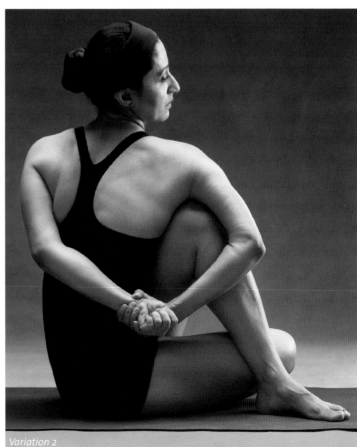
Variation 2

43. NATARAJASANA
DRISHTI – Sama or Hastagrai

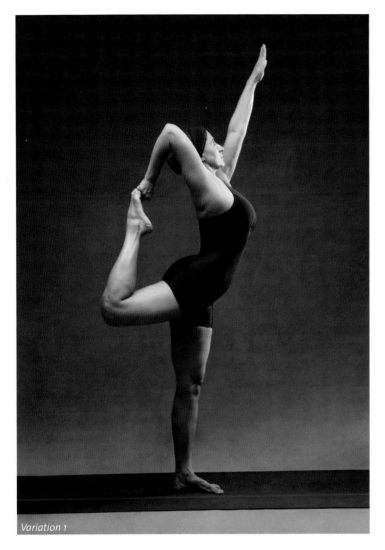

Variation 1

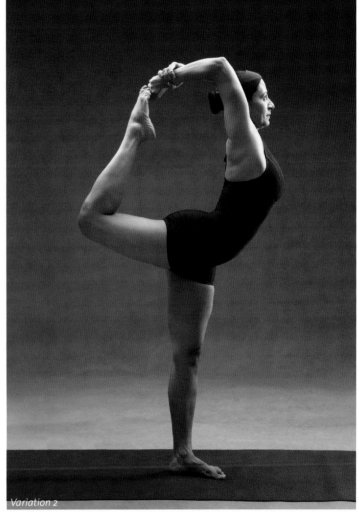

Variation 2

TIPS
- Keep both the knees bent while in the process of establishing the backward leg stretch, which would help in easing the stretch.
- Keep the back of the head and the shoulders relaxed throughout the stretch.
- Keep the shoulder socket flexible to accommodate the movement of the elbow.

BENEFITS
- A very good contraction for the spine.
- The shoulder blades rotate freely thus increasing flexibility of the shoulders.
- The chest expands fully which works on postural alignment.
- Challenges the balance which builds up focus and concentration.

CAUTION
- Do not attempt this asana if you have a spinal problem.
- Do not snap out of the asana. Come out of it slowly.
- Relax the elbows and the arms first by unwinding them and then gently place them by the side of the hip.
- Master Dwi Pada Kapotasana, Eka Pada Raja Kapotasana, Urdhva Dhanurasana and other back-bending asanas well before attempting this asana.

ENERGY FLOW
- Strengthens the Muladhara Chakra and engages all the chakras to maintain a balanced flow of energy.

44. NAVASANA
DRISHTI – Angushtagrai

TIPS
- Keep the spine straight, with the chest lifted in the position.
- Relax the neck and shoulder muscles.
- Keep the lower abdomen strong with Mula Bandha to keep the position steady.
- Breathe in equal ratio (5:5).

BENEFITS
- Strengthens the abdominal muscles.
- Reduces fat around the waist and torso.

CAUTION
- Do not attempt this asana if the back is weak.
- The stomach should be completely empty before attempting this asana.

ENERGY FLOW
- Energises the Muladhara Chakra, benefits the Svadhisthana Chakra and builds focus in the Ajna Chakra.

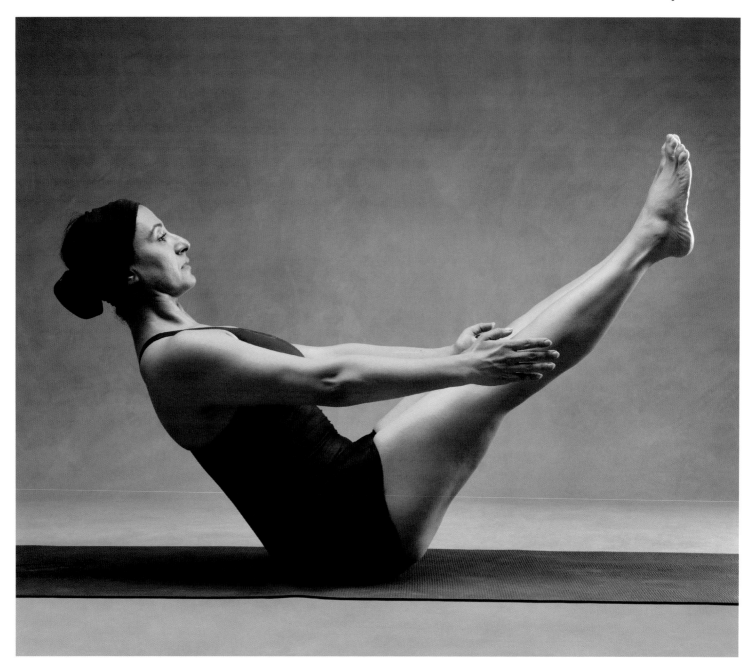

45. PADANGUSTASANA / PADA HASTASANA
DRISHTI – Nasagrai

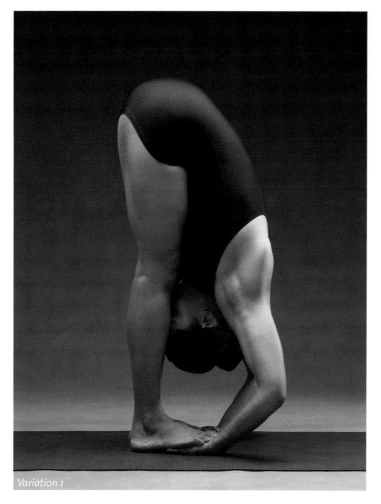

Variation 1

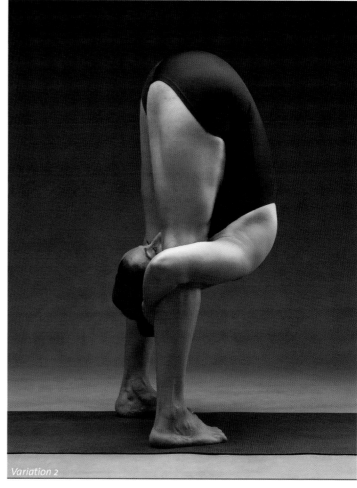

Variation 2

TIPS

- Raise the hip high up towards the ceiling.
- Further extend by tilting the pelvis upward while dropping the head downwards.
- Press the toes and feet into the floor and relax the length of the back by drawing the shoulders away from the ears and releasing the tension in the neck.

BENEFITS

- Abdominal organs are toned and digestive juices increase, while the liver and the spleen are activated.
- Benefits people suffering from a bloating sensation and gastric troubles.
- Relieves exhaustion, both physical and mental.

CAUTION

- If there is a spinal disc disorder, avoid this asana. However, you could try this position by keeping the knees slightly bent, with the back concave.
- People with problem of blood pressure should avoid this asana or be very cautious. If you are trying it do nonetheless, make sure not to bring the head between the knees.
- This asana could lead to dizziness due to the rush of blood.

ENERGY FLOW

- Try doing a Mula Bandha and feel the energy flow down the spine towards gravity. You could also progress to do the Uddiyana Bandha. (Make sure you have practised the bandhas well before you engage them along with the asanas.)
- Energy flows along the length of the spine all the way from the Muladhara Chakra to the Sahasrara Chakra at the top.
- All the chakras are vitalised.

46. PADMASANA
DRISHTI – Nasagrai

TIPS
- Place the seat bones firmly on the floor.
- Yield the weight of the body firmly to the floor and release all tension from the spine.
- Press the knees in towards one another to ensure your feet are sufficiently placed across the thighs.
- Keep the knees pointed towards the floor to eventually touch the ground.

BENEFITS
- Padmasana is one of the most relaxing poses.
- The asana does not allow the spine to slouch, which benefits smooth flow of energy though the spine.
- Aids concentration and keep the mind alert and attentive.
- Releases stiffness in the knees and the ankles.

CAUTION
- Practise half Padmasana by placing one foot first, e.g. the right one on the root of the left foot, and flap to loosen the knee and ankle. Repeat the same with the left foot. This exercise would help release the tightness in the knees.

ENERGY FLOW
- Energises and aligns all the chakras.

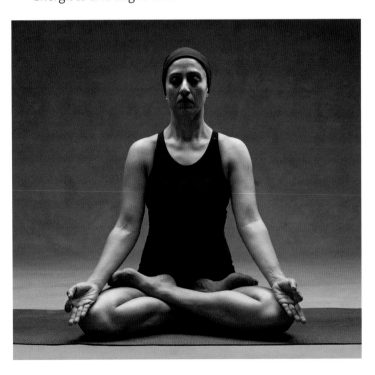

47. PARIVRTTA ARDHA CHANDRASANA
DRISHTI - Hastagrai

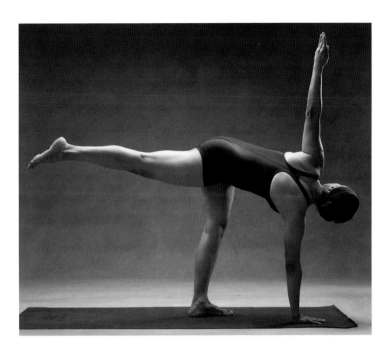

TIPS
- Focus on the balance and then tilt into the asana. Stay still until the body adjusts itself to gravity.
- Step by step, strengthen the muscles to hold the asana for as long as it is comfortable with equal ratio (5:5) breathing.

BENEFITS
- Good hip opener that creates space in the hip area, thus benefiting all the organs around.
- Frees the organs of the body for sideward movement which encourages peristaltic movement in the walls of the organs.

Once the asana is in balance it is important to relax the neck muscles before attempting the challege of lifting head up towards the ceiling.

CAUTION
- When in the asana, if there is a feeling of blood rush or if breathing becomes difficult, the asana should released and reconstructed.
- Do not attempt this asana with tired legs or knees.

ENERGY FLOW
- All the chakras benifit from this asana.

48. PARIVRTTA HANUMANASANA
DRISHTI – Urdhva

TIPS
- Same as Hanumanasana.
- Turn the torso to one side till you get Purva Drishti.
- Once the drishti is achieved, start reclining the length of the torso towards the front leg and clasp the feet.

BENEFITS
- Same as Hanumanasana.

- Stretches the length of the torso, benefiting the upper body and its organs.
- Releases the shoulders and the neck into a stretch.

CAUTION
- Make sure that the hip and the leg area are well warmed up.
- To achieve this asana, flexibility of the groin is important.

ENERGY FLOW
- Same as Hanumanasana but the twist in this asana creates a sideward energy pattern rather than an upward one.

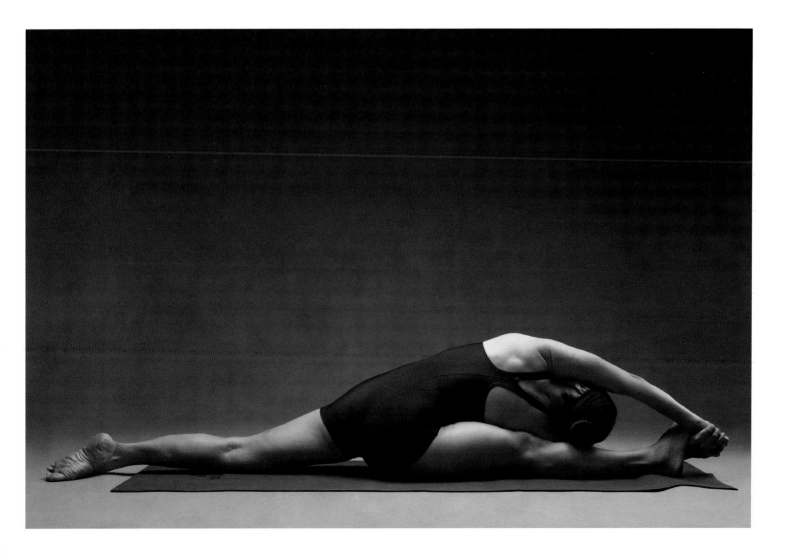

49. PARIVRTTA JANU SHIRSASANA
DRISHTI – Hastagrai

TIPS
- Sit firm without tilting.
- The chin should face upward, with the chest open.
- Widen the elbows; initiate the entire stretch from the armpit.
- The angle between the bent knee and the stretched leg should be obtuse.
- While extending the trunk, inhale and lift the ribs up so that more space is created in the abdomen.
- Stretch the knee that is touching floor even further, to maximise the extension of the trunk.
- The knees and the calf are to be pressed firmly into the ground, avoiding feet tilting towards the floor.

BENEFITS
- Balances and tones the liver and spleen.
- Aids digestion, activates the kidneys and tones the abdominal organs.
- Benefits people with enlarged prostate.
- Benefits people suffering from prolonged fever.
- Relieves stiffness in the legs, knees, hips, pelvis and develops suppleness around these areas.
- Eases the effects of stress on the heart and mind.
- Eases stiffness in the shoulders, hips, elbows and wrists.
- A good stretch to stimulate blood circulation to the spine.
- Relieves backaches and neck pains.
- Opens up the back and chest, benefiting respiration.

CAUTION
- If the trunk is not extending sufficient, do not jerk or over-stretch it. Instead, relax in the stretch and progress gradually.
- If the asana is difficult to achieve, use a strap to prevent the rounding of the shoulders and back. It will also aid to keep the spine straight and erect.
- Do not allow the knees to tilt and keep them evenly stretched on both sides to avoid injury along the hamstrings.

ENERGY FLOW
- The Muladhara Chakra, Manipura Chakra, Anahata Chakra and Vishuddha Chakra benefit from this asana.

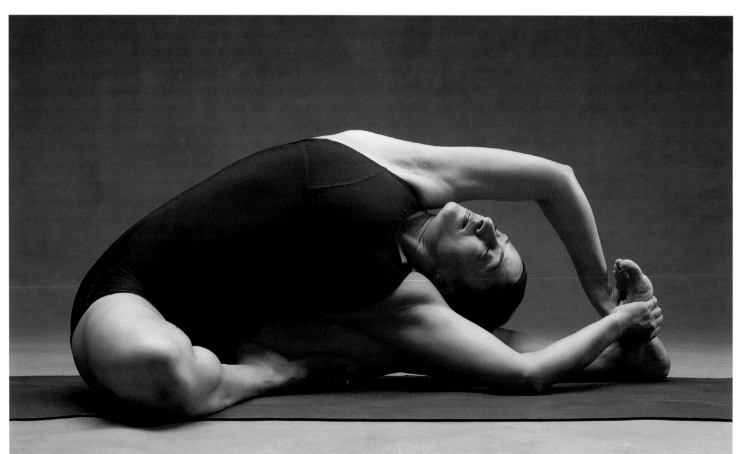

50. PARIVRTTA PARSVAKONASANA
DRISHTI – Hastagrai

TIPS
- Exhale completely before twisting the torso.
- Extend the arm from the armpit while placing it on the outer side of the opposite knee.
- Aim at crossing the arm and shoulder completely over the opposite thigh.
- Extend and rotate the chest upward, making sure the spine is stretched.
- Keep the gaze calm and forehead relaxed.

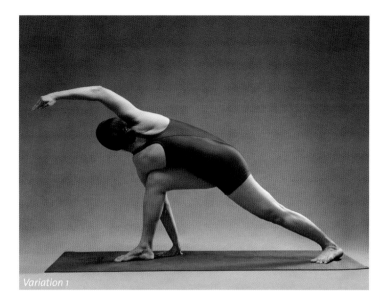

Variation 1

BENEFITS
- The lunge on one leg and deep stretching of the other leg creates a dynamic balance of strength and flexibility. It tones ankles, knees, and thighs.
- Reduces fat around the waist and hip.
- Contracts the abdominal organs which increases blood supply around them and the spinal column, thus rejuvenating the region.
- Increases peristaltic activity and aids elimination.

CAUTION
- Avoid this asana if you are feeling week in your knees.
- Avoid looking up in this asana if you have cervical spondylitis.
- Do not practise this asana if you have high blood pressure, a cardiac condition, palpitation, heartburn or dysentery.

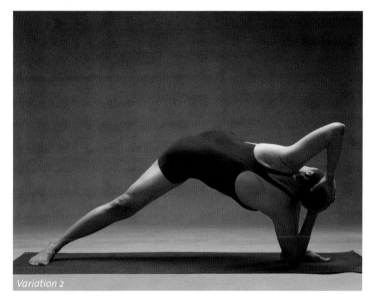

Variation 2

ENERGY FLOW
- The twisted position of the torso has major benefits on the Muladhara Chakra and Svadhisthana Chakra. The main flow of the energy, however, begins from the Muladhara Chakra, squeezing and rushing all the way to the Sahasrara Chakra, which, in this case, has an energising effect on the body.

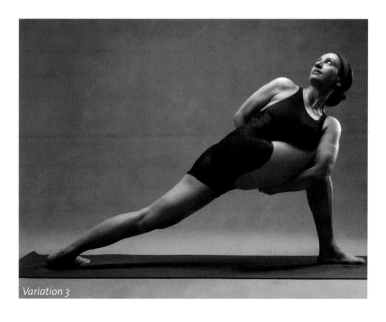

Variation 3

51. PARIVRTTA PRASARITA PADOTTANASANA
DRISHTI – Nasagrai

TIPS

- Bend the knees slightly to ease into the stretch and to release any strain, pain or pressure in the lower back. Straighten them gradually by tilting the hip towards the ceiling.
- Exhale slowly and pull the thighs deeply into the hip sockets.
- Free the neck muscles and drop the head towards the floor.
- Open the shoulders square and pull them away from the ears.
- Let the left hand grab the right toe and the right hand grab the left toe.
- Gently rotate the chest as if to point towards on side.

- To complete the asana, come up, change the crossing of hands and rotate the chest to the other side.

BENEFITS

- Helps develop hamstring and abductor muscles.
- Increases flexibility along the length of the trunk.
- Increases shoulder and neck flexibility.

CAUTION
- Avoid this asana if there is a problem of blood pressure.
- Do not attempt this asana after an upset stomach or dysentery.

ENERGY FLOW
- This asana activates the Manipura Chakra , Vishuddha Chakra and Svadhisthana Chakra.

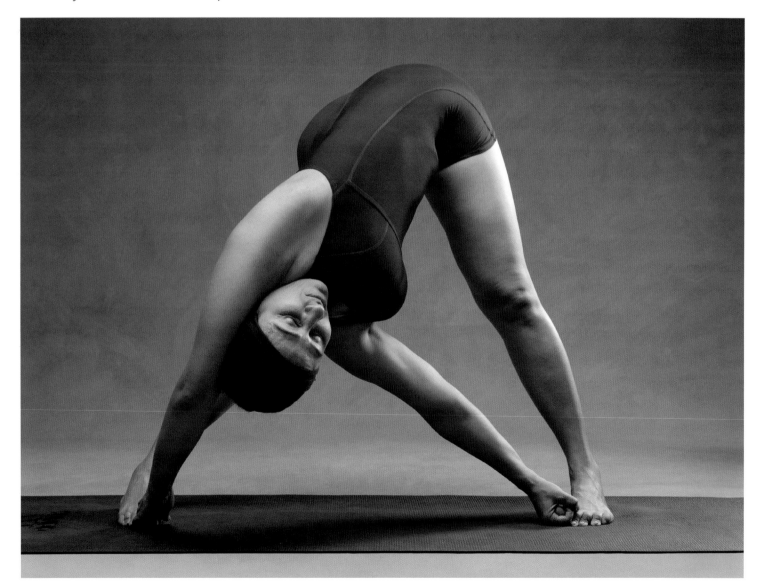

52. PARIVRTTA TRIKONASANA
DRISHTI – Hastagrai

TIPS
- While bending towards the right side, turn the left foot and hip to a 60° angle inward. Similarly, the right foot would turn in while bending towards the left side.
- The thigh muscles should be rotated inwards to ensure proper muscular support.
- Root the feet to the ground firmly.
- Keep the knee cap and the thigh muscles to be pulled, gently upward.
- Open / lengthen the chest skywards instead of stretching the arm backward.

BENEFITS
- Improves spinal health.
- Increases blood supply around the lower part of the spinal region.
- Invigorates the abdominal organs.
- Strengthens the leg and thigh muscles.
- Relieves pain in the back, invigorates the abdominal organs and strengthens the hip muscles.

CAUTION
- Do not practise this asana if you are recovering from dysentery or a stomach problem.
- Avoid this asana if you have a headache, migraine or cold.
- Do not look up in the asana if you are feeling tired.

ENERGY FLOW
- Energy is drawn up from the floor towards the twist of the torso into the chest and flows through the length of the arms.

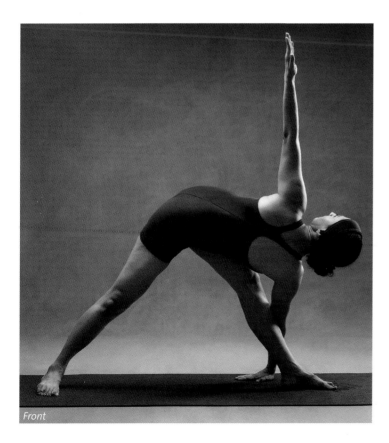
Front

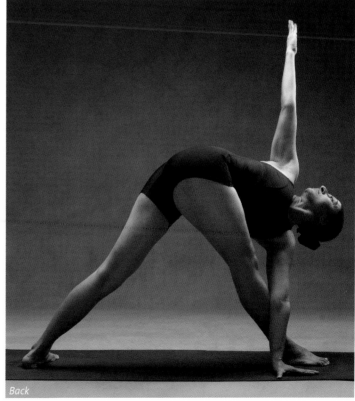
Back

53. PARIVRTTA UTKATASANA
DRISHTI – Urdhva

TIPS
- Stabilise the position of the hip.
- Swing open the chest and place the arm on the floor firmly.
- Pay attention to the length of the back and do not curve the back.
- Look up and away from the shoulder to the centre of the palm.

BENEFITS
- Corrects minor deformities in the legs.
- Removes stiffness from the shoulders.
- Makes ankles and calves strong.
- The diaphragm is lifted and makes space in the abdominal area which improves the peristaltic movement.
- Tones the abdomen and the abdominal organs.
- Benefits the heart as chest is completely open.

CAUTION
- Do not practise this asana with an upset stomach or just after a bout of dysentery
- Avoid the asana if you have a headache, migraine or cold.
- Do not look up in the asana if you are feeling lack of balance

ENERGY FLOW
- The energy required in holding this stretch is generated from the Muladhara Chakra. The energy thus produced benefits both the upper and the lower regions of the body. The Muladhara Chakra and Anahata Chakra enjoy maximum benefit of this asana.

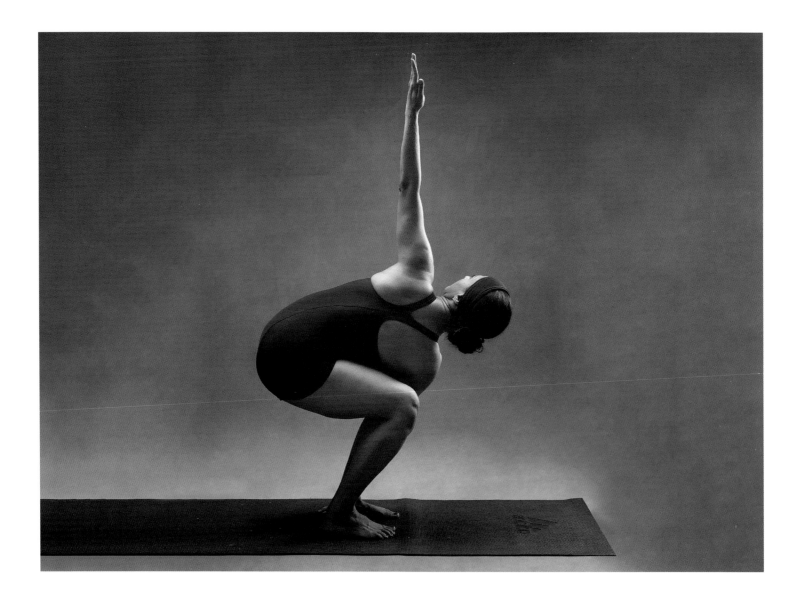

54. PARSVAKONASANA
DRISHTI – Hastagrai

TIPS
- Make sure the knee does not bend beyond the ankle limit; it should be in line with the back of the heel.
- Work the legs evenly, releasing them from the pelvis and the inner groin, stretching them away from one another to create a balance of energy in the posture.
- The length of the trunk should slowly be reclined on to the length of the thigh before placing the palm on the ground.
- Keep the chest expanded and the shoulders relaxed.

BENEFITS
- The lunge on one leg and deep stretching of the other leg creates a dynamic balance of strength and flexibility. It also tones ankles, knees and thighs.
- Stretches the chest and develops its width, thus benefiting the lung capacity and muscles around the heart.
- Reduces fat around the waist and hips and relieves sciatic and arthritic pain.
- Increases peristaltic activity and aids elimination.

CAUTION
- Avoid this asana if you feel weak in the knees.
- Avoid looking up in this asana if you have cervical spondylitis.
- Do not practise this asana if you have high blood pressure, a cardiac condition, palpitation, heartburn or dysentery.

ENERGY FLOW
- The stretched position of the torso and the open chest benefits all the chakras. The main flow begins from the Muladhara Chakra and goes all the way to the Sahasrara Chakra, which has a calming effect on the body.

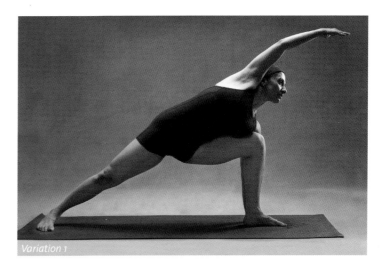

Variation 1

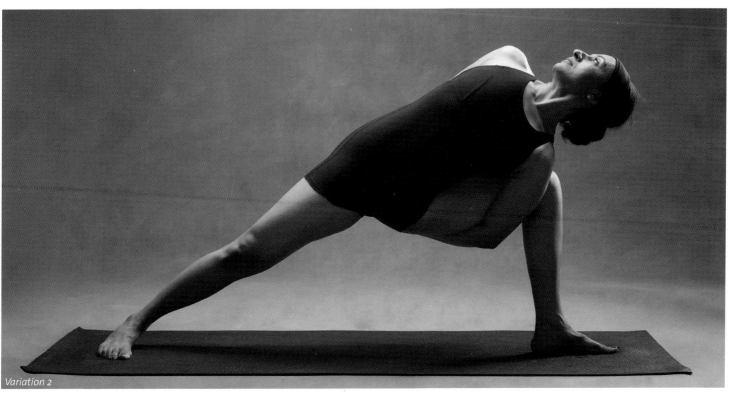

Variation 2

55. PARSVOTTANASANA
DRISHTI – Nasagrai

TIPS

- Open the soles of the feet and align them parallel to the one another.
- Turn the body in a coordinated motion along with rotation of the hips for perfect alignment.
- The hip, body, chest and face should be turned in the direction of the foot in the front.

BENEFITS

- Cools the brain and soothes the nerves.
- Relieves tightness in the hamstrings, strengthens leg muscles.
- Helps improve symmetry and balance of the pelvis and hips while strengthening them.
- Deepens the breathing and releases arthritic tension in the neck, shoulder area and wrist.
- Tones the liver and spleen.
- Reduces menstrual discomfort, especially in the back and abdominal region.

CAUTION

Do not attempt this asana if you have:
- Blood pressure or hernia.
- Just recovered from dysentery.

ENERGY FLOW

- Smooth flow of energy from the Muladhara Chakra to the Sahasrara Chakra is experienced in this asana.

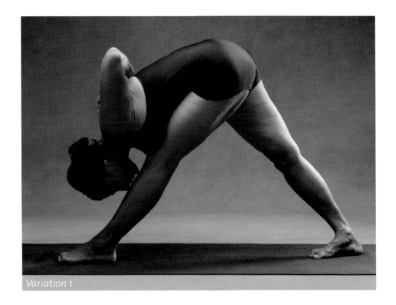
Variation 1

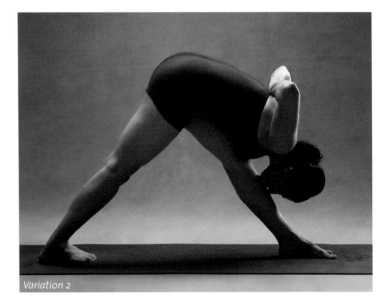
Variation 2

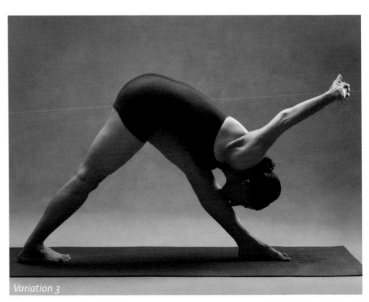
Variation 3

56. PARYANKASANA
DRISHTI – Nasagrai

TIPS
- Knees and ankles should have attained good flexibility to handle the stretch of this asana.
- Lean backward (recline) and place the elbow on the floor. The knees should remain touching the floor.
- Raise the chest up, expanding it towards the ceiling and stretch the neck backward and allow the crown to reach the floor slowly.
- Position the buttocks pushed towards the thighs and lengthen the trunk so that the stretch is well distributed.

BENEFITS
- The dorsal region is completely expanded, benefiting the lungs.
- The stretch in the neck energises the thyroid and parathyroid glands.

CAUTION
- Beginners could keep their knees apart until the knee caps and ankles achieve flexibility.
- If the asana is not comfortable on the floor, prepare by practising this asana on a soft base like a mattress. If this stretch is tried out on a hard floor, it could be injurious.
- Master Vajrasana and Veerasana before attempting this asana.

ENERGY FLOW
- The Vishuddha Chakra governs the function of the throat region, and the thyriod glands benefit from the energy produced by this chakra. This asana also relaxes the Ajna Chakra.

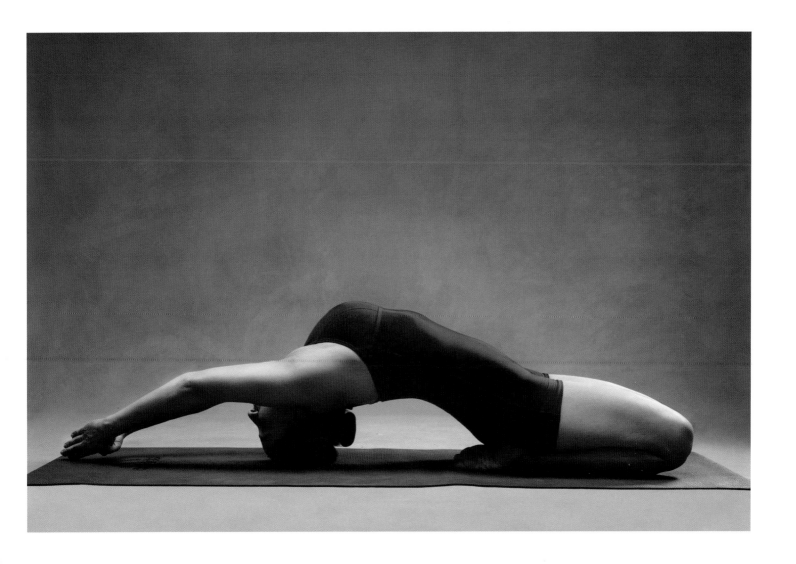

57. PASCHIMOTTANASANA
DRISHTI – Sama

TIPS
- Keep the spine straight while sitting with the legs stretched.
- Gently fold the body to rest along the length of the thigh.
- Do not pull the body forward as it will result in tension.
- Try not to hunch the back.
- Progress slowly to reach the nose to the knee.
- Keep tucking in the lower abdomen which lengthens the abdominal region, thus creating space for the fold.
- Exhale completely while bending forward.

BENEFITS
- Stretches the entire length of the back, making it the most important forward-bending asana.
- Prepares the spine for all forward-bending asanas.
- Benefits the abdominal organs as the length of the abdomen is maintained.
- Helps flexibility along the length of the legs.

CAUTION
This asana is an intense stretch for the back.
- Do not attempt this asana if the back is strained or weak.
- Do not pull the body forward as it results in injury of the lower back.
- Make sure this asana is done after loosening up the body with other asanas.
- Do not attempt this asana at the beginning of the day's practice.

ENERGY FLOW
- Activates all the chakras releasing a powerful flow of energy along the length of the spine. This asana, as it progresses into perfection, brings tranquility in the body.

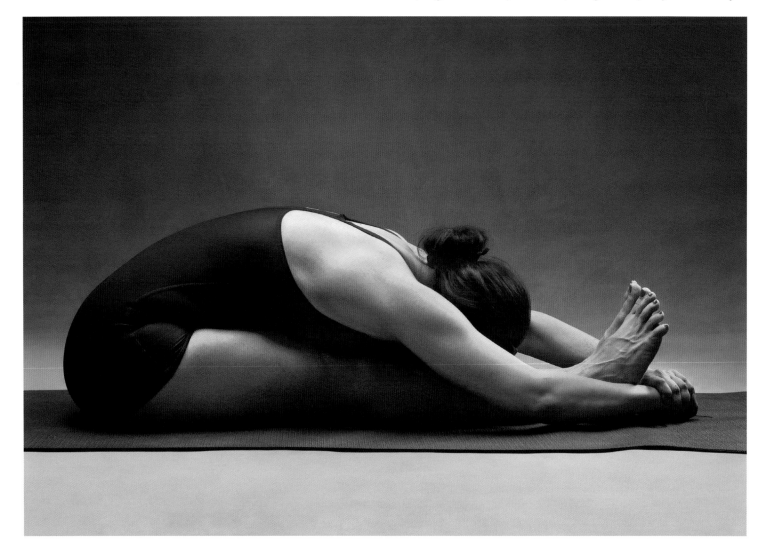

58. PASHASANA
DRISHTI – Parsva

TIPS
- Make sure the soles of your feet are completely rooted to the ground.
- Maintain balance by keeping the calves tight.
- Lean forward and keep the seat free so that twisting becomes comfortable.
- Keep the abdomen tucked in and the chest lifted up with the collarbones free for the twist.

BENEFITS
- Gives strength and balance to the feet.
- The ankles gain elasticity.
- Stretches the shoulders freely and expands the chest fully, benefiting the heart.
- Benefits the liver, spleen and the pancreas.
- Helps in reducing fat around the areaby compressing the abdomen.
- Massages the organs around the stomach area, which aids in digestion.

CAUTION
- Do not attempt this asana if the knees are weak.
- If the feet are not resting on the floor, keep a prop under the heels so that the asana does not strain the knee.
- Keep the back straight and not tilted forward.

ENERGY FLOW
- The twisted position of the body constricts the flow of energy while in the asana. Once the asana is released, it floods the chakras with strong prana energy.

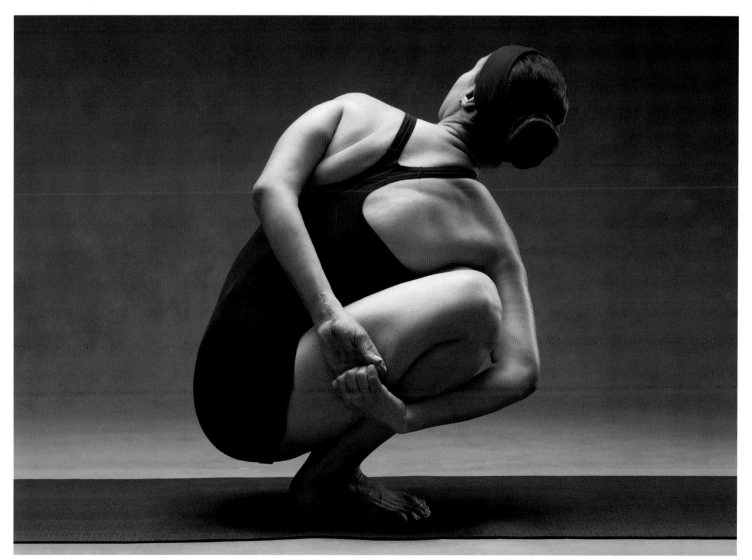

59. PINCHA MAYURASANA
DRISHTI – Nasagrai

TIPS
* When attempting the asana for the first time, face the wall and place the palm on the floor about a foot away, so that swinging the leg up would be against the wall. The wall will help check the momentum of the lifting legs.
* Once the balance is established in the above manner, practise this asana with no wall support.

BENEFITS
* Along with the benefits of an inverted asana, develops strength in the shoulders and the back.
* An entire body stretch that also tones the abdominal area.
* Builds focus and concentration.

CAUTION
* This is an extreme asana for the back, so make sure it is held steady.
* Attempt this asana closer to the wall until the asana becomes steady.

ENERGY FLOW
* All the chakras benefit from this asana.

NOTE
This challenging asana has lots of benefits but requires proper preparation. After adequate practice of all the basic asanas, the body gets tuned and ready for the Vishesha or extreme asanas. Master the Preceding asanas and Succeeding asanas mentioned below before attempting this asana.

Preceding asanas
Surya Namaskara, Natarajasana, Chakrasana, Adho Mukha Tadasana, Pincha Mayurasana

Succeeding asanas
Janu Shirsasana, Gomukhasana, Bharadwajasana, Sarvangasana , Halasana, Matsyasana

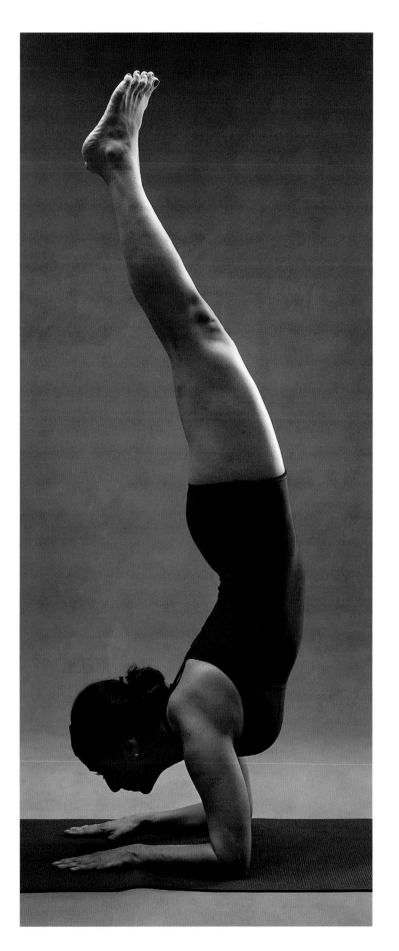

60. PINDASANA

DRISHTI – Nasagrai

TIPS

- From Karna Peedasana, release the knees and get into Padmasana. Use the hands to tuck in the feet.
- Once the balance is achieved by holding Mula Bandha, pull in the lower abdomen and wraps the hands around the Padmasana.

BENEFITS

- Same as in Halasana.
- However, the spine is stretched more as the knees are bent and this helps more circulation of the blood around the area.
- The sacrum opens up, thus relaxing it and the muscles around the area.
- Greatly benefits the abdominal organs.

CAUTION

- Breathing could be difficult in this challenging asana. However, it is very important to focus on breathing while in the asana.
- Do not attempt to wrap the hands around the legs until the balance is achieved. Otherwise the neck could get injured.

ENERGY FLOW

- Same as Karna Peedasana.

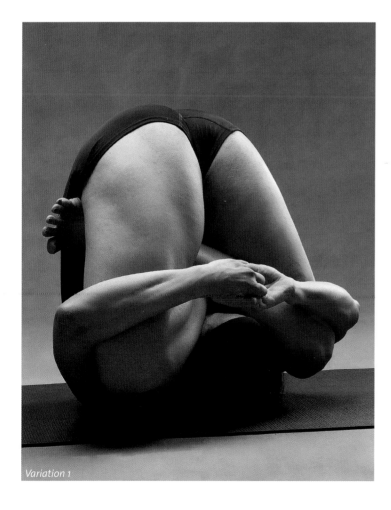

Variation 1

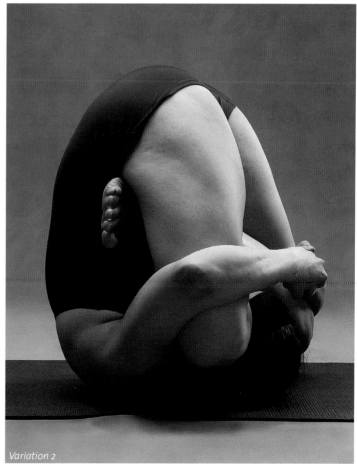

Variation 2

61. PRASARITA PADOTTANASANA
DRISHTI – Nasagrai

TIPS
- Bend the knees slightly to ease into the stretch and to release any strain / pain / pressure in the lower back.
- Straighten them gradually by tilting the hip towards the ceiling.
- Exhale slowly and pull the thighs deeply into the hip sockets.
- Free the neck muscles and drop the head towards the floor.
- Open the shoulders square and pull them away from the ears.
- Lengthen the spine, focusing on opening the chest and stretching forward.
- Stimulates digestive power and internal cleansing.

BENEFITS
- Helps develop hamstring and abductor muscles.
- Helps blood flow to the brain as in Shirsasana.

CAUTION
- Avoid this asana if there is a problem of blood pressure.
- Do not attempt this asana after an upset stomach or dysentery.

ENERGY FLOW
- All the chakras from the Sahasrara Chakra to the Muladhara Chakra benifit from this asana.

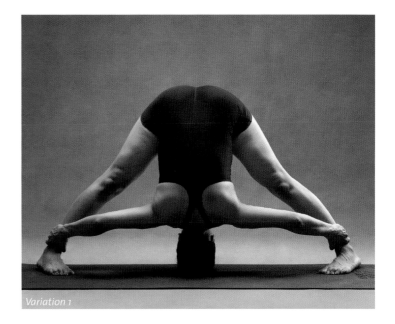
Variation 1

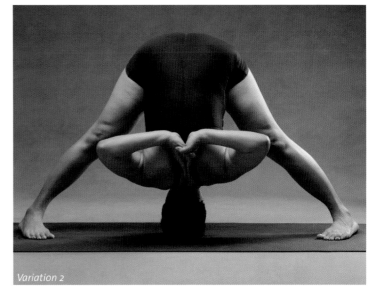
Variation 2

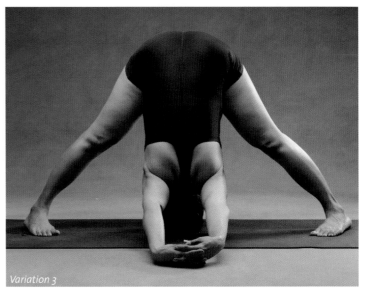
Variation 3

62. PURVOTTANASANA
DRISHTI – Sama

TIPS
- Make sure that the palms are placed shoulder-width apart and keep the fingers open for a good grip and support.
- If lifting the hip gets difficult, bend the knees, place the soles of the feet on the floor and then attempt to lift the hip.
- Keep the elbows and knees stretched to keep the asana steady.
- Keep the abdominal area tucked in and glutes tightened to strengthen the stretch.
- Strongly lift the chest up as it should be completely open and the neck comfortably thrown back.
- Breathing should be deep, calm and steady throughout the stretch.

BENEFITS
- A counter-asana for most of the forward-bending asanas.
- Strengthens the arms and the wrists.
- Stretches the entire length of the leg and spine.
- Lengthenes and stretches the front of the body, thus lifting the heart above the level of the spine, improving circulation around the area.
- Strengthens the muscles of the chest, shoulders and the back.
- Tones the abdominal organs.

CAUTION
- Avoid this asana if you have a cardiac condition, constipation or gastric issues.
- Do not attempt this asana in the advanced stages of pregnancy.

ENERGY FLOW
- All the chakras are highly activated in this asana.

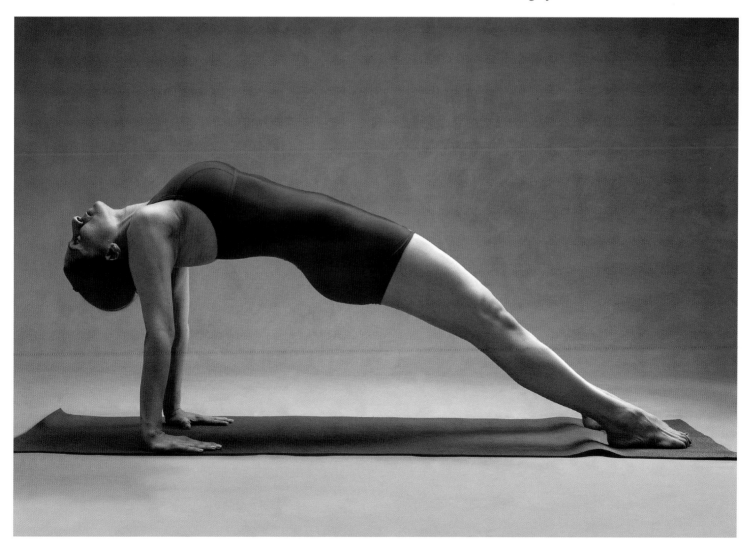

63. SAMASTHITI
DRISHTI – Sama

TIPS
- Stand straight with folded hands.
- Keep the face calm and eyes closed.
- Focus on distributing equally the weight of the body around the mounds of the feet and the centre of the heel while engaging the arches.
- Pay attention to the line of your ankles, knees, hipbones, which should be in alignment with the collarbones.
- Also, focus on the lower abdomen and pull the pelvis in and up.
- Once the position is formed, release the tension from the length of the body and breath deep and easy.

BENEFITS
- Marks the point of preparation for any asana.
- Builds focus, concentration and mindful preparation.
- Centers and roots the body to earth.
- Focuses on straightening and lengthening every area of the body and tones the muscles of the body.
- The slow build-up of the asana helps memorise the correct alignment of the body.

CAUTION
- Close your eyes once the balance in the body is established and the feet are rooted.
- If there is a problem of balance, stand close to a wall and practise this asana.

ENERGY FLOW
- Aligns and arranges all the chakras.

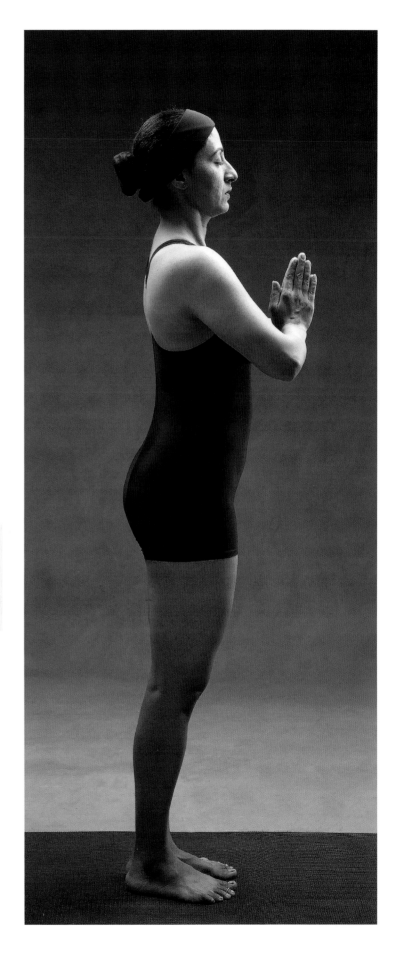

64. SANTULANASANA
DRISHTI – Hastagrai

TIPS

- Open the soles of the feet and align them parallel to each other.
- 'Santulana' means balance and poise.
- Fold the right leg backward, gently pulling it towards the buttocks and point the knees towards the floor.
- Gently stretch the hand upward towards the ceiling. Fix the gaze to the centre of the palm.

BENEFITS

- Helps build focus.
- Grounding of the toes to the floor aids in establishing balance and poise.

CAUTION
- Do not look up if you have a head ache or a migraine
- Keep hip position in a straight line.

ENERGY FLOW

- When the hand is lifted and the gaze points towards the tip of the fingers, it energises the Vishuddha Chakra.
- Balancing asanas align the body and, therefore, all the chakras align themselves, creating steadiness in the body and mind.

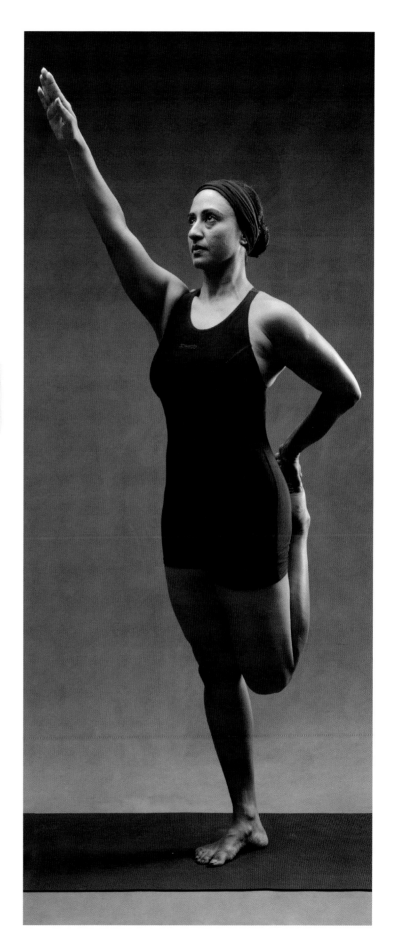

65. SARVANGASANA
DRISHTI – Nasagrai

TIPS
* Keep the knees and the feet together.
* Keep the buttocks tight to help hold the hip position steady.
* If there is difficulty in breathing, it could be because the torso is not aligned to the chest and neck. If so, push the waist, hip and thighs upward, then adjust the shoulder and chest and do not allow the hip to drop down.
* Keep the elbows close to the body so that they support the chest better.
* Press the palm firmly into the back if the torso can be stretched further.
* Feel the lift of the body from the back of the neck.

BENEFITS
* The inversion of the body boosts the circulatory and the respiratory systems.
* Nourishes the cells and the nervous system of the body.
* Helps relieve insomnia and soothes the nerves.
* Improves the functioning of the thyroid and parathyroid glands.
* Relieves breathlessness and throat disorders.
* Helps treatment for allergies like colds and sinus.
* Improves bowel movements.
* Alleviates urinary disorders.
* Helps treat problems pertaining to the uterus and reduces uterine fibroids.
* Relieves blockages and heaviness in the ovaries. Benefits in the treatment of ovarian cysts.
* Reduces menstrual cramps and helps regulate menstrual flow.

CAUTION
* If holding the asana for more than a minute, make sure to place a blanket under the shoulders
* Only the back, shoulders and the back of the neck should be in contact with the blanket.
* Do not practise this asana with an upset stomach or diarrhoea, as this asana helps relieve constipation.
* People suffering from high blood pressure should avoid this asana.

ENERGY FLOW
* The energy from the Muladhara Chakra directly flows through all the other chakras to the Vishuddha Chakra.

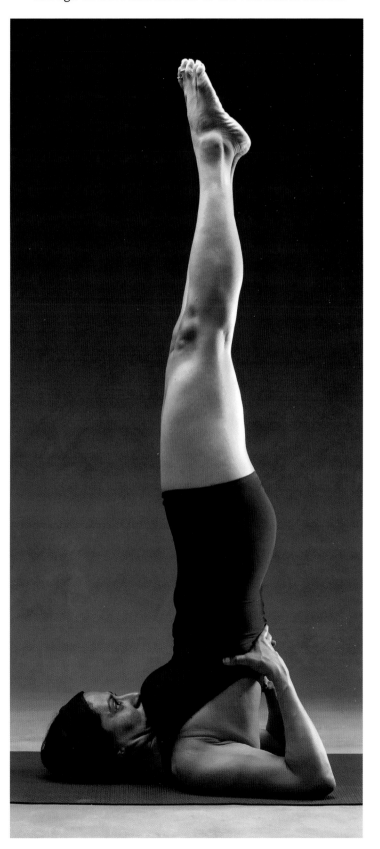

66. SETHUBANDHASANA
DRISTHI – Nasagrai

TIPS

- It is possible to lessen the weight of the body on the elbows and the wrists by stretching the spine towards the neck, keeping the heels firmly on the ground.
- Keep the chin tucked firmly into the chest.
- Keep the sternum lifted up.
- Draw the spine up and in.

BENEFITS

- Gives an intense spinal stretch which helps prepare the back for a Dhanurasana.
- Strengthens the neck, dorsal, lumber, sacral and back thigh muscle
- The expansion of the chest and front ribs opens the heart to stimulate circulation and increases the lung capacity.
- Helps promote healthy blood circulation along the length of the body.
- Tones the spine.
- Strengthens the abdominal and pelvic organs.
- Stimulates the pituitary, pineal and thyroid glands.
- Regular practice before the menstrual cycle will help prevent excess menstrual flow and eases menstrual cramps.
- Prevents prolapse of the uterus.

CAUTION

- Do not practise this asana with an injured neck.

ENERGY FLOW

- This asana benefits the Muladhara Chakra, Svadhisthana Chakra, Manipura Chakra, Anahata Chakra, Vishuddha and Ajna Chakra. The downward flow of the chakra energy from the Muladhara Chakra benefits all the glands of the body.

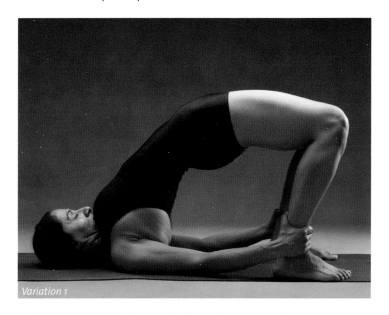
Variation 1

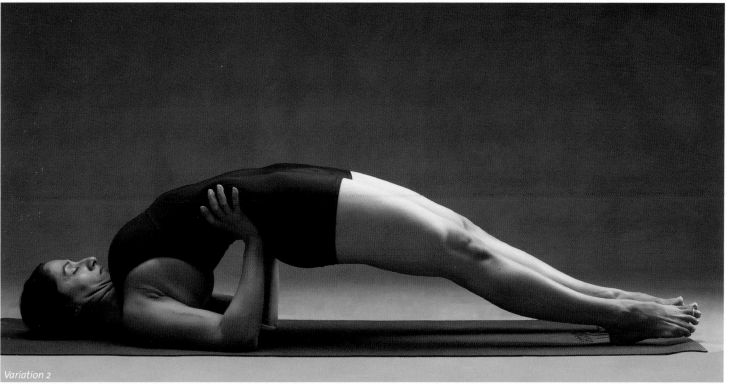
Variation 2

67. SHALABHASANA
DRISHTI – Nasagrai

TIPS
- Ease into the stretch with the legs slightly bent and then extend the legs powerfully from the glutes to hold in the position.
- A slight inward push of the glutes would help a better lift of the thigh.
- Strengthen the abdominal muscles by breathing out completely and pressing the navel right into the ribs.
- Press the forehead to the floor to achieve balance and then lengthen the chest up.
- Take support of your fist or palms under the thigh to hold in position.

BENEFITS
- Aids in digestion and relieves gastric trouble and flatulence.
- The spine is stretched backward which increases blood circulation and strengthens the spine.
- Benefits people suffering from slip disc.
- Benefits the bladder and the prostate gland.
- Relieves back pain.
- Builds stamina.

CAUTION
- Do not force the lift too much as it effects breathing.
- This asana cannot be practised during pregnancy.

ENERGY FLOW
- The Muladhara Chakra, Svadhisthana Chakra, Manipura Chakra and Anahata Chakra benefit from this asana.

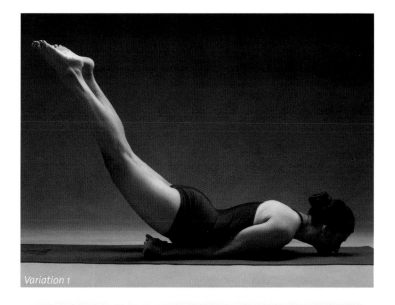
Variation 1

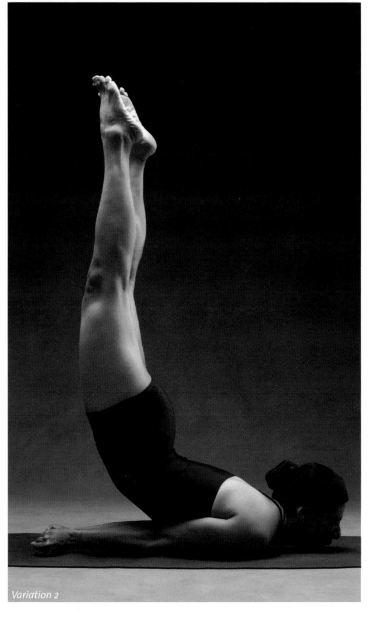
Variation 2

68. SHAYANASANA
DRISHTI – Sama

TIPS

- Lie face down on the floor. Stretch the entire length of the body with a forward movement before turning to the side.
- Carefully bend the knee and grab the toes. Extend the leg towards the ceiling until the leg is completely stretched upward.
- Constantly stabilise the hip by tucking the pelvis in and keeping the navel tucked in.

BENEFITS

- The stretch in the pelvic region relaxes the muscles of the area.
- The organs around the area get good blood supply, thus benefiting the reproductive and digestive organs.
- Relieves menstrual cramps and leg cramps.

CAUTION

- Make sure the hip bones are in line with the shoulders and not tilted either forward or backward.
- Keep the abdominal muscles pulled in to keep the hip strong.

ENERGY FLOW

- The Muladhara Chakra freely releases energy to other chakras, especially the Svadhisthana Chakra.

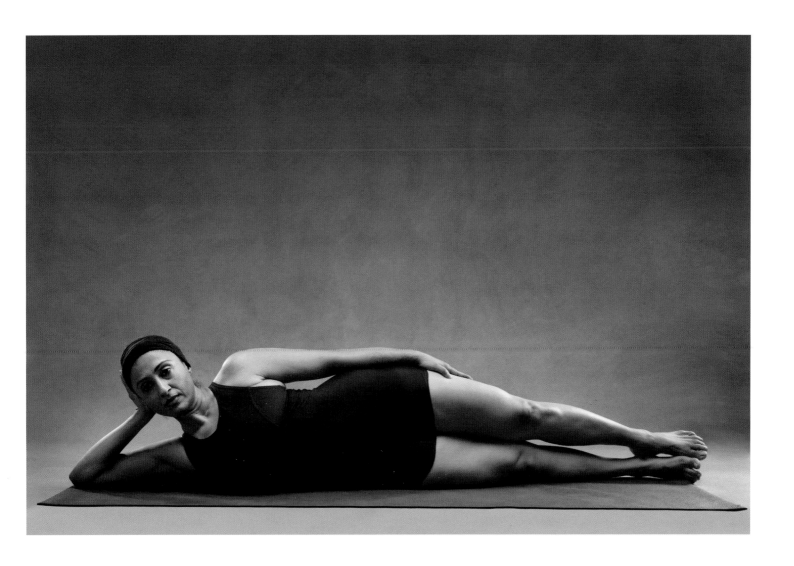

69. SHIRSASANA
DRISHTI – Sama

TIPS
- Keep the elbows shoulder-distance apart and the entire forearms pressed firmly to the ground.
- Keep the shoulders drawn away from the ears to release the weight of the body from the crown, which then naturally shifts to the forearms.
- Swing the legs off the ground with the knees bent; both the feet should leave the ground simultaneously.
- The whole body should remain perpendicular to the ground.
- When practising this asana while taking the support of the wall, make sure you are not too far from it. Leave only 2 to 3 inches space between the wall and the head. If the distance is greater, the spine shall curve and the stomach shall protrude.
- Once the proper head stand is achieved, it is advisable to come down to the floor with the legs straight, without bending the knees, which helps gauge the Mula power. Do not fear the fall as it is not as bad as we imagine.

BENEFITS
- Makes healthy, pure blood flow through the brain cells.
- Ensures proper blood supply to the pituitary and pineal glands in the brain.
- Increases the haemoglobin content in the blood.
- Improves conditions like insomnia, memory loss, etc.
- The lungs gain the power to resist climatic changes

CAUTION
- The head should not feel too heavy. If this occurs, the face will become flushed and the eyes may turn red. This will happen only when the centre of the head is not placed properly and the weight of the body may be more towards the front or the back of the head.
- Beginners, who fall in this asana, should practise it only once a week and then progress to a regular practice once the balance is achieved.
- A wrong posture may lead to aches and pains in the head, neck, shoulders and back.
- Do not practise this asana if you have high or low blood pressure.
- Avoid the asana if you have a regular condition of headaches, migraines, shoulder ache or spondylitis.
- The asana is dangerous if you have a cardiac condition.

- Provides relief from cold, cough, tonsillitis, foul breath and palpitations.
- Relieves digestive and eliminatory problems.

ENERGY FLOW
- The Sahasrara Chakra benefits from this asana.

NOTE
Do not practise the variations if the basic Shirsasana is not steady and is causing pain in the neck. The head should not feel all the weight of the body. The weight of the body has to be distributed along the length of the forearm, triceps, the entire length of the neck along with the shoulders.

Practise the basic Shirsasana for at least 5 months before you start attempting the variations.

Try one at a time and hold the position for at least 1 minute.

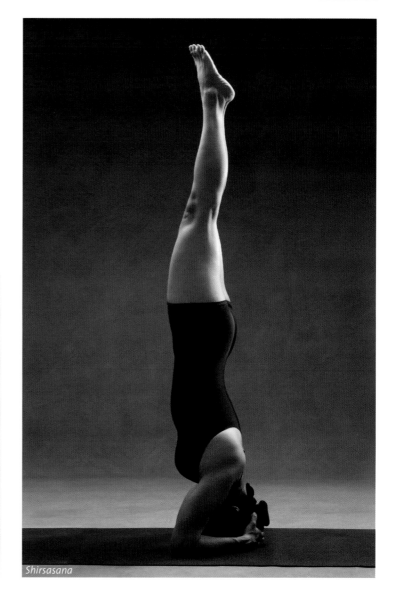
Shirsasana

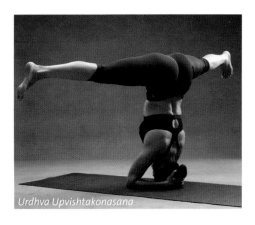

Urdhva Upvishtakonasana

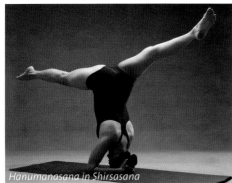

Hanumanasana in Shirsasana

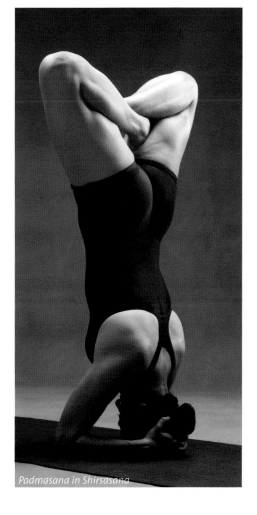

Padmasana in Shirsasana

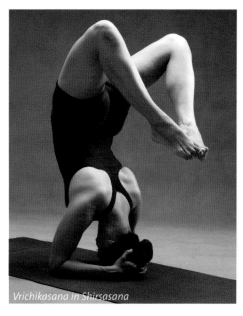

Vrichikasana in Shirsasana

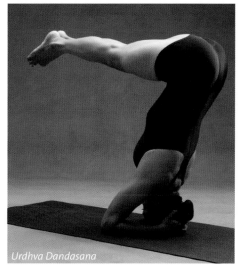

Urdhva Dandasana

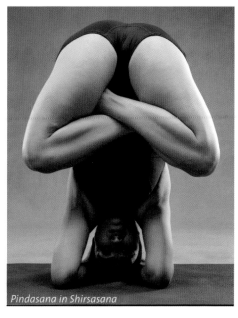

Pindasana in Shirsasana

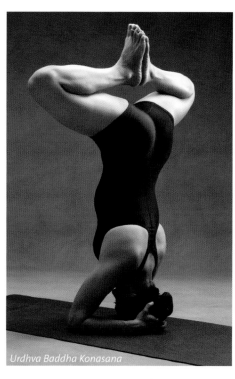

Urdhva Baddha Konasana

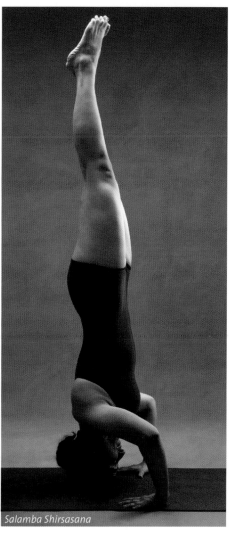

Salamba Shirsasana

70. SIMHASANA
DRISHTI – Sama

TIPS
- Lift the hip up and slide the body forward while maintaining Padmasana.
- The hip bones should remain parallel to the ground.
- Lift the chest up and keep the palm pressed to the ground.
- Inhale and exhale in equal ratio (5:5) deep breathing in Ujjayee.

BENEFITS
- Breathing out from the mouth, making the sound of a roar or a storm, releases stress from the body.
- Expands the chest for deep breathing.
- Expands the hip bones, benefiting the abdomen and intestines.
- Helps the liver function better, as the asana lifts the midriff up, releasing stress from the area around the liver.

CAUTION
- Do not attemp this asana if you are not comfortable in Padmasana.

ENERGY FLOW
- All chakras are activated in this asana. The body expands, allowing good energy movement.

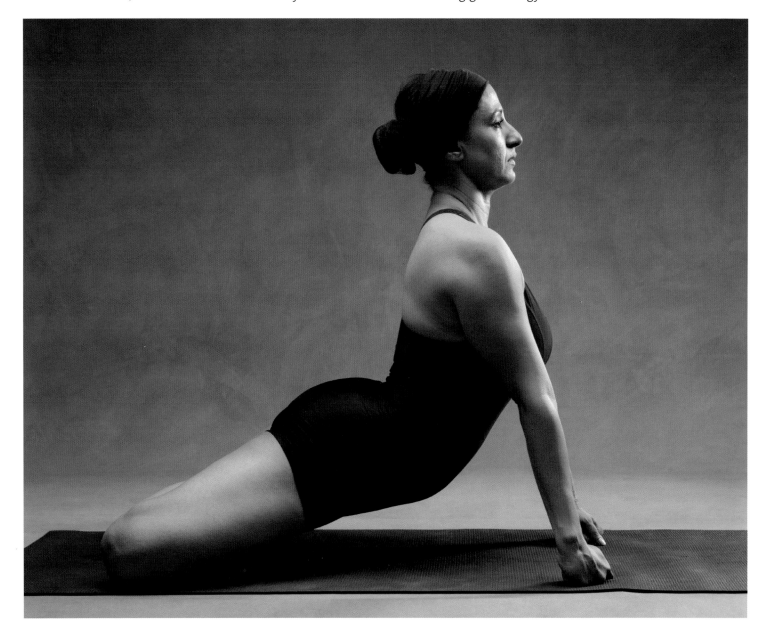

71. SUPTA PADANGUSTASANA
DRISHTI – Padayoragrai

TIPS
- Keep the shoulders pressed to the floor, with the chest open and the back of the head resting on the floor comfortabley.
- As you progress in the stretch, engage the Uddiyana Bandha by flattening the abdominal wall down, while the chin is brought closer to the shin.
- As in all the asanas, both sides of the body have to be worked on with equal strength and flexibility.
- Keep the bandhas in place all through the asana. This will help in stabilising the asana.

BENEFITS
- The intense stretch of the legs increases blood circulation along the leg muscles.
- The lift and the rotation of the leg promote balance, flexibility and strength.
- Helps maintain stillness of the mind, as the focus of this stretch is intense.

CAUTION
- Prepare well for this asana with the Preceding asanas so that the muscles of the legs are warmed up sufficient.
- If you have suffered a back injury, this asana can be a little challenging as you will have to be sure that your back has regained its alignment. Try by keeping the knee bent and pressed towards the chest for a few sessions until you feel confident of the abdominal length and realignment of the hip.

- Helps harness sexual energy.
- Benefits people suffering from sciatica and paralysis of the legs.
- The nerves around the hip and back receive ample blood circulation, making them very strong and supple.

ENERGY FLOW
- All the chakras are relaxed in this asana.

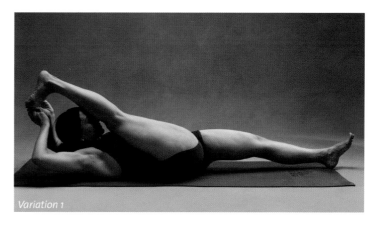
Variation 1

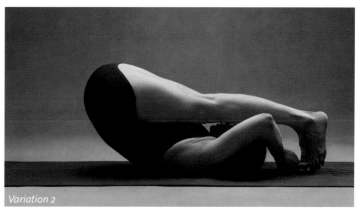
Variation 2

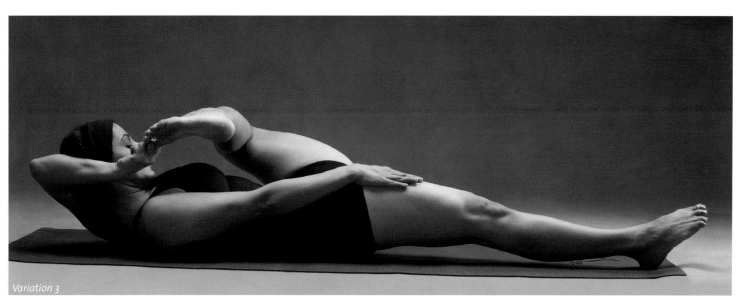
Variation 3

72. SUPTA TRIVIKRAMASANA
DRISHTI – Sama

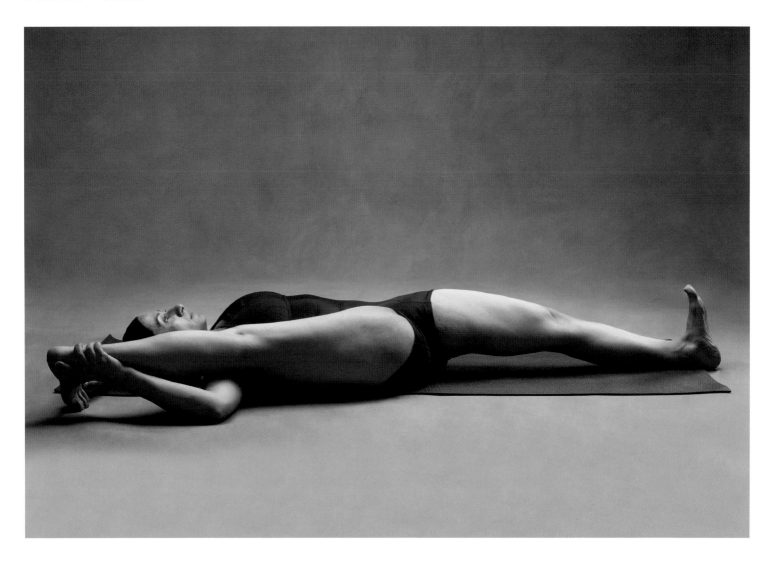

TIPS
- The inner side of the lifted leg's calf should stay along the length of the right ear.
- Ease into the stretch slowly and gradually.
- Keep breathing in the stretch.

BENEFITS
- Stretches the legs fully.
- Prevents hernia and sciatica pains.
- Improves flexibility and strength along the area of the groin and keeps them healthy.
- Lessens sexual desire, if you are preparing for meditation.

CAUTION
- Sufficient warm-up and preparations have to be done before attempting this asana.

ENERGY FLOW
- This asana energises the Muladhara Chakra and Svadhisthana Chakra the most, while the other chakras also benefit from this stretch.

73. SUPTA VEERASANA
DRISHTI – Sama

TIPS
- From Veerasana, recline backward with elbow support towards the floor and rest the shoulders on the floor.
- If there is a curve in the lower back, slide the buttocks towards the thighs and relax the muscles of the shoulders, legs and thighs.

BENEFITS
- Relaxes strained muscles and tones them.
- Stretches the hip bone and benefits the digestive system and reproductive organs.
- Relaxes the glutes.

CAUTION
Do not attempt this asana if:
- The lower back is strained.
- The knees are strained.

ENERGY FLOW
- The backward stretch is highly beneficial for all the chakras of the body as it relaxes them and rejuvenates their task of producing optimum energy.

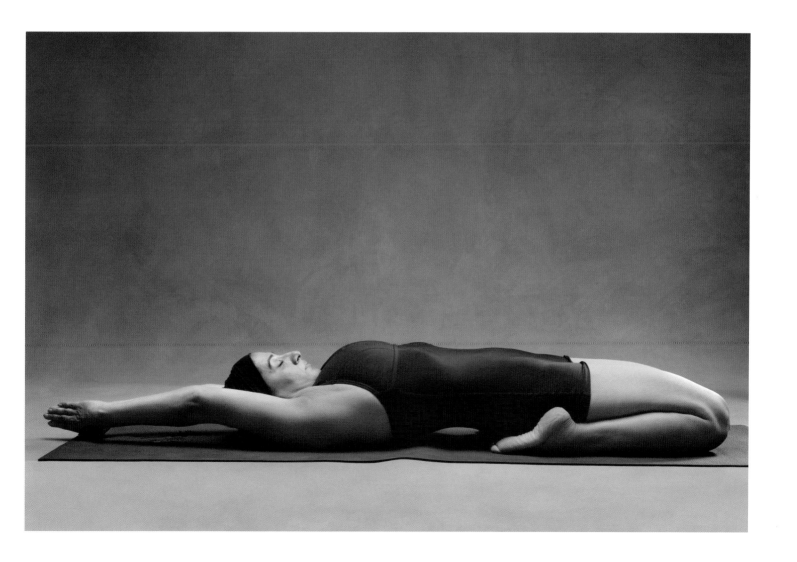

74. TADASANA
DRISHTI – Sama

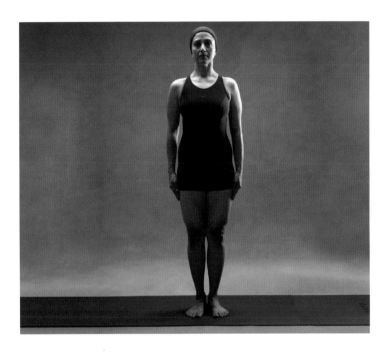

TIPS
* Focus on placing the weight of the body on the arches of the feet.
* Pay attention to the line of your ankles, knees and hip bone, which should be in alignment with the collarbones.
* Pay attention to the lower abdomen and pull it in and up.

BENEFITS
* The body is centered and rooted to earth, thus making the body aware of gravity.
* Focuses on straightening and lengthening every area of the body and tones the muscles of the body.
* The slow build-up of the asana helps memorise the correct alignment of the body.

CAUTION
* Do not close eyes if the balance of the body is not established or if the feet do not feel rooted.
* If there is a problem of balance, stand close to a wall and practise this asana.

ENERGY FLOW
* This asana energises the Muladhara Chakra and Svadhisthana Chakra the most, while the other chakras also benefit from this stretch.

75. TANDAVASANA
DRISHTI –Sama

TIPS
* Try getting into this asana after Prasarita Padottanasana.
* Open the feet and rotate the thigh muscles before lowering the hip to be in line with the knees.
* Tuck in the sacrum and then attempt straightening the spine tall towards the ceiling.
* Keep the thighs and calves strong and do not lift the body along with the torso.

BENEFITS
* Strengthens the groin, legs and the lower back.
* The floor muscles are challenged with the weight of the body, which benefits the reproductive and digestive organs.

CAUTION
* Do not attempt this asana from a Tadasana position to avoid strain on the knees.
* Keep the Muladhara Chakra pulled in as it is a complete stretch of the groin. Therefore, the floor muscles play an important role in strengthening the position.
* Do not attempt this asana in the beginning stages of pregnancy.

ENERGY FLOW
* In this asana, the Muladhara Chakra releases energy flow along the spine, thus benefiting all the chakras.

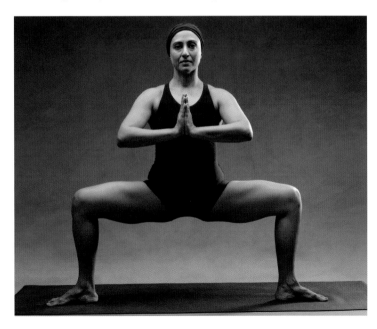

76. TITTIBASANA
DRISHTI – Sama

TIPS

- Start this asana from Adho Mukha Svanasana and then jump closer to the palms and wrap the legs around the palms.
- Do not lift the hip too high while trying to position the body.
- Keep the abdominal muscles contracted and maintain the length of the front of the body.
- Try to release the hunch in the back while lifting the legs forward off the floor to get in a straight line with the shoulders.

BENEFITS

- Strengthens the arms and shoulders.
- Tones the abdominal muscles.
- Especially beneficial to the intestines, making them stronger and function better.
- Provides flexibility along the length of the legs.

CAUTION

- Do not attempt this asana if the arms and wrists are not strong.
- Do not allow the head to droop down from the spine. That could make the body topple while attempting the lift.
- To avoid a fall, keep the drishti fixed to a point all the time.

ENERGY FLOW

- From the Muladhara Chakra, the source, energy flows to all chakras that immensely benefit from this asana.

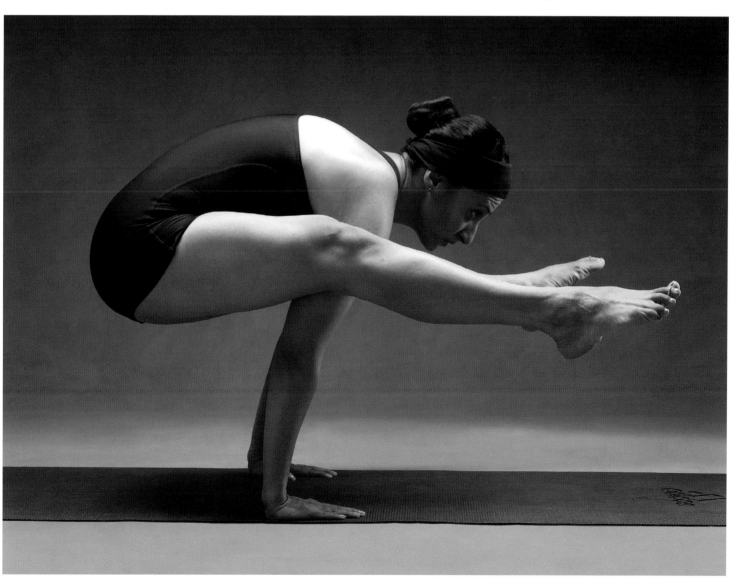

77. TOLASANA / UTH PLUTHI
DRISHTI – Nasagrai

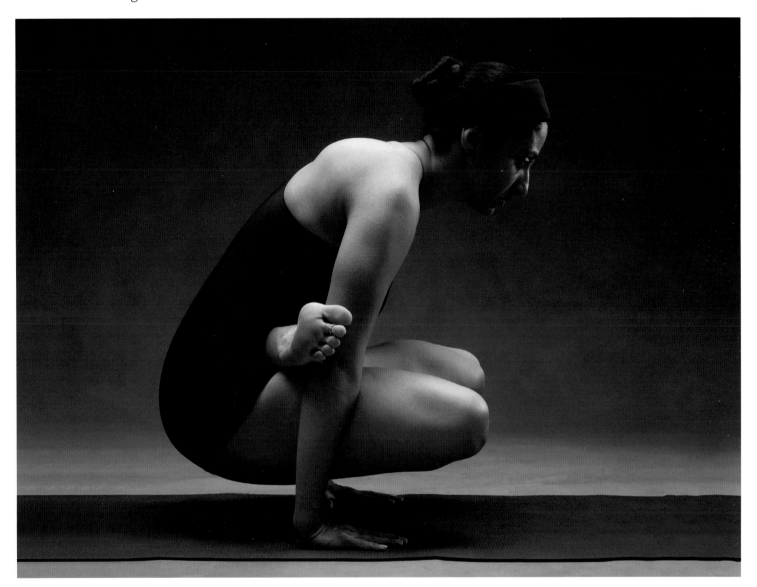

TIPS
- The point of lift in this stretch is the core. Maintain Uddiyana Bandha just before you lift the buttocks off the floor.
- Keep the breathing deep in Ujjayee as the strength and the energy flow are increased, which helps the hip float. (The swinging movement makes Uth Pluthi the Tolasana.)

BENEFITS
- Strengthens the arms, wrist and hands.
- Builds strength along the abdominal wall, increasing the core power.

CAUTION
- Get comfortable in Padmasana before you practise Tolasana.
- The strength in the arms and wrists have to be worked on before attempting this asana.
- Master Navasana to build up the core strength as that is the power behind this asana.

ENERGY FLOW
- The energy is bound to the inner body to help get the power to lift and swing. However, once the asana is released, the energy rushes to all parts of the body giving a sense of great calm and serenity. The Muladhara Chakra and the Svadhisthana Chakra benefit from these asanas.

78. TRIANGA MUKHAPEEDA PASCHIMOTTANASANA
DRISHTI – Bhoomigrai

TIPS

- Push the trunk forward from the length of the chest and try to press the entire body on to the length of the leg.
- Do not rest the elbows on the floor.
- Keep the buttocks squarely pressed to the ground. If the body naturally tilts, try keeping the torso strong in place which would control the tilt. Eventually, as the flexibility increases, the hip will be stable sufficient not to tilt.

BENEFITS

- Helps straighten the drooping curvature of the back.
- Relieves stiffness in the legs, knees, hips, pelvis and develops suppleness around the area.
- Balances and tones the liver, spleen and kidney.
- Benefits people with an enlarged prostate.
- Benefits people suffering from prolonged fever.

CAUTION

- A sharp pain in the knee indicates that you are not prepared for this level of deep stretch. If this occurs, sit on a cushion and try this stretch until the knee gets used it. If the asana is difficult to achieve, use a strap to prevent rounding of the shoulders and back. It will also help to keep the spine erect.
- Do not allow the knees to tilt and keep them evenly stretched on both sides to avoid injury along the hamstrings.

ENERGY FLOW

- All the chakras benefit from this stretch.

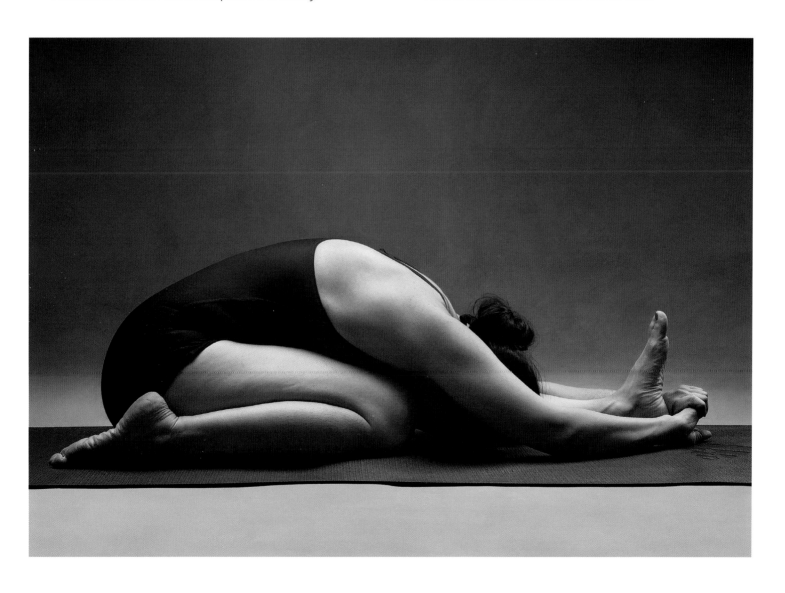

79. TRIANGA MUKOTTANASANA
DRISHTI – Urdhva

TIPS
- Stand comfortably with the feet a foot apart.
- Keep Sama Drishti throughout the contraction of the spine backward.
- Start with opening the hip and leaning backward.
- Then work on expanding the chest by completely stretching the hand downwards to take support in the back of the calves or thigh.
- After the chest is completely lifted up, look up, stretching the neck backward.

BENEFITS
- Prepares the spine to curve backward.
- A good asana to practise before attempting advanced back-bending asanas.
- Expands the chest completely.

CAUTION
- It is important to do a forward bend after this asana (Prasarita Padottanasana).
- Do not bend the knees in an attempt to get more curve at the back as this asana does not need intense curve. It is more about working on strength rather than flexibility.
- Monitor that the breathing is comfortable throughout the asana build-up and during the hold.

ENERGY FLOW
- The Manipura Chakra opens up, benefiting the Anahata chakra.
- The Muladhara Chakra senses a control which optimises the chakra functions once the asana is released.
- The Vishuddha Chakra is energised with deep breathing.

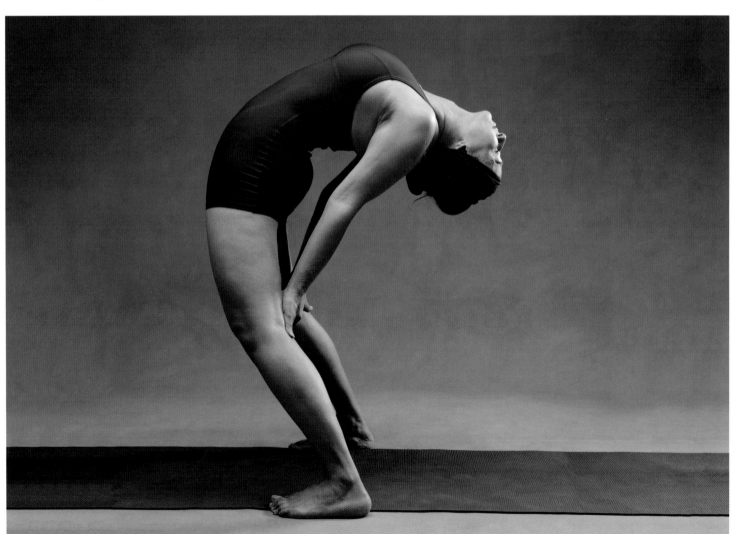

80. TRIKONASANA
DRISHTI – Hastagrai

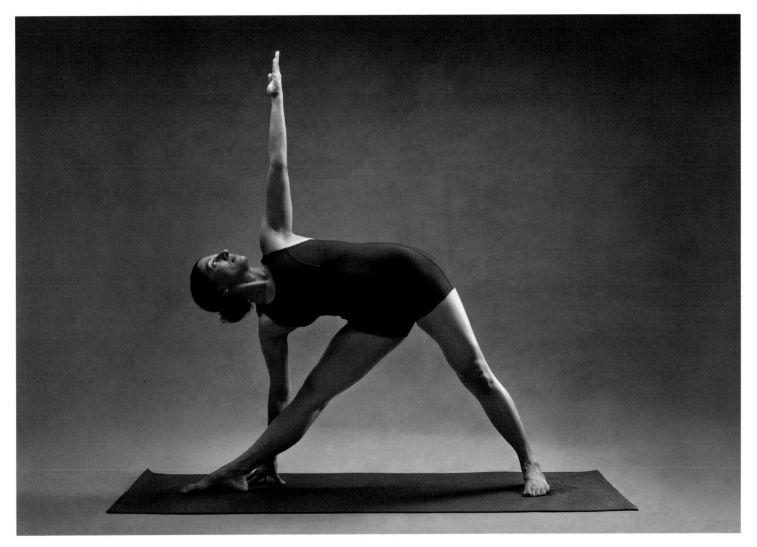

TIPS
- Keep the chest open and not tilted forward or inwards.
- Maintain the arms in a straight line towards the sky.
- Keep the sacrum tucked in and the hip rotated backward.
- Do not rest your body weight on the arm stretched towards the floor.

BENEFITS
- The lateral stretch in this asana improves flexibility of the hip, torso and the spine.
- Tones the leg muscles, removes stiffness in the legs and corrects any minor deformity of the legs.
- Relieves tightness in the neck.
- Stretches the shoulders and aligns the length.
- Provides relief from gas and flatulence.
- Reduces menstrual cramps.

CAUTION
- Do not look up if you experience slight dizziness due to the lateral rush of blood.
- Do not look up if you suffer from vertigo / blood pressure too should avoid looking up.
- Do not hold the position for too long.

ENERGY FLOW
- The leg feels rooted to the ground. The energy is drawn up from the floor towards the stretch of the torso into the distance of the arms. It energises and creates ample space for the rotation of all the chakras and strengthens the body, preparing it for challenging asanas.

81. TRIVIKRAMASANA
DRISHTI – Sama

TIPS
- Slightly bend the knee of the standing leg to ease the lift and once achieved, gently straighten it.
- Gradually progress into this asana, as it is a powerful stretch on the hamstrings.
- Keep both the legs and torso evenly engaged.
- Stretch the back of the lifted leg long and strong.

BENEFITS
- Fully stretches the legs.
- Helps in flexibility of the hip and the torso area.
- Prevents hernia.
- Helps achieve balance and concentration.
- Lessens sexual desire and thereby stills the mind.

CAUTION
- Master leg stretching asanas such as Parsvakonasana, Prasaritha Padottanasana, Utthita Hasta. Pandangushtasana etc. before attempting this asana.
- Trying the same asana lying down (Supta Trivikramasana) would help loosen the leg muscles.
- The hip and torso should be in line and equally engaged – not overstretched or tilted to one side of the body, which would make the other side underactive.

NOTE
This challenging asana has lots of benefits but requires proper preparation. After adequate practice of all the basic asanas, the body gets tuned and ready for the Vishesha or extreme asanas. Master the Preceding asanas and Succeeding asanas mentioned below before attempting this asana.

Preceding asanas
Veerabhadrasana (Series), Ardha Chandrasana, Trianga Mukhottasana, Prasarita Padottanasana, Utthita Hasta Padangustasana Series

Succeeding asanas
Ardha Badha Padangustasana, Utkatasana

ENERGY FLOW
- This asana aligns all the chakras and activates them. The downward flow of energy from all the chakras towards Sahasrara Chakra is highly beneficial for mental well-being.
- Thae Vishuddha Chakra is energised with deep breathing.

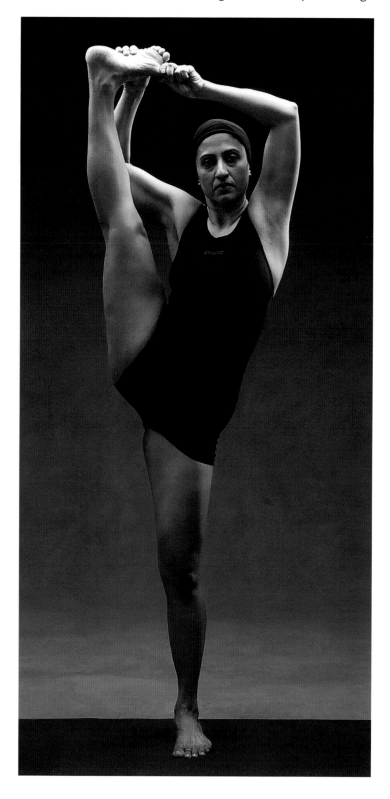

82. UBHAYA PADANGUSTASANA
DRISHTI – Padayoragrai

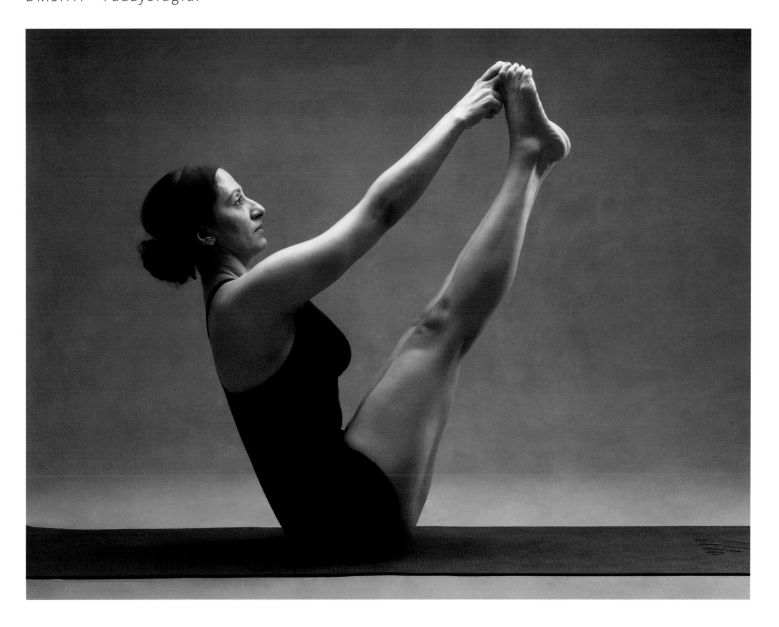

TIPS
- This asana could be a little difficult in the beginning till the balance on the seat bones is established.
- Once this balance is achieved, begin to focus on the length of the back first and then the further extension of the legs.
- If the back flops during the process, do not release the asana. Instead, bend the knees slightly and reestablish the length of the spine by straightening it again.

BENEFITS
- Benefits the length of the legs with flexibility.
- Tones abdominal muscles and the organs in the area.
- Stretches the shoulder and arms and releases stress from the upper back.
- Benefits the hips by increasing the supply of blood into the area.

CAUTION
- This asana requires a great sense of balance. Therefore, carefully establish the stretch of the body from both sides and avoid the curving of the back.

ENERGY FLOW
- This asana benefits the Muladhara Chakra.

83. UBHAYA PASCHIMOTTANASANA
DRISHTI – Sama

TIPS

- Attempt this asana from Navasana.
- Maintaining Sama Drishti helps balance.
- Engage in Mula Bandha only after the legs are fully lifted.
- Maintain balance by keeping the chest wide and strong.

BENEFITS

- Excellent for abdominal strength.
- Benefits the intestines with a rich supply of blood.
- Provides flexibility and strength to the muscles along the length of the legs and back.
- Helps build focus, poise and balance.
- Helps relieve severe backache.

CAUTION

- Do not attempt this asana if you have an upset stomach or indigestion.
- If the stomach feels tight and bloated with gas or if there is water retention, avoid this asana as it leads to muscle cramps around the back and leg area.
- While bringing the chest close to the thighs, make sure that both sides of the chest are evenly stretched.
- Keep the mind alert and focus on the point of balance.

- Simulates the ovaries, uterus and the entire reproductive system.

ENERGY FLOW

- This asana energises the Muladhara Chakra and improves functions around the area of Muladhara Chakra and Svadhisthana Chakra.

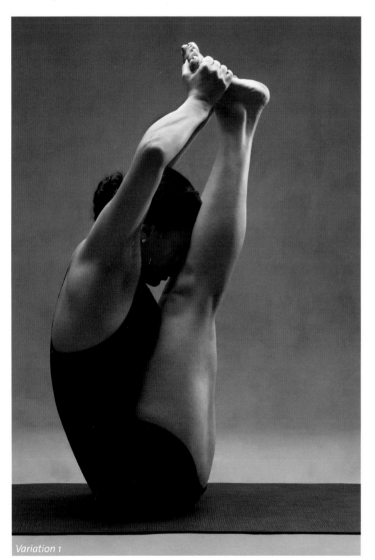

Variation 1

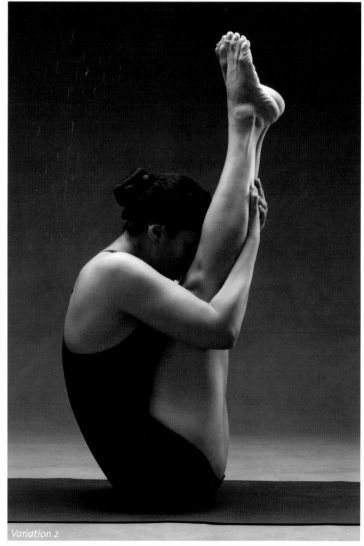

Variation 2

84. UBHAYA UPAVISHTAKONASANA
DRISHTI – Urdhva / Sama

TIPS
- Similar to Upavishtakonasana.
- From Upavisthakonasana, keeping the legs straight, lift them off the floor.
- Draw in the lower abdomen and adjust the pelvis to achieve balance.
- Lift the chest up and look straight ahead or up.
- Try engaging both Mula Bandha and Uddiyana Bandha in this asana.

BENEFITS
- Similar to Upavishtakonasana.
- Provides a good supply of blood to the spinal column, lower back and waist, thus benefiting all the abdominal organs.
- Increases the sense of balance in the body and mind.

CAUTION
- Practise Prasarita Padottansasana to be comfortable in this asana.
- The sciatica nerve is intensely stretched in this asana. If there is a problem in the sciatica nerve, please do not attempt this asana.
- After regular practice of Prasarita Padottanasana, try this asana and stop if still there is discomfort.

ENERGY FLOW
- The Muladhara Chakra and the Svadhisthana Chakra benefit from this asana.

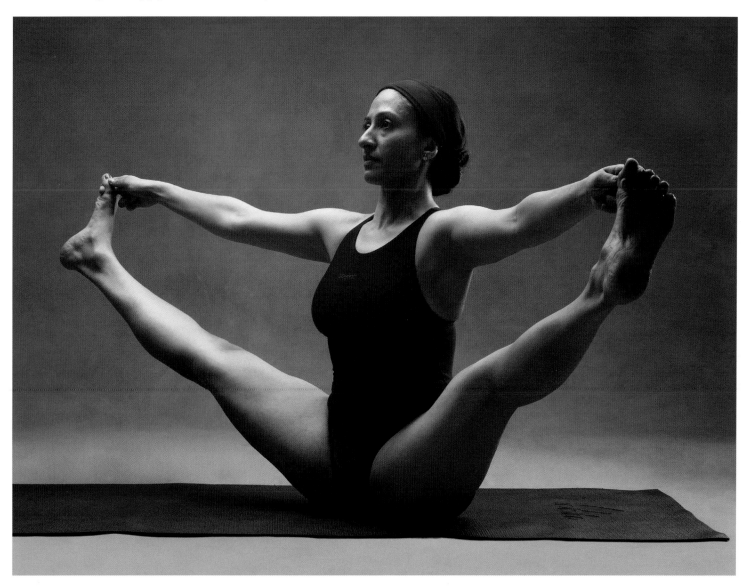

85. UDDIYANA BANDHA
DRISHTI – Nasagrai

TIPS
* Visualise and feel like you are making the entire stomach disappear, leaving a huge hollow at the bottom of the rib cage.

BENEFITS
* A good massage for the organs of the chest and the abdomen.
* Increases the elasticity of the diaphragm.
* Strengthens the lungs by exercising them while reducing the content of the air.
* The pulling up of the abdomen into the rib cage invigorates the area by a providing a good supply of blood to the abdominal organs and stimulating the digestive system.
* Helps in regulating the activities of the nerves.

CAUTION
* For this bandha to be effective, you must not have eaten for at least 5 hours. The stomach and colon too should be completely empty.
* Make sure that all the air is exhaled out.
* Do not breathe in until the stomach is released completely and gently.
* The lungs might get damaged if you gasp for breath with a sudden jerk.

ENERGY FLOW
* This asana activates the Manipura Chakra and the Anahata Chakra the most, while the Muladhara Chakra is the energy source for achieving this bandha.

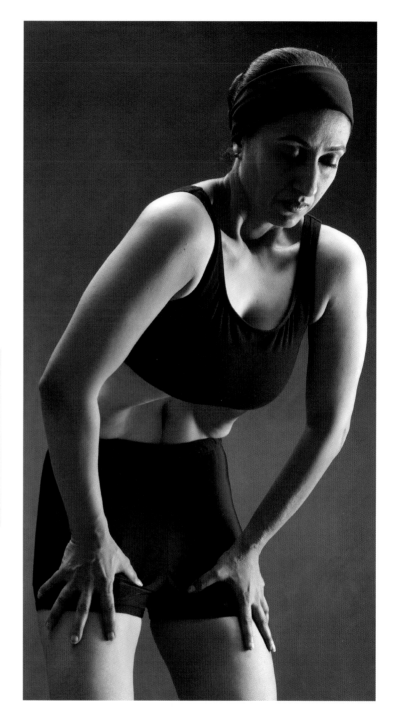

86. UPADASANA
DRISHTI – Nabigrai

TIPS
- Keep the position of the hip and torso well-balanced, so as to not overstretch or overwork one side of the body.
- While stretching the leg up, keep the toes pointed and do not tilt the hip too much.
- While stretching the arms towards the feet, initiate the stretch from the armpit, consciously feeling the ribs stretch all along.
- Keep the grounded foot open for better support and grip. The toes should feel extended from the arches while raising the other foot.
- The hip should be parallel to the floor as in pointing to the ceiling and not leaning backward or forward.

BENEFITS
- A good asana to practise when there is mental or physical strain.
- Tones the abdominal organs and increases the digestive juices, while activating the liver and spleen.
- Benefits persons suffering from a bloating sensation in the abdomen or from gastric troubles.
- Relieves stomach ache, backache and abdominal cramps during menstruation.

CAUTION
- Do not attempt this asana if you suffer from a spinal disc problem.
- The spine should remain concave throughout the asana.
- Do not force this stretch. Wait till the hamstrings and spine feel flexible sufficient to take up this challenge. Keep attempting.

ENERGY FLOW
- The energy flows in a downward movement from the Muladhara Chakra to the Sahasrara Chakra. It stimulates the nervous system and regular practice will keep the whole body rejuvenated.

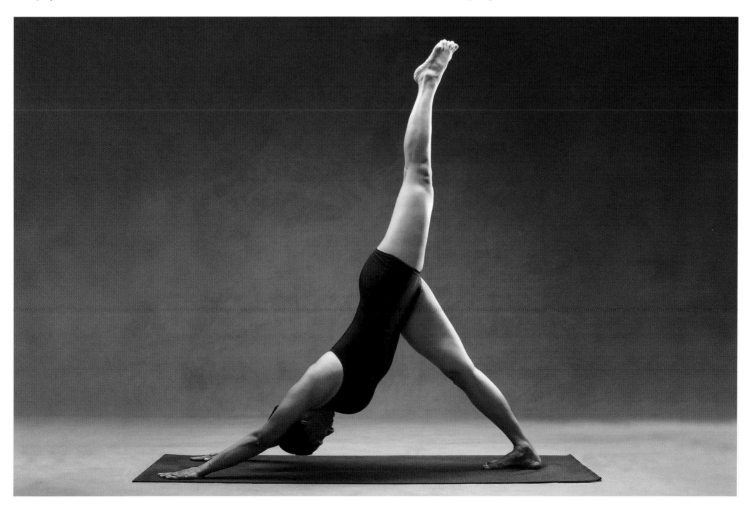

87. UPAVISHTAKONASANA
DRISHTI – Nasagrai

TIPS

- Fold your body into the stretch carefully step by step, by gently releasing all the points of resistance.
- Adjust the tailbone to ease the stretch by tilting it upward.
- Keep the chest open at all times.
- Extend the chin to the floor.
- Maintain Uddiyana Bandha.
- Maintaining Mula Bandha will help in the opening of the hips and thighs, as it extends the torso.

BENEFITS

- Stretches the hamstrings, providing it with a good supply of blood.
- Keeps the pelvic region healthy.
- Prevents hernia and also cures mild cases of sciatic pains.
- Regularises menstrual flow and also stimulates the ovaries.

CAUTION
- This is a very safe asana with hardly any contraindications. Keep trying regularly till you achieve it.

ENERGY FLOW
- Similar to that of the Baddha Konasana. In this asana, the flow of energy extends towards the length of the legs from the Muladhara Chakra.

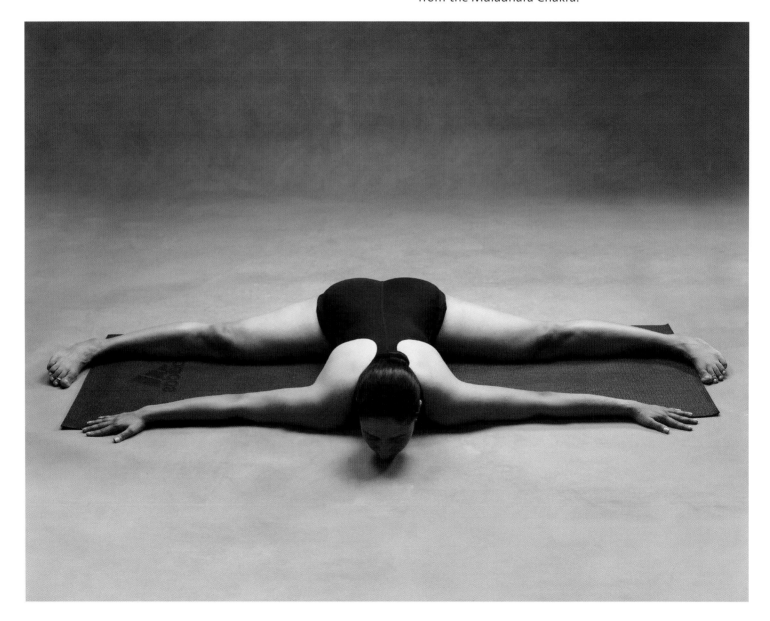

88. URDHVA DHANURASANA / CHAKRASANA
DRISHTI – Purva

TIPS
- Try this asana from Sethubandhasana.
- First lift the hip up, then expand the chest and widen the armpits to get a perfect curve.
- Release the chest gently towards the head in the curve, to ensure proper breathing.
- While achieving the curve, ensure that the weight of the body shifts to the thighs and feet.
- Once the curve is achieved, make sure that the body weight is evenly distributed on the palms and feet.
- Keep the feet parallel to each other.
- Keep the inner edges of the feet pressed to the ground.

BENEFITS
- Tones the spine and makes it flexible.
- Expands the chest completely which is very beneficial to the heart.
- Strengthens the abdominal and pelvic organs.
- Improves blood circulation along the entire length of the body.
- Stimulates the thyroid glands.
- Keeps the uterus healthy and strong and prevents its prolapse.

CAUTION
Do not do this asana if:
- You are tired or stressed.
- You have high blood pressure or low blood pressure.
- You have headache / migraine.
- You have an upset stomach, constipation or diarrhoea.
- You have a stiff back.
- You have just recovered from a shoulder injury or a back pain.

ENERGY FLOW
- The energy moves from the Muladhara Chakra to all the parts of the body.

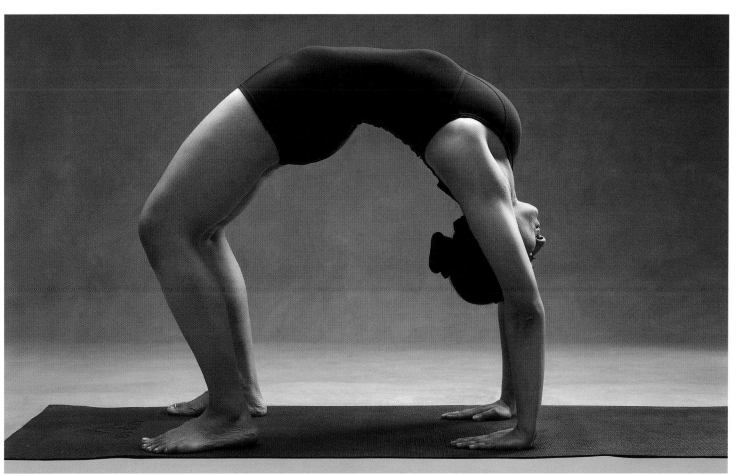

89. URDHVA TADASANA
DRISHTI – Sama

TIPS
- Focus on placing the weight of the body on the metatarsals (the front mounds of the feet).
- Pay attention to your ankles, knees, hipbones, which should be in line with the collarbones.
- Focus on the lower abdomen and pull the pelvis in and up.
- Feel tall and stretched towards the sky.

BENEFITS
- Same as Tadasana.
- Tones especially the calves, ankles and the arches of the feet.

CAUTION
- While releasing the asana, gently bring the feet down.
- Make sure the 5 points of the metatarsals are evenly placed on the floor.
- If you lose balance, first soften the knees, before the heels drop to the ground.

ENERGY FLOW
- This asana helps all the chakras to align.

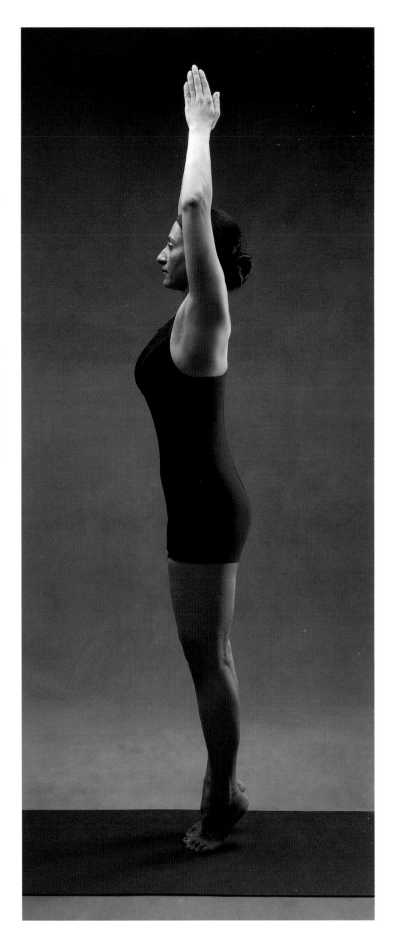

90. URDHVA MUKHA PASCHIMOTTANASANA
DRISHTI – Nasagrai

TIPS
- Make sure the entire back is resting on the floor.
- Lift the legs up to Sarvangasana position.
- Then slowly bring the pelvis down while the legs are stretched along the length of the abdomen.
- Aim at taking the length of the legs back and way beyond the head.

BENEFITS
- Has all the benefits of Paschimottanansana.
- Additionally, stretches and tones the abdominal walls, supplying the area with ample blood.
- The legs get a full stretch thus toning them and the calves.
- Helps relieve severe backache.
- Soothes the adrenal glands.
- Simulates the ovaries, uterus and the entire reproductive system.

CAUTION
- Do not lift the upper body towards the knee, instead lower the pelvis towards the length of the abdomen.
- Attempt this asana slowly and progress into the deep Mulabandha to reap maximum benefit of the asana.

ENERGY FLOW
- The energy from Muladhara Chakra energises all the chakras. This asana encourages downward flow of the energy into the bases of the chakras along the length of the spine.

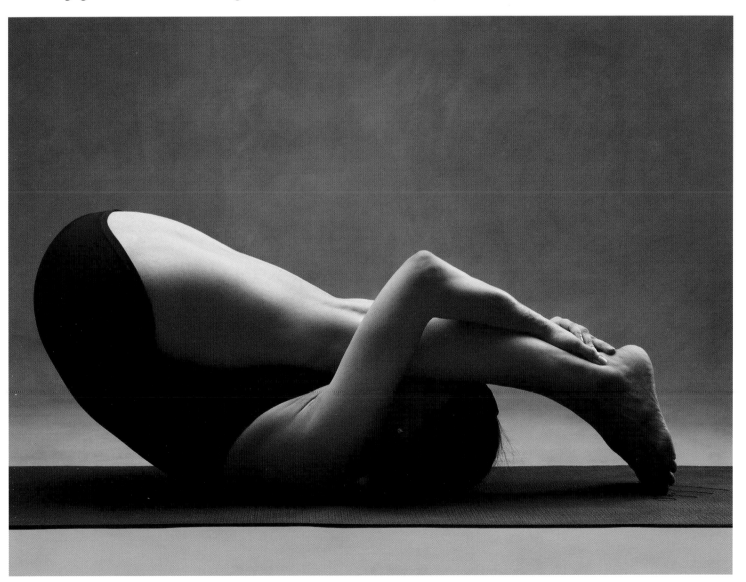

91. URDHVA MUKHA SVANASANA
DRISHTI – Urdhva

TIPS

- Always flow and slide forward from Chaduranga Dandasana into Urdhva Mukha Svanasana.
- Straighten the arms and lift the chest up, while the shoulders drop backward and away from the ears.
- Lift the chin up towards the ceiling, keeping the neck long and make sure the breathing is comfortable. An overstretched neck makes breathing uncomfortable.
- Maintain strong legs, keep abdomen tucked in and glutes firm, so as to support the lower spine.

BENEFITS

- Strengthens back muscles.
- Releases back strain and stiffness in the back.
- Challenges the hip and thighs, thus strengthening them.
- Fully expands the lungs which help increase their capacity and their elasticity.

CAUTION

- The junction where the spine meets the head should not be compressed.
- Focus should be on breathing rather than expanding the stretch to an uncomfortable breathing position.
- Use the pectorals instead of the shoulder muscles.

ENERGY FLOW

- The flow of energy is along the length of the spine. The chakras get a natural release, thus accelerating their circular movement.

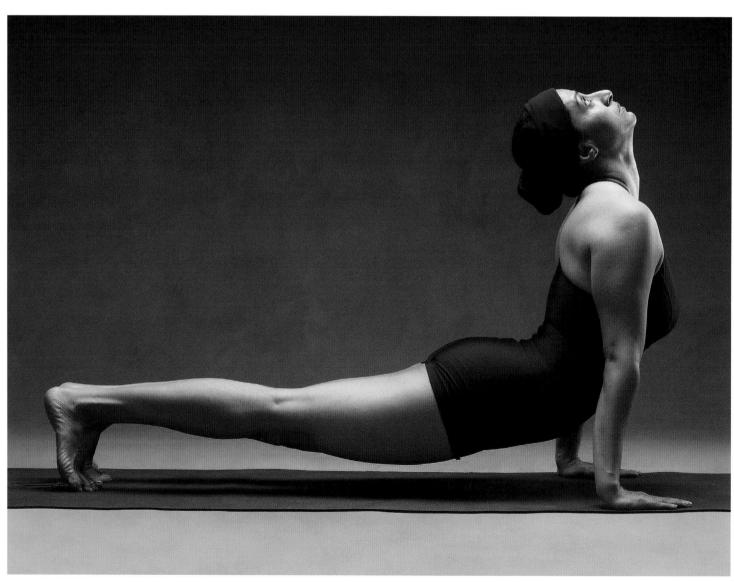

92. URDHVA MUKHA TADASANA
DRISHTI – Urdhva

TIPS
- Stand straight, with folded hands stretched above the crown of your head.
- Keep the face calm and the eyes staring at the thumb.
- Focus on placing the weight of the body on the arches of the feet.
- Pay attention to your ankles, knees, hipbones, which should be in alignment with the collarbones.
- Pay attention to the lower abdomen and pull them in and up.
- Focus on the length of the torso.
- Once the asana is achieved, release tension from the length of the body and breath deep and easy.

BENEFITS
- Marks the point of preparation for any asana.
- Builds focus, concentration and mindful preparation.
- The body is centered and rooted to earth, thus making the body aware of gravity.
- Focuses on straightening and lengthening every area of the body and tones the muscles of the body.
- The slow build-up of the asana helps memorise the correct alignment of the body.

CAUTION
- Close the eyes once the balance in the body is established and the feet feel rooted.
- Try not to curve the lower back, which usually happens when you try to stretch the hands above too much. Instead, pay attention to the length of the torso.
- If there is a problem of balance, stand close to a wall and practise this asana.

ENERGY FLOW
- This asana aligns and arranges all the chakras.

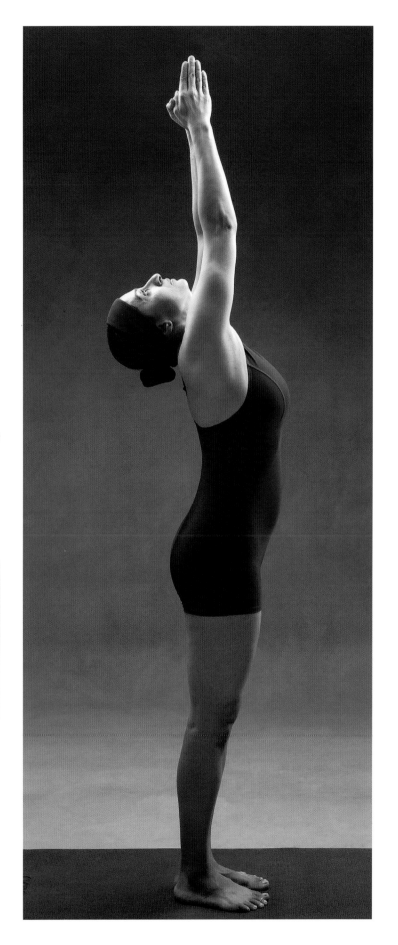

93. URDHVA MUKHA UPVISHTAKONASANA
DRISHTI – Sama

TIPS
- Attempt this asana from Baddha Konasana.
- Keep the groin strong and stretched while attempting the lift of the leg to form an upward stretch.
- Keep the drishsti in Sama to establish a good balance.

BENEFITS
- Benefits the legs with flexibility and length.
- Tones abdominal muscles and the organs in the area.
- Stretches the shoulders and arms releasing stress from the upper back.
- Benefits the hip by increasing the supply of blood into the area.

CAUTION
- This asana requires a great sense of balance. Therefore, carefully establish the stretch of the body from both sides and avoid the curving of the back.

ENERGY FLOW
- This asana benefits the Muladhara Chakra which in turn benefits all the the other chakras with a powerful flow of energy.

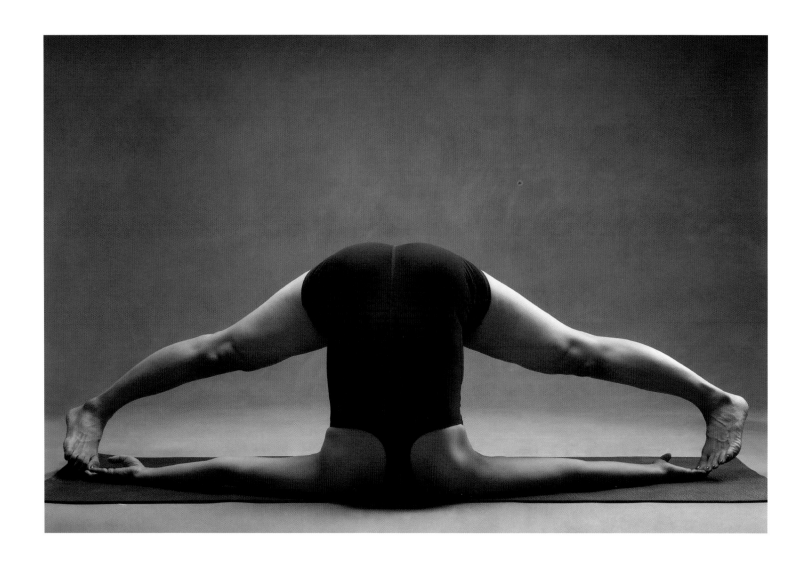

94. USHTRASANA
DRISHTI – Purva

TIPS

- Pull the thigh muscles upward towards the hip bones and lengthen the spine.
- With the hip under control, curve the spine backward to achieve maximum stretch of the chest.
- Open the collarbones to release the stretch of the neck.
- Once comfortable in this position, push the lower back deep inwards, which would relax the length of the spine, making it easy to position the back parallel to the ground.
- The impetus for the upward movement while releasing the asana should come from the thighs and chest.

BENEFITS

- Benefits people with drooping shoulders.
- Stretches the spine completely, increasing the blood supply along its length.
- Tones the back and the spine.
- Increases lung capacity.
- Oxygenates the organs of the body.
- Removes stiffness in the shoulders, back and ankles.
- Relieves abdominal cramps and regulates menstrual flow.

CAUTION
Do not:
- Overstretch your back.
- Practise this asana if you have migraine, hypertension or are recovering from a heart problem.
- Practise this asana in case of severe constipation.

ENERGY FLOW

- The vital flow of energy is from the Anahata Chakra towards the Sahasrara Chakra and also from Anahata Chakra to the Muladhara Chakra.

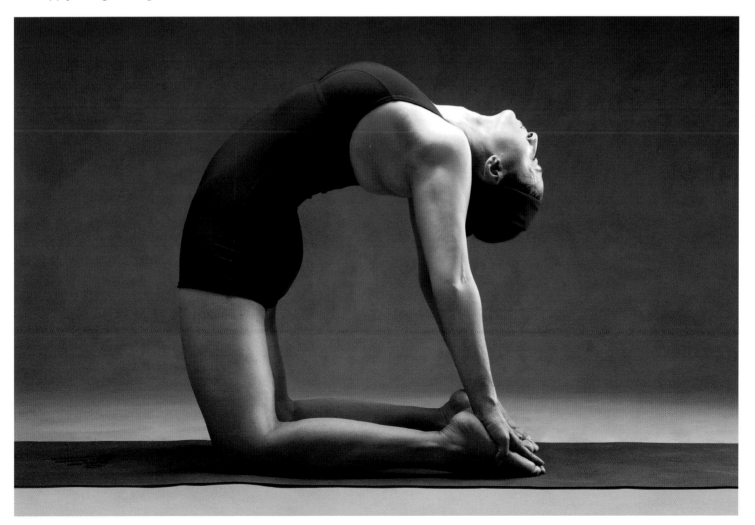

95. UTTHITA HASTA PADANGUSTASANA
DRISHTI – Angushtagrai

TIPS
- Root the standing leg firmly on the floor and pull the leg muscles strongly upward.
- Do not focus too much on lifting the leg high. Instead, concentrate on keeping the back straight.
- Protect your back by engaging the core.
- Do not worry if the lifted leg is not straight, as it will eventually be straight.

BENEFITS
- Tones the lower region of the spine and the nerves connected to the legs.
- Strengthens the knees.

CAUTION
- Those who find this asana very difficult and exhausting can try doing it lying down – Supta Utthita Hasta Padangustasana.
- The practice of Trikonasana and Parsvakonasana will strengthen and prepare the legs to do this asana.

ENERGY FLOW
- This asana activates the Muladhara Chakra for balance and intense stretch along the length of the legs. It also increases balance and focus, thus benefiting the Vishuddha Chakra as well.

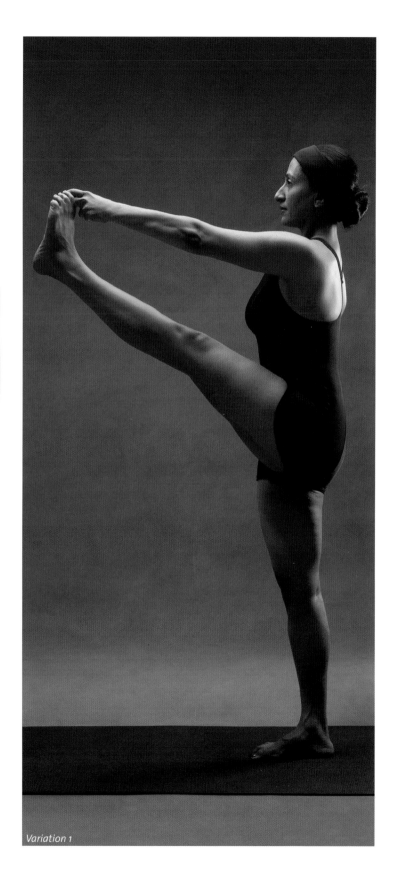

Variation 1

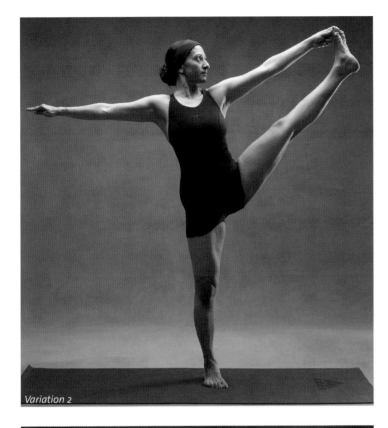

Variation 2

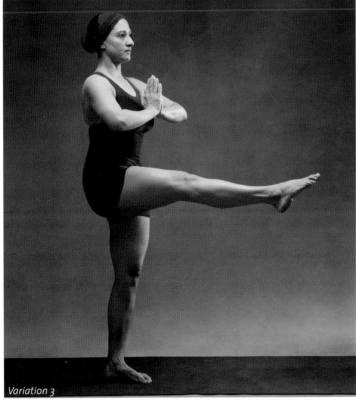

Variation 3

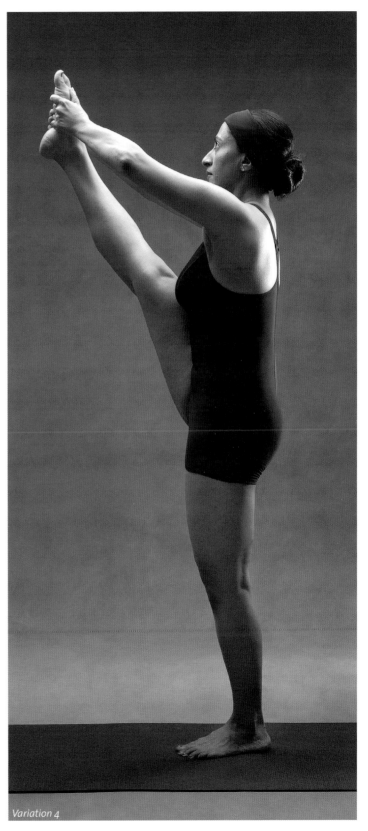

Variation 4

96. JUMP FORWARD, BACKWARD
DRISHTI – Bhoomigrai

TIPS
- This jump-momentum is best achieved form Padangustasana.
- Distribute the weight of the body from your feet to the arms.
- Bend your knees to avoid unwanted pull in your hamstrings.
- Tip forward and exhale.
- With the body's weight shifting completely into the hand as the foundation, jump with both legs and bottom up in the air.
- Lengthen the legs as you land into Chaduranga Dandasana.

BENEFITS
- Pushes the body up in the air, making it supple, releasing all tensions.
- Reduces abdominal tension and stiffness in the back.
- Cures stomach aches and tones the liver, spleen and the kidneys
- Relieves mental and physical exhaustion.
- Rejuvenates the spinal nerves.

CAUTION
Do not attempt this jump if you:
- Have a weak back.
- Have a slipped disc.
- Have heaviness in the head.
- Suffer from acidity or dizziness.

ENERGY FLOW
- The vital flow of energy is from the Muladhara Chakra to the Sahasrara Chakra.

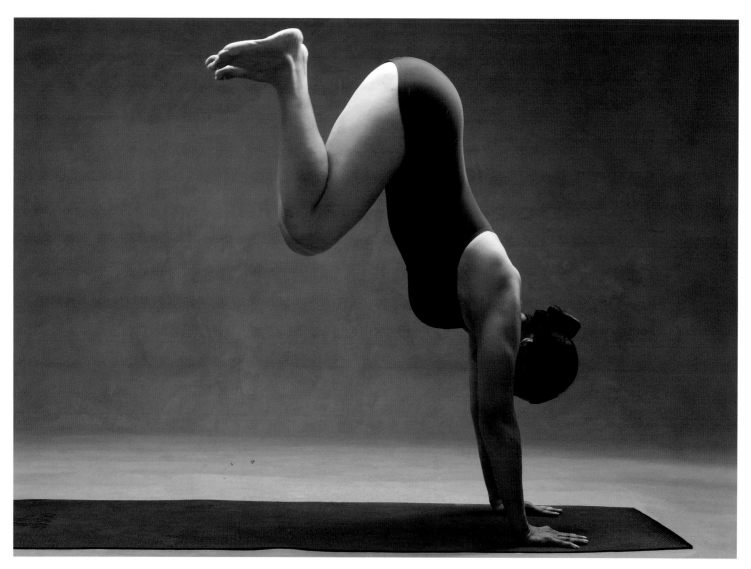

97. UTTANASANA
DRISHTI – Bhoomigrai

TIPS
- Make sure the pelvis is tilted so that the hip is pointed towards the ceiling.
- Lengthen the spine and keep it is straight.
- To ease into this asana, bend the knees slightly, then lengthen the spine towards the floor. Once the maximum stretch of the spine is achieved, slowly tilt the pelvis upward while the knee is gradually straightened.

BENEFITS
- Reduces abdominal and back pain.
- Helps ease menstrual cramps.
- Cures stomach aches and tones the liver, spleen and the kidneys.
- Relieves mental and physical exhaustion.
- Rejuvenates the spinal nerves.
- Slows down the heartbeat.
- Benefits brain cells
- Cools the eyes.

CAUTION
Do not attempt this asana if you:
- Have a weak back.
- Have a slipped disc.
- Have heaviness in the head.
- Suffer from acidity or dizziness.

ENERGY FLOW
- The vital flow of energy is from the Muladhara Chakra to the Sahasrara Chakra.

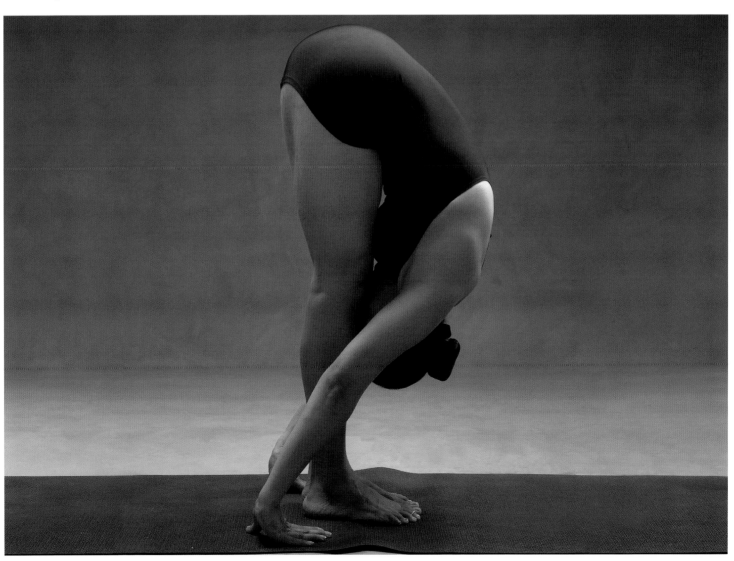

98. UTKATASANA
DRISHTI – Angushtagrai

TIPS

- Lower the hip like you are about to sit on a low stool. Pay attention to the dropping of the hip rather than bending the knees to bring the hip down.
- If namaste makes it difficult to relax the shoulders, then open the arms and drop the shoulders away from the ears.
- Do not stoop forward. Instead, lift the chest up. This will release any constriction in the back of the neck and shoulders, and also aid deeper and easier breathing in the asana.

BENEFITS

- Removes stiffness in the shoulders and neck.
- Opens knee joints and removes stiffness in the ankles.
- Develops leg muscles evenly.
- Lifts the diaphragm to release space in the abdominal area.
- Tones the abdomen and the back.
- Fully expands the chest, thus benefiting the heart.

CAUTION

- If you have cervical spondylitis, keep your gaze straight in the front (Sama Drishti). Also, hold the hands stretched forwards in line with your shoulders.
- If there is pain in the knees:
  - Avoid this asana or
  - Start the asana from half-squat position rather than bending your knees from standing position or
  - Hold on to a pillar in the front for support before going down so that the knee does not bear the entire weight of the body.

ENERGY FLOW

- A wave of energy flows through the stretch releasing strong energy both upward and downwards. The Muladhara Chakra and the Anahata Chakra enjoy maximum benefit of this asana.

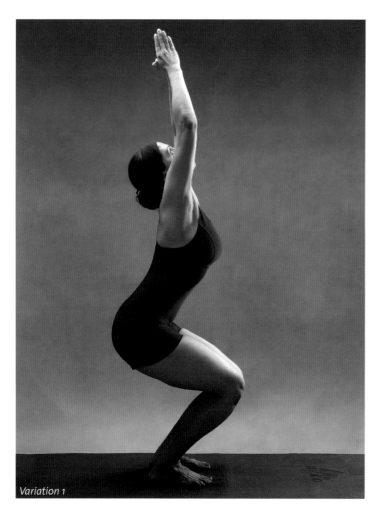
Variation 1

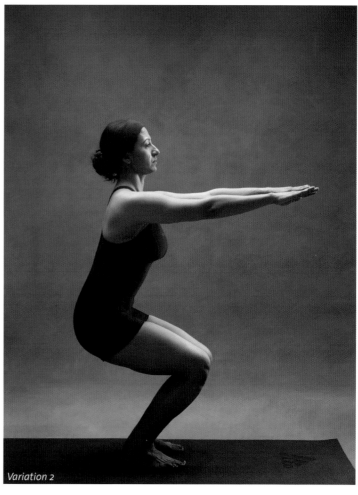
Variation 2

99. VAJRASANA
DRISHTI – Sama

TIPS
- Position the buttocks to be pushed more towards the thighs and sit comfortably on the heels.
- Release the curve of your lower back to feel relaxed and straight.
- Keep the navel tucked in, creating depth in the lower abdomen.
- Stay in this position while breathing deep.

BENEFITS
- Relaxes the tailbone.
- Very beneficial when back is strained.
- Helps digestion and, therefore, could be practised even after meals.
- Helps flex the feet, thus relaxing them.
- Relaxes the leg muscles and calms the body.

CAUTION
- Do not practise this asana if your knees are strained due to long periods of standing or walking.
- People with varicose veins should be very careful attempting this asana. Props, like cushion or a blanket, should be placed between the calf and the thigh to avoid straining or damaging the veins.

ENERGY FLOW
- This asana aligns all the chakras and relaxes their movement. Therefore, this asana has a calming effect on the body.

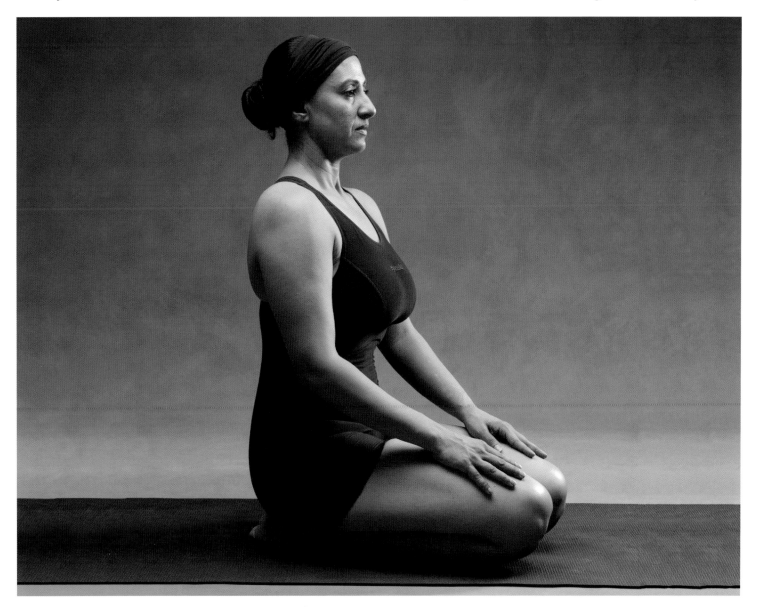

100. VASHISTASANA
DRISHTI – Hastagrai

TIPS
- Make sure that the outer side of the foot touching the ground is rested firmly on the floor.
- Keep the body absolutely straight, with the tail bone tucked in.
- Grip your toe with your index and middle fingers.
- Use the same technique like the Supta Padangustasana.

BENEFITS
- Fantastic asana to strengthen the wrists.
- Exercises the length of the legs and the spine.
- Exercises the sides of the abdomen.

CAUTION
- Do not attempt this asana if the wrists are not strong.

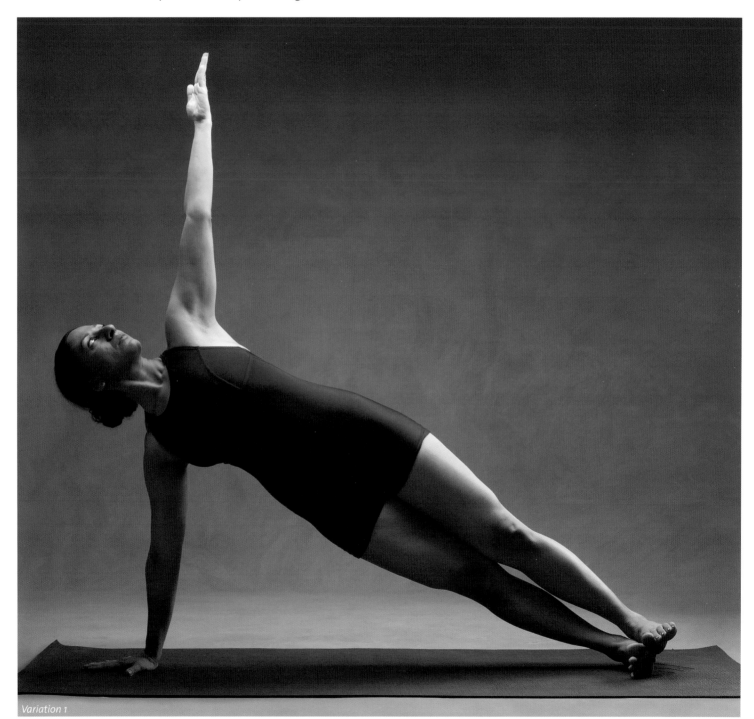

Variation 1

ENERGY FLOW

- The lateral alignment of all the chakras when in this asana covers a different dimension of the body, benefiting the flow of energy along the sides.

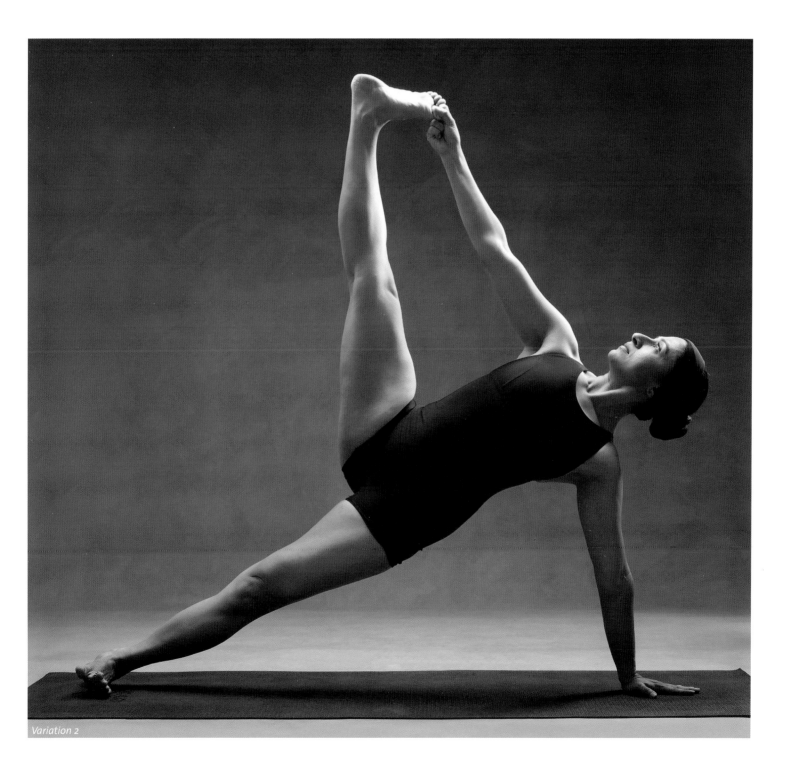

Variation 2

101. VATAYANASANA
DRISHTI – Nasagrai

TIPS
- Make sure that the Ardha Padma is firm on one side of the leg.
- Push the knee of the Padmasana leg to a backward stretch before bending the other leg's knee.
- In the beginning, this would seem to be a very difficult asana. With practice, it will be achieved.

BENEFITS
- Increases circulation in the hip joints, making them strong and flexible.
- Rectifies minor deformity in the thighs and calves.
- Releases stiffness in the arms, forearms and wrists through the entwining of the hands.
- Increases elasticity in the groin.

CAUTION
- Do not attempt this asana if you have an injured knee or recovering from a hip injury.
- People who have back problems should be very careful while attempting this asana, as the back could be further injured if it is not kept straight.

ENERGY FLOW
- The Muladhara Chakra is the activated in this asana while the other chakras get automatically aligned and energised.

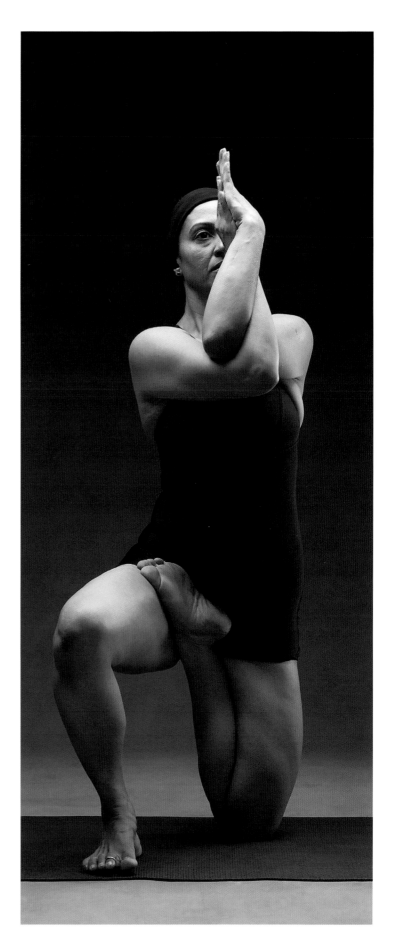

102. VEERABHADRASANA
DRISHTI – Bhoomigrai

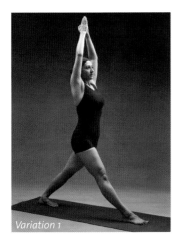
Variation 1

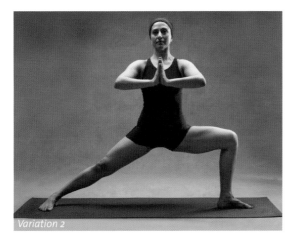
Variation 2

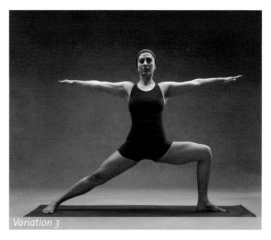
Variation 3

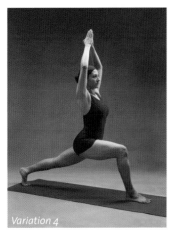
Variation 4

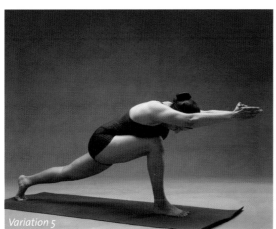
Variation 5

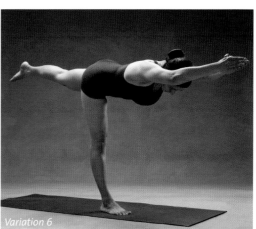
Variation 6

TIPS
- From the position of a lunge, bend and slide the body forwards to the extent possible.
- Lift the back leg up and stretch it so that the body is kept parallel to the ground.
- From this position of readiness, straighten the grounded foot, so as to achieve steadiness and alignment.

BENEFITS
- Trains the body to balance and to increase stamina and strength.
- Helps contract and tone the abdominal muscles.
- Opens the hip joints, thus increasing blood circulation to the region.
- Makes the leg muscles sturdy and strong.

CAUTION
- Do not practise this asana if your knees are weak or tired.

ENERGY FLOW
- The energy of this asana flows from the Muladhara Chakra into the two ends of the body – the head and the foot rooted to the floor.

103. VEERASANA
DRISHTI –Sama

TIPS
- Adjust the position of the buttocks from Vajrasana and rest them on the floor.
- Release the curve of the lower back to feel relaxed and straight.
- Keep the navel tucked in, thus creating depth in the lower abdomen.
- Stay in position while breathing deep.

BENEFITS
- Relaxes the tailbone.
- Very beneficial when back is strained.
- Helps digestion and therefore could be practised even after meals.
- Relaxes the leg muscles and calms the body.

CAUTION
- Do not practise this asana if the knees are strained due to long periods of standing or walking.
- People with varicose veins can comfortably practise this asana.
- Props like a cushion or a blanket should be placed between the floor and the buttocks if the knees are stiff.

ENERGY FLOW
- This asana aligns all the chakras and relaxes their movement. Therefore, this asana has a calming effect on the body.

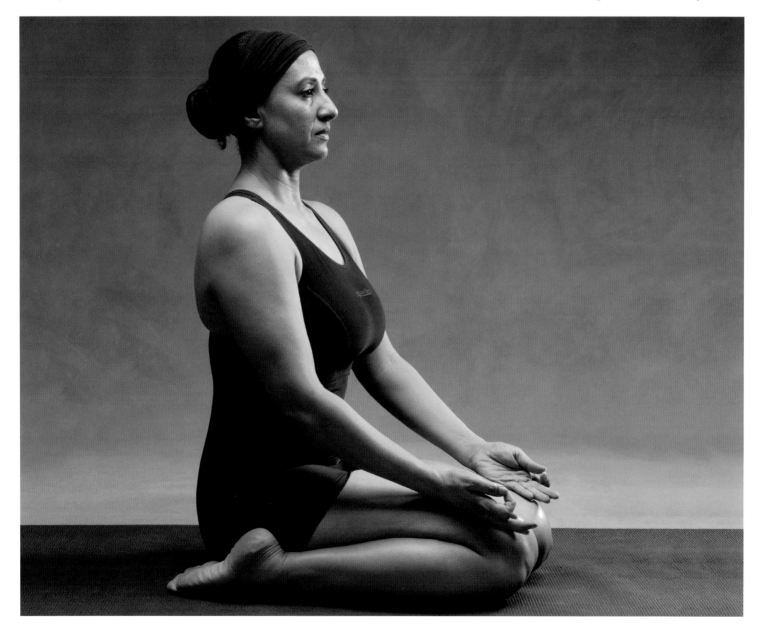

104. VIPARITA DANDASANA
DRISHTI – Nasagrai

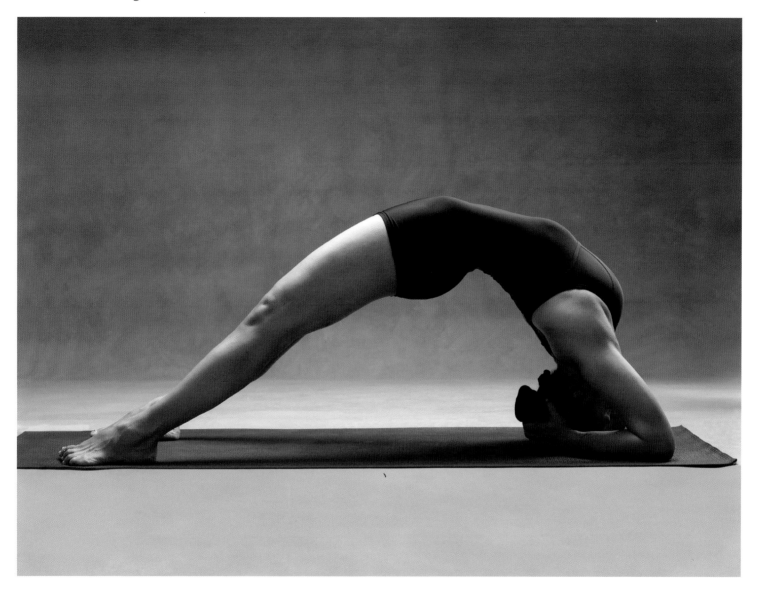

TIPS
- When the head is reclined to get it on the floor, the diaphragm is contracted and the breathing will feel short. At this point, exhale and raise the shoulders as high as possible and along with it, intensify the curve of the back.
- Keep the feet parallel to each other.

BENEFITS
- An exhilarating asana to keep the spine healthy while the chest is completely open. The spine becomes well-toned and flexible.
- Beneficial to the heart since it completely expands the chest.
- Strengthens the abdominal and pelvic organs.
- Improves blood circulation along the entire length of the body.
- Stimulates the thyroid glands.
- Has a soothing effect on the brain.

CAUTION
- Same as Urdhva Dhanurasana, but it further challenges the upper body.

ENERGY FLOW
- All the chakras are energised in this asana.

105. VISHWAMITRASANA
DRISHTI – Sama

TIPS
- Get into Parsvakonasana, then attempt to tuck the shoulder under the back of the bent knee.

NOTE
This challenging asana has lots of benefits but requires proper preparation. After adequate practice of all the basic asanas, the body gets tuned and ready for the Vishesha or extreme asanas. Master the Preceding asanas and Succeeding asanas mentioned below before attempting this asana.

Preceding asanas
Utthita Hasta Padangustasana, Ardha Chandrasana, Veerabhadrasana, Chaduranga Dandasana, Vashistasana

Succeeding asanas
Vajrasana, Veerasana, Krounchasana, Akarna Dhanurasana, Gomukhasana, Supta Utthita Hasta Padangustasana, Sarvangasana, Halasana, Matsyasana

- Using support from the palm on the floor and the strength in the hip, start stretching and lifting the leg that is beside the shoulder.
- Do not allow the body to flop until the leg is fully stretched.
- Keep the chest expanded and strong throughout the asana.

BENEFITS
- Challenges the balance.
- Tones abdominal muscles.
- Stretches and strengthens the thigh muscles.
- Increases strength and circulation around the hip area.

CAUTION
- Do not try this asana unless you have mastered Hanumanasana, Upavishtakonasana and Vashistasana.
- This is an advanced asana, so do not force the stretch in the very first attempt.

ENERGY FLOW
- All the chakras benefit from this asana.

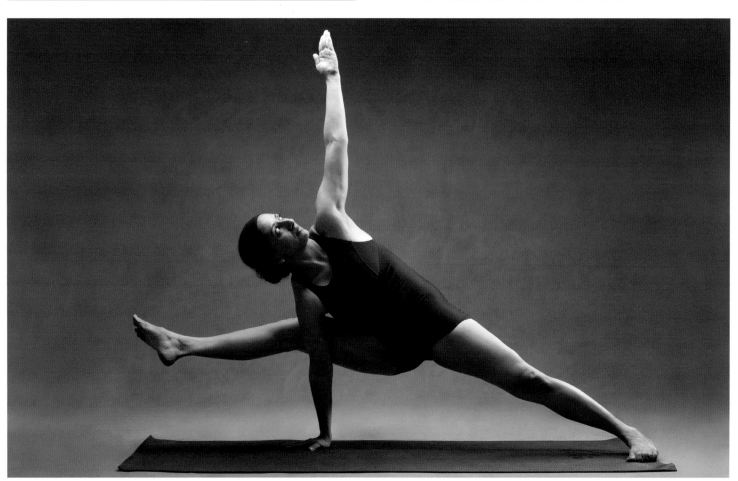

106. VRIKSHASANA

DRISHTI – Sama

TIPS

- Keep the hip bones in line with each other. This will help with balance in the asana.
- Distribute the weight of the body along the length of the feet and press the big toe firmly on the ground.
- Focus the gaze to a point and do not get distracted from that point if you lose balance.
- Keep the folded leg's knee pointed towards the floor.

BENEFITS

- Aligns the body and builds up sense of balance and poise.
- Helps in proper alignment of the body and builds concentration.
- Lengthens and strengthens the leg muscles and also makes the hip steady and strong.

CAUTION

- Avoid this asana if the knees are not feeling strong.

ENERGY FLOW

- This asana aligns and balances all the chakras.

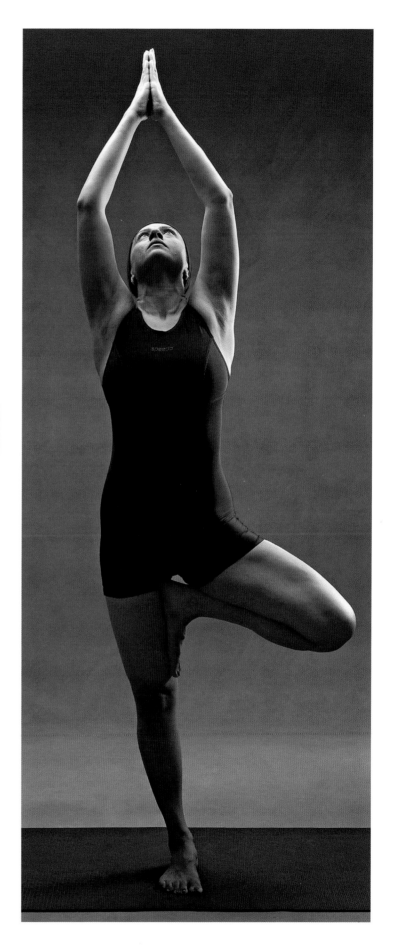

107. YOGA MUDRASANA
DRISHTI – Nasagrai

TIPS
- Yield the weight of the body firmly to the floor and release all tension from the spine.
- Inhale deeply and expand the chest, feeling the shoulder blades drop into the body, while opening the entire area of the collarbones.
- Secure the hands in a tight grip.
- Lengthen the spine, adjusting the hip position by tucking it more towards the thigh and not towards the back.

BENEFITS
- Expands the chest and lungs to release tension and stiffness from the shoulders.
- Prepares the practitioner to get comfortable with Padmasana as it engages the bandhas.
- Opens up the hip and knees, improving flexibility and aligns the vertebrae of the spine as the back is drawn straight.
- Keeps the entire length of the abdomen and the spine toned and healthy.
- Releases stiffness in the knees and ankles.
- Benefits the entire lumbar regions.
- Engages all the bandhas in this asana to further benefit the body due to their binding energy.

CAUTION
- People who are not used to sitting on the floor might find this asana challenging on the knees.
- Try to practise Padmasana sitting on a pillow for the first few times.
- Practise half Padmasana by placing one foot first, for eg. the right one on the root of the left foot and flap to loosen the knee and ankle. Repeat the same on the left. This exercise would help release the tightness in the knees.

ENERGY FLOW
- Benefits and energises all the chakras of the body.

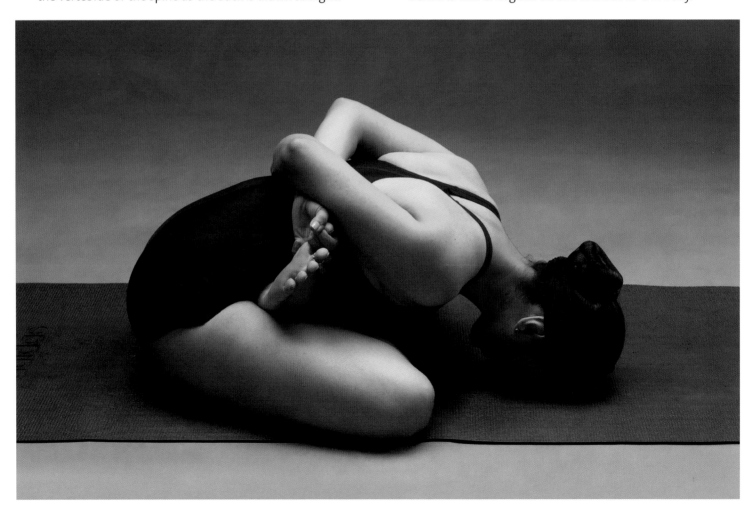

108. YOGA NIDRASANA
DRISHTI – Dhyana

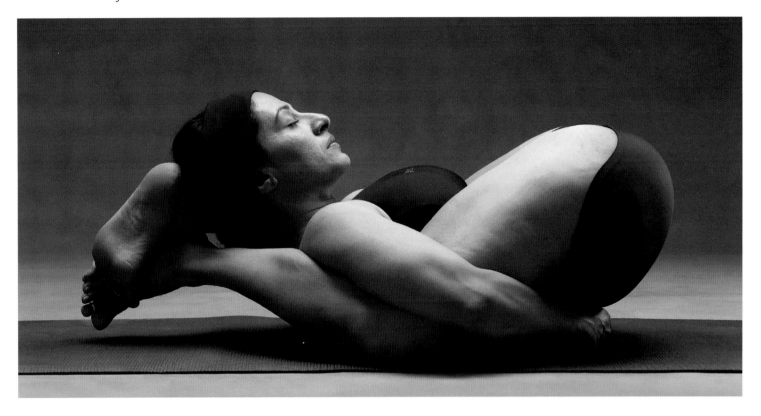

TIPS
- Inhale deeply and completely exhale in each step attempted in this asana.
- Expand the chest and elbows and raise the chest.
- Cross both the legs first, then take them behind the head to place them on the back of the neck (like a pillow).
- Before resting the legs under the neck, lift the neck up, then the dorsal region to adjust the shoulders until they are comfortable.
- Breathe normally once in the asana.

NOTE
This challenging asana has lots of benefits but requires proper preparation. After adequate practice of all the basic asanas the body gets tuned and ready for the Vishesha or Extreme asanas. Master the below mentioned Preceding asanas and Succeeding asanas before attempting this asana.

Preceding asanas
Baddha Konasana, Upavistakonasana, Krounchasana, Akarna Dhanurasana, Supta Utthita Hasta Padangustasana, Kapilasana

Succeeding asanas
Sarvangasana Halasana Karna Peedasana Urdhva Dhanurasana

BENEFITS
- Thoroughly stretches the entire length of the spine.
- Completely contracts the lungs and the abdomen, which tones the kidneys, lungs, liver, spleen, intestine, gall bladder. Practised regularly, this asana protects these organs from diseases.

CAUTION
- Carefully work into this intense asana and progress gradually.
- Flexibility of the groin and the hamstrings has to be well-established before attempting this asana.
- Master Baddha Konasana, Supta Utthita Hasta Padangustasana, Eka Pada Shirsasana, Kapilasana before attempting this asana.

ENERGY FLOW
- This asana relaxes all the chakras.

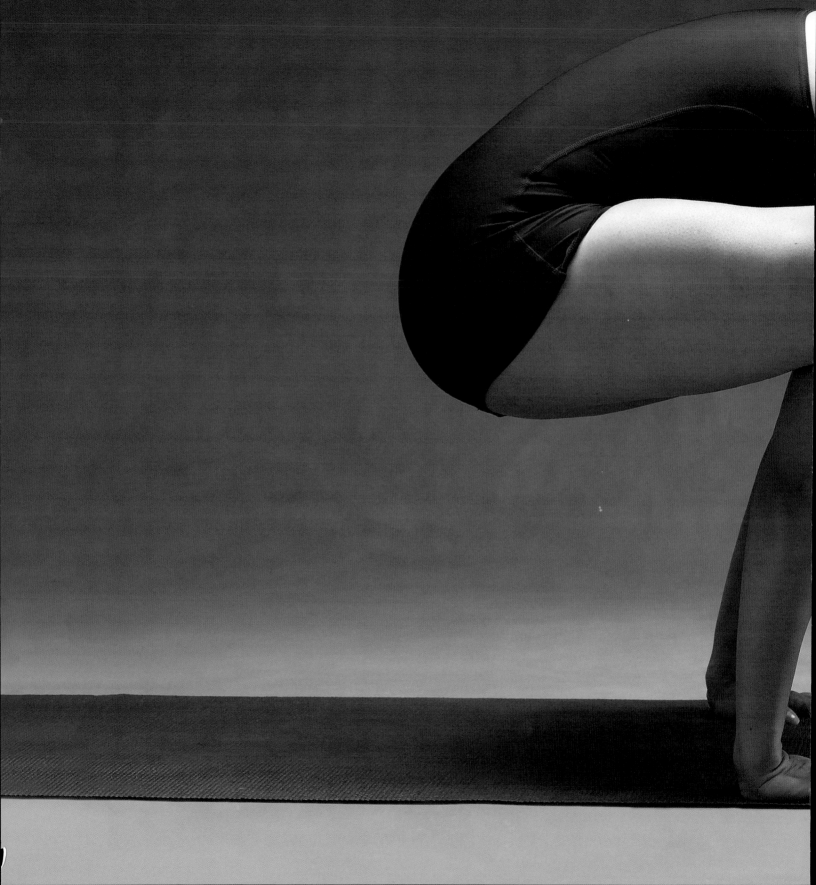

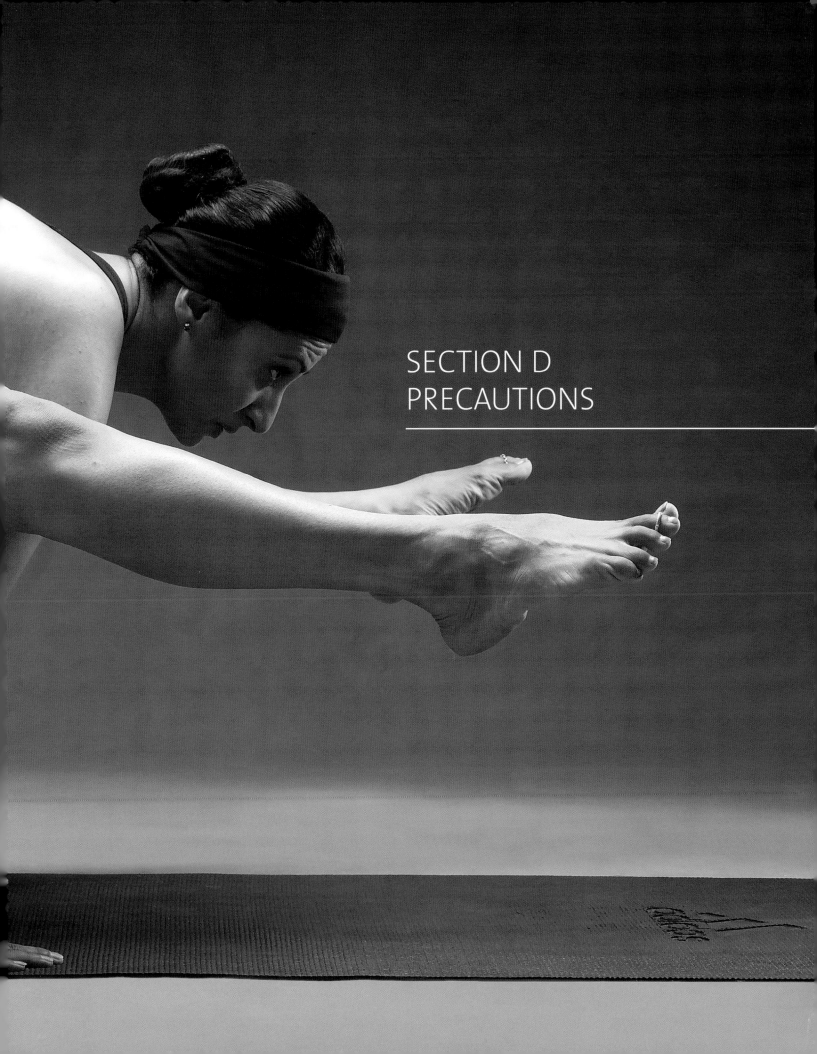

SECTION D
PRECAUTIONS

CHAPTER 10
COMMON INJURIES

The body's response to any kind of injury is pain. Pain is a reaction of the mind to any impact or damage to the body. The intensity of pain depends on the mind-body relationship – the mind's ability to manage the stress that the body is going through and to prepare the body to combat the pain with total awareness. This helps reduce the intensity of pain to a great extent.

IDENTIFYING COMMON INJURIES DUE TO FAULTY PRACTICE

FEET ARCHES

REASONS
Weak arches could be the main reason for chronic pain in the calves and soles of the feet, further straining the knees and hip. Eventually, the ill effect would transfer to the lower back, neck and shoulders too. The strain in the arches is mainly due to the lack of toning in the ligaments of the feet or due to the lack of strength around the supporting muscles.

CARE
* Consciously avoid inversion and rotation of the foot.
* Root the centre of the heel and the ball of the toe to the ground, thus creating a gentle arch in the feet.
* Observe the muscles of the feet lifting upward while the bones are grounding downwards.
* Observe an immediate sense of lightness, firm connect to the ground and a feeling of stability.

A targeted asana practice will help build strength and alignment of the feet. On a more subtle level, it will also improve other body functions like breathing, blood circulation, health of the vital organs and create an overall feeling of balance and well-being.

ASANAS THAT BENEFIT THE FEET
Note: The suggested asanas help strengthen the area. These should not be practised if the area is already injured or is in the process of healing.

Standing Asanas
Tadasana
Vrikshasana
Santulanasana
Utittha Hasta Padangustasana
Ardha Padma Padangustasana
Vatayanasana

Floor Asanas
Vajrasana
Veerasana
Gomukhasana
Malasana
Supta Utittha Hasta Padangustasana
Sethu Bandhasana (Purna)

KNEES

REASONS
Though a complex joint, the knee has a very delicate structure and even a slight jerk could trigger pain. The cause of a knee problem could be a torn ligament, cartilage damage, a runner's knees or an athlete's knees. Yoga practice is unlikely to damage the knee, as asanas do not create an impact on the knee unlike in sports. However, if there exists a previous problem like bone chip, tendonitis or meniscus tear, repeated bending, folding, stretching or twisting the knees in yoga, could irritate the nerves around the knee cap and also overstretch the tendons.

CARE
* Holding the asana without the knowledge of proper alignment results in one of the bones or muscles being

slightly out of alignment. This could cause physical stress due to uneven distribution of weight which sometimes leads to a slight shift in the position of the knee cap, making the knee region prone to injuries.

- Flat feet or fallen arches is another condition which could cause knee pain.
- When the muscles along the thighs are not rotated properly while constructing an asana, it could lead to pain in the knees (a common oversight by many yoga asana practitioners). Practitioners should pay attention to the IT band that runs along the length of the thighs on its sides. Often, the hip muscles attached to this IT band become tight (common in runners and weight lifters), creating tension along the band. The band might also lose its ability to glide over the underlying muscles in the thigh, which then inhibits knee movement. In these circumstances, some asanas could cause the tissue to thicken and bind, which pull the knee and cause pain.

ASANAS THAT BENEFIT THE KNEES
The following asanas help strengthen the area. These should not be practised if the area is already injured or is in the process of healing. These asanas are basically for the hip and thigh muscles that are attached to the IT band and keep the surrounding tissues flexible and pliable to reduce friction and further injury.

Standing Asanas
Tadasana
Santulanasana
Parsvatanasana (keep knees soft)
Prasarita Padottanasana (with knees slightly bent)

Floor Asanas
Shalabhasana
Paschimottanasana
Setu Bandhasana
Gomukhasana
Akarna Dhanurasana
Supta Utthita Hasta Padangustasana
Halasana
Urdhva Mukha Paschimottanasana

HAMSTRINGS

REASONS
Hamstrings are the muscles that constantly work to hold us upright. They help us walk and are the power behind a run. The nature of their work is heavy-duty, hence they are tough. Tightness in the hamstrings could be mainly due to the following reasons:

A. The hip pushed forward, hyper-extends the knees. This posture also makes the upper back rounded which makes the weight of the body fall below the hips, straining the hamstrings.
B. Bending forward too much and constantly overstretching the back, leads to not only tight hamstrings but also a deep chronic pain in the gluteus along with tension in the upper and the lower back.
C. The foot and knees become weak when a lot of athletic activities like running, jumping, etc., are involved. When the foot is strained, a sudden movement or forward stretch causes a lot of strain which may involve a tear, slowing down healing.

CARE
- Progress into a forward bending stretch without forcing it. Work on comfortably releasing the hamstrings' tightness by preparing them for the stretch and by giving them enough time to progress.
- While attempting a forward-bending asana, start with keeping the knees bent and working only on straightening the spine. The bent knee gives a comfortable resistance while stretching.

ASANAS THAT BENEFIT THE HAMSTRINGS
The following asanas help strengthen the area. These should not be practised if the area is already injured or is in the process of healing.

Standing Asanas
Urdhva Tadasana
Santulanasana
Parsvakonasana
Parsvatanasana
Utkatasana
Vatayanasana

Floor Asanas
Ardha Badha Paschimottanasana
Vajrasana
Supta Vajrasana
Baddha Konasana
Krounchasana
Akarna Dhanurasana
Supta Utthita Hasta Padangustasana (lying down)

Tip: To progress into a straight-legged forward stretch, first press the heel to the ground and draw the thigh muscles (especially the quads – the front of the thighs) upward towards the seat bones. This helps keep the back straight and comfortable instead of rounding and straining it.

HIP

REASONS
Generally, hip muscles tend to be tight. To understand this it is important to study the anatomy of the hip. The hip area is governed by two important muscles – the muscles of the inner thighs and groin whose function is to draw the leg to the centre line of the body (adductor muscles) and the muscles of the outer hip, which moves the thighs apart and away from the body's centre line (abductor muscles). The functions of both these muscles are heavy-duty and, therefore, tend to get easily strained. However, the groin is especially tight as its function is to pull the heads of the thigh bones (femur) together, keeping them centered in the socket. These are further stabilised by the abductors which oppose the groin muscles. Simple factors such as walking, jogging, climbing, etc., contribute to stress and strain in the hip joints. In fact, yoga practitioners can also strain the hips if the asanas are practised without sufficient preparation or warm-up.

CARE
- The groin muscles are two sets of muscles extending on each side of the pubic bone, reaching into the inner thighs.
- These muscles are more susceptible to injuries as the muscles around this area are often tight due to prolonged hours of sitting, driving or postural imbalance.
- Any sudden forceful stretching causes these muscles and tendons to tear, causing tightness and pain.
- The other muscle drops from the gluteus, which has the main task of stabilising the thigh bones and keeping

them secure in the hip joint. When these muscles are tense, the pain around this area extends from the gluteus into the lower back.

ASANAS THAT HELP HIP ALIGNMENT
The following asanas help strengthen the area. These should not be practised if the area is already injured or is in the process of healing.

Standing Asanas
Vrikshasana
Adho Mukha Svanasana
Parivrtta Trikonasana
Ardha Chandrasana (with support)
Parivrtta Ardha Chandrasana (with support)
Trianga Mukhottasana
Prasarita Padottanasana
Vatayanasana

Floor Asanas
Dhanurasana
Ananta Shayanasana
Urdhva Pada Ananta Shayanasana
Vajrasana
Veerasana
Bharadwajasana
Baddha Konasana
Mandukasana
Bekasana
SuptaUtthita Hasta Padangustasana
Sarvangasana
Shavasana

SACRUM

REASONS
The sacrum and hip form the centre of the body. The very function, structure and shape of the bones around the sacrum and hips make them very susceptible to misalignments. They consist of 5 fused vertebrae at the base of the spine. The sacrum is triangular in shape and acts as a gravitational centre of the body, which helps the body twist, turn and even remain motionless.

CARE

- Wrong posture causes stress in the joints as they get overused.
- Postural imbalance due to defective arches of the feet, where the balance of both the legs differ, can cause misalignment.
- It is important to identify the cause of strain in the sacrum and around the hips. It is usually experienced as a stinging pain on the sides of the lower back immediately after a Parivrtta Asana, such as Parivrtta Trikonasana (twisting and bending), or sitting or walking for a long period.
- Avoiding certain forward-bending asanas that the practitioner can identify over time would prevent further damage. (Lying on the floor and testing the alignment of the hip would help observe the improvement.)

ASANAS TO HELP STRENGTHEN AND ALIGN THE SACRUM

The following asanas help strengthen the area. These should not be practised if the area is already injured or is in the process of healing.

Standing Asanas
Vrikshasana
Adho Mukha Svanasana
Parivrtta Trikonasana
Ardha Chandrasana (with support)
Parivrtta Ardha Chandrasana (with support)
Trianga Mukhottasana
Prasarita Padottanasana
Vatayanasana

Floor Asanas
Dhanurasana
Ananta Shayanasana
Urdhva Pada Ananta Shayanasana
Vajrasana
Veerasana
Bharadwajasana
Baddha Konasana
Mandukasana
Bekasana
Supta Utthita Hasta Padangustasana
Sarvangasana
Shavasana

GLUTEAL MUSCLES

REASONS
Strong gluteal muscles are key to good posture. Good posture prevents joint pains and muscular aches. A common habit of forward-tilted hip automatically leads to a rounded upper back. This kind of posture under-develops the gluteal muscles, causing problems.
A. The main task of the gluteal muscles is to provide movement of the thigh back and forth (e.g. walking).
B. They help stabilise the thigh bone in the hip socket when shifting weight from one leg to another (e.g., in Vrikshasana).

CARE
- When you notice the heels of your shoes are worn out at the edges, it is time to take this as a warning signal to align your posture.
- Attention should be paid to aligning foot position. Adjust the foot in such a way so as to feel the centre of the heel rooted to the ground.
- Align the torso to position in line with the hips and shoulders. Tucking in the lower abdomen helps this alignment. The above-mentioned alignment immediately takes away the tension from the knees and ankle, indicating proper gluteal alignment.

ASANAS TO STRENGTHEN THE GLUTEAL MUSCLES
The following asanas help strengthen the area. These should not be practised if the area is already injured or is in the process of healing.

Standing Asanas
Tadasana
Urdhva Tadasana
Vrikshasana
Surya Namaskara B
Ardha Chandrasana
Veerabhadrasana
Utthita Hasta Padangustasana
Utkatasana
Vatayanasana

Floor Asanas
Shalabhasana
Ananta Shayanasana
Urdhva Pada Ananta Shayanasana
Ushtrasana
Baddha Konasana
Mandukasana
Akarna Dhanurasana
Sarvangasana
Urdhva Dhanurasana
Eka Pada Urdhva Dhanurasana
Shavasana

LOWER BACK

REASONS
Strain in the lower back is a warning for a check-up. It is important to understand the lower back pain. Some medical reasons could be:
A. Herniated or degenerated disk
B. Scoliosis
C. Tilted pelvis
D. Urinary tract infection
E. Undigested food
Note: Please consult a doctor before you begin therapy.

CARE
While doing asana practice:
- Do not bend forward, keeping your knees straight. If an asana needs bending forward, bend with knees bent.
- Work on strengthening the legs and shoulders, build up body alignment before addressing the problem area of the lower back.
- Keep the spine tall by engaging the core (lower abdominal area).
- Keep the abdomen elongated while doing any seated asana, thereby ensuring a straight spine.
- Do not walk briskly if you have a strained back; instead, walk at a slow and steady pace while swinging the arms.

ASANAS THAT BENEFIT THE LOWER BACK
The following asanas help strengthen the area. These should not be practised if the area is already injured or is in the process of healing.

Standing Asanas
Tadasana
Trikonasana
Prasarita Padottanasana
Vatayanasana

Floor Asanas
Bhujangasana
Shalabhasana
Dhanurasana
Ananta Shayanasana
Veerasana
Ushtrasana
Gomukhasana
Bharadwajasana
Sarvangasana
Shavasana

SHOULDERS

REASONS
The problem in the shoulders mainly starts with bad postural habits or overuse of the shoulder muscles that support the arms. The muscles closest to the neck and along the shoulder blades take the brunt of these issues. When the shoulders are in a perpetual slouch, tension builds up, pulling the inner corner of the shoulder blades up towards the ears, causing the back to round and shoulders to hunch, creating a chronic muscle tension not only around the shoulders but also in the neck. Shoulders are delicate and have a unique structure, which is easily susceptible to injuries.

CARE
- The most common shoulder injury happens at the outermost corner of the shoulder, beneath the deltoid (a large muscle used to lift the arm).
- Keep the shoulder blades tucked into the back while the midriff is firmly lifted up, lengthening the torso.
- Observe the position of the neck to avoid shoulder injuries.
- To avoid shoulder injury, make sure the chin is positioned pointing towards the chest all the time.

ASANAS THAT BENEFIT THE SHOULDERS
A variety of asanas can help restore balance and strength to the shoulder muscles and increase mobility to the shoulder

blade. The following asanas help strengthen the area. These should not be practised if the area is already injured or is in the process of healing.

Standing Asanas
Surya Namaskara
Trikonasana
Parsvakonasana
Vashistasana
Utkatasana
Vatayanasana

Floor Asanas
Bhujangasana
Dhanurasana
Ushtrasana
Bharadwajasana
Sarvangasana
Halasana
Setu Bandhasana
Urdhva Dhanurasana

UPPER BACK AND CHEST

REASONS
The most common cause for a tight upper back is the tendency to slouch the shoulders. Slouching causes the shoulder blades to droop away from the spine and point outwards, thus straining the muscles around them. This also weakens the front of the body especially the upper chest. In both the cases (upper chest and back), the shoulders roll forward and down, forming a hunch and the muscles around the hunch cease to support the functioning of the shoulders. Shoulders work as a foundation to a lot of yoga asanas. It is very important to rectify any tightness in the upper chest or back, which could otherwise make the practice difficult.
Note: It is important to rectify postural defects before practising any yoga asana to avoid discomfort or injuries. These can be corrected with awareness and focus on those specific areas. Without proper postural alignment, if the asanas are forced on the body, in due course, injury sets in.

CARE
* Maintain a proper alignment of the shoulder joints so that the chest feels fully opened and broad.

* The tips of the shoulders should stay firm and comfortable inside the back.
* The neck should experience a free range of movements.
* The arms lift up full length without pain or discomfort.

ASANAS THAT BENEFIT SHOULDERS, UPPER BACK AND CHEST
Asanas which would aid in the progress and the practice of this opening of the chest should be done carefully and progressively. The following asanas help strengthen the area. These should not be practised if the area is already injured or is in the process of healing.

Standing Asanas
Surya Namaskara
Trikonasana
Parsvakonasana
Vashistasana
Utkatasana
Vatayanasana

Floor Asanas
Bhujangasana
Dhanursana
Ushtrasana
Bharadwajasana
Sarvangasana
Halasana
Setu Bandhasana
Urdhva Dhanurasana

NECK

REASONS
The neck has large muscles that converge at its back and are attached to the base of the skull. These include the muscles along the spine as well as those running along the sides of the neck to the base of the head. Neck tension can frequently be caused by:
A. The habit of thrusting the neck forward.
B. Tightness in the shoulders due to tension.
C. Disc herniation.
D. Lower back problems.
It is important to understand the causes of the neck tension. If it is postural (habit), rectify the posture before getting into

therapy. There could be a number of forces at work that can misalign the neck positions.

CARE

- If any misalignment is noticed at the neck, the first step is to pull the chin in and back towards the base of the skull. Observe the tension relax along the length of the neck and collarbone.
- Adjust the breast bone upward while you drop the shoulder blades into your body.

ASANAS FOR RELAXING AND ALIGNING THE NECK

The following asanas help strengthen the area. These should not be practised if the area is already injured or is in the process of healing.

Standing Asanas
Trikonasana
Parivrtta Trikonasana
Parshavkonasana
Parivrtta Parsvakonasana
Ardha Chandrasana
Vatayanasana

Floor Asanas
Bhujangasana
Ananta Shayanasana
Urdhva Pada Ananta Shayanasana
Ushtrasana
Paryankasana
Bharadwajasana
Dwi Pada Rajakapotasana
Gomukhasana
Marichyasana (all 4)
Supta Utthita Hasta Padagushtasana
Sarvangasana
Matsyendrasana
Shavasana

RESTORATIVE YOGA ASANAS

- It is important to plan and sequence – a set of yoga asanas – which would help heal an injury in a particular part of the body. Such asanas are referred to as restorative asanas – asanas that release tension and stress from the area of the pain. These gentle asanas should be practised with consciousness and focused breathing. Restorative asanas should be held for at least 30 seconds in stillness, with total awareness of the pain in the area of the injury. Deep breathing in these asanas adds on to the process of healing. Therefore, it is important to select the asanas that one is comfortable with. If required, take help of props like chairs, pillows, bolsters, blankets, etc.
- Restorative asanas are always non-challenging and are done to rest the body yet engage the mind. A relaxed breathing helps the mind focus on changing the experience of physical pain and moving beyond it.

TIPS TO PREPARE THE BODY TO FOCUS ON RESTORATIVE ASANAS:

- De-stress – any kind of mundane stress takes a toll on the body, breath and mind. Eventually, it contributes to a faulty practice which means practice without focus. Stress creates an imbalance in the doshas (p. 18).
- Consciously monitor your thoughts. That will help reduce stress in the body and mind. Mindfully observe your thoughts and your reaction to those thoughts. This helps deal with the intensity of the reactions to thoughts, which in turns helps analyse the source of stress and prepares the body and mind to cope with it better.

NOTE ON PRACTICE (SADHANA) FROM THE YOGA SUTRAS

CHAPTER 2: SADHANAPADAH

II.1
Tapahsvadhyayesvarapranidhanani kriyayogah

The practice of yoga intends to reduce both physical and mental impurities. It aids in
developing our ability for self-analysis and helps us understand that in the final
analysis, we are not the masters of everything we do.

II.2
Samadhibhavanarthah klesatanukaranarthasca

With an understanding...then, such practices will be certain to remove the obstacles to clear perception.

GLOSSARY

ahamkara	ego
ahimsa	non-violence
ajna	brow
akasha	sky; ether; space
anahata	heart
ananda	bliss
anandamaya	of pure joy
angushtagrai	tip of the thumb
annamaya	physical
antara	breath held after inhalation
anuloma	with the natural order
aparigraha	non-covetousness
ardha chandra	half-moon
asana	posture
ashtanga	eight-limbed
ashteya	honesty
ashwini	horse
asmita	pride
avidya	ignorance
Ayurveda	ancient indian medicinal science
bandha	bond
bhakti	devotion to god
bhastrika	bellows
bahya	breath held after exhalation
bhrumadhya	centre of the bows
bhujangini	cobra
bija	seed
brahmacharya	knowledge of everything; later to mean celibacy
brahmari	bee
buddhi	intellect
chakra	energy centre
chandra	moon
chitta	mind
dharana	focus; concentration
dharma	righteousness
dhyana	meditation
dosha	characteristic; psychobiological functioning
drishti	gaze; point of focus
ekagra	deep concentration; single-point focus
guna	human tendencies
guru	revered teacher
hastagrai	hand; palm
Hatha Yoga	balancing the lunar and solar energy channels of the body with physical postures
hrdaya	region of the heart along with the rib-cage
ida	energy channel of the moon (lunar)
ishvara	god; supreme being
jalandhara	chin
jnana	knowledge
kaivalya	freedom from bondages to achieve total bliss
kaki	crow
kanda	junction where the sushumna nadi is connected to the muladhara chakra
kapala	head
kapha	phlegm
karma	action; law of actions
kechari	tongue-swallowing
klesha	suffering
kosha	layer of energy
kriya	technique or practice within a yoga discipline, meant to achieve a specific result
kshipta	distressed
kumbhaka	holding; retention
kundalini	coiled
maha vedha	great-variation lock
mandala	geometric drawing of the cosmos
manduka	frog
manipura	solar plexus

manomaya	of thought energy	sama	straight
mantra	holy sound or chant	samadhi	peace; absorption; freedom from ailments
matangi	tantric name of Saraswati (Goddess of Knowledge)	santosha	content
maya	worldly desires	sattvic	peaceful; wise; knowledgeable
mudra	seal	satya	truthful
mugdha	confused; perplexed	shakti chalana	circulation of energy
mula	root	shanmukhi	six-mouthed
muladhara	base or root chakra	smriti	memory
nabho	turning the underside of the tongue up	soucha	clean
nabi	navel	surya namaskara	sun salutation
shuddhi	cleansing	sushumna	central energy channel
nadi	energy channel	svadhisthana	sacral or navel chakra
nasagrai	tip of the nose	svadhyaya	self study
nirudha	balanced state of mind	tadaka	bottom; bed of a pond; pond; lake
niyama	rules / principles	tamasic	lethargic; fatigued; dull
pada	step	tapas	austerity
padayoragrai	tip of the toes	uddiyana	upward-moving energy locks
parivrtta	twists	ujjayee	victorious
parsva	side (left or right); lateral	urdhva	upward
paschimottana	forward	vajroli	thunderbolt
pingala	energy channel governed by the sun (solar)	vata	air / wind
pitta	bile	vayu	air current
prajna	complete knowledge	vibhuti	accomplishments as a result of a practice
prana	inner breath of life	vidya	proper knowledge
pranamaya	of life energy	vijnanamaya	comprising intellect, the power of judgement
pranayama	breathing exercise		
pratyahara	self-assessment; gaining mastery over sensory stimuli	vikshipta	distracted
		viloma	against the natural order
purvattana	backward	vinyasa	flow of breath along with flow of asanas
rajasic	dynamic of character		
rishi	sage	viparita	inverted
sadhak /sadhaki	practitioner	viparita karani	half-shoulder
sadhana	constant practice	vishesha	extreme
sahasrara	crown	vishuddha	throat
salamba	head-supported	vrtta	fluctuations of the mind
		yama	moral restraints

108 ASANAS: ENGLISH TRANSLATION

Adho Mukha Svanasana	downward-facing dog pose	Janu Shirsasana	head-on-knee pose
Adho Mukha Shavasana	downward-facing rest pose	Kala Bhairavasana	pose named after Sage Kalabhairava
Adho Mukha Tadasana	downward-facing tree pose	Kapilasana	pose named after Sage Kapila
Akarna Dhanurasana	archer's pose	Kapotasana	pigeon pose
Ananta Shayanasana	relaxing Lord pose	Karna Peedasana	knee-to-ear pose
Ardha Padma Padangushtasana	half-lotus hand-to-toe pose	Krounchasana	heron pose
		Kurmasana	tortoise pose
Ardha Padma Paschimottanasana	half-lotus forward-bend pose	Malasana	garland pose
		Mandukasana	big-frog pose
Ardha Chandra Natarajasana	half-moon Dancing Lord pose	Marichyasana	pose named after Sage Marichyasana
Ardha Chandrasana	half-moon pose	Matsyasana	fish pose
Baddha Padmasana	bounded-lotus pose	Matsyendrasana	named after Sage Matsyendra (half spinal-twist)
Baddha Konasana	bounded-angle pose		
Bakasana	crane pose	Natarajasana	Dancing Lord pose
Bekasana	frog pose	Navasana	boat pose
Bharadwajasana	pose named after Sage Bharadwaj	Padangushtasana / Padahastasana	hand-to-feet forward-bend pose
Bhujangasana	snake pose		
Chaduranga Dandasana	four-limbed staff pose	Padmasana	lotus pose
Chakorasana	wing pose	Parivrtta Ardha Chandrasana	twisted half-moon pose
Chakrasana / Urdhva Dhanurasana	wheel pose / lifted-bow pose	Parivrtta Hanumanasana	twisted Monkey Lord pose
		Parivrtta Janu Shirsasana	twisted head-to-knee pose
Dhanursana	bow pose	Parivrtta Parsvakonasana	twisted side-angle pose
Dwi Pada Koundinyasana	pose named after Sage Koundinya	Parivrtta Prasarita Padottanasana	twisted wide-legged pose
Urdhva Shalabhasana	lifted-locust pose		
Eka Pada Bakasana	one-legged crane pose	Parivrtta Trikonasana	twisted triangle pose
Eka Pada Kapotasana	one-legged pigeon pose	Parivrtta Utkatasana	twisted chair pose
Eka Pada Shirsasana	one leg-on-head pose	Parsvakonasana	stretched side-angle pose
Eka Pada Urdhva Dhanurasana	one-leg lifted-bow pose	Parsvottanasana	intense forward-stretch pose
		Paryankasana	couch pose
Eka Pada Uttanasana	one-legged intense-lifted pose	Paschimottanasana	seated forward-bend pose
Garbha Pindasana	embryo pose	Pashasana	noose pose
Gomukhasana	cow-face pose	Pincha Mayurasana	peacock pose
Halasana	plough pose	Pindasana	embryo pose
Hanumanasana	pose named after Lord Hanuman	Prasarita Padottanasana	wide-legged pyramid pose

Purvottanasana	lifted-upward plank pose
Samasthiti	relaxed-and-steady pose
Santulanasana	balance pose
Sarvangasana	complete-body pose
Setu Bandhasana	bridge pose
Shalabhasana	locust pose
Shayanasana	pose named after Lord Vishnu's pose
Shirsasana	headstand pose
Simhasana	lion pose
Supta Padangushtasana	supine hand-to-feet pose
Supta Trivikramasana	supine leg-lift named after Sage Trivikrama
Supta Veerasana	supine diamond pose
Tadasana	steady pose
Tandavasana	Lord-of-Dance pose
Tittibasana	firefly pose
Tolasana / Uth Pluthi	balance-scale pose
Trianga Mukhapeeda Paschimotannasana	three-limbed forward-bend pose
Trianga Mukhottasana	backward-facing pose
Trikonasana	triangle pose
Trivikramasana	pose named after Sage Trivikrama
Ubhaya Padangustasana	lifted hand-to-feet pose
Ubhaya Pashchimottanasana	both-legs-lifted upward-stretch pose
Ubhaya Upavistakonasana	both-legs-lifted seated-angle pose
Uddiyana Bandha	upward abdominal-lock pose

Upadasana	lifted-leg pyramid pose
Upavistakonasana	seated stretched-angle pose
Urdhva Dhanurasana / Chakorasana	lifted-bow pose
Urdhva Tadasana	lifted-stand pose
Urdhva Mukha Paschimottanasana	upward-facing forward-stretch pose
Urdhva Mukha Svanasna	upward-facing dog pose
Urdhva Mukha Tadasana	upward-facing steady pose
Urdhva Mukha Upavistakonasana	upward-facing stretched-angle pose
Ushtrasana	camel pose
Utthita Hasta Padangustasana	elevated / standing hand-to-feet pose
Uttanasana	forward-bend pose
Utakatasana	fierce pose / thunderbolt pose
Vajrasana	adamantine pose
Vashistasana	pose named after Sage Vashishta
Vatayanasana	pose named after Sage Vatayana
Veerabhadrasana	warrior pose
Veerasana	hero pose
Viparita Dandasana	intense-curve pose
Vishwamitrasana	pose named after Sage Vishwamitra
Vrikshasana	tree pose
Yoga Mudrasana	bounded pose
Yoga Nidrasana	yogic-sleeping pose
Shavasana	complete-rest pose

INDEX